A FRAMEWORK FOR Assessing Mortality and Morbidity After Large-Scale Disasters

Ellen J. MacKenzie, Scott H. Wollek, Olivia C. Yost, and Daniel L. Cork, *Editors*

Committee on Best Practices for Assessing Mortality and Significant Morbidity Following Large-Scale Disasters

Board on Health Sciences Policy

Health and Medicine Division

A Consensus Study Report of

The National Academies of
SCIENCES · ENGINEERING · MEDICINE

THE NATIONAL ACADEMIES PRESS
Washington, DC
www.nap.edu

THE NATIONAL ACADEMIES PRESS 500 Fifth Street, NW Washington, DC 20001

This activity was supported by a contract between the National Academy of Sciences and the Federal Emergency Management Agency (Contract No. HSHQDC-17-A-B0001/70FBTX19F00000007). Any opinions, findings, conclusions, or recommendations expressed in this publication do not necessarily reflect the views of any organization or agency that provided support for the project.

International Standard Book Number-13: 978-0-309-68025-7
International Standard Book Number-10: 0-309-68025-5
Digital Object Identifier: https://doi.org/10.17226/25863
Library of Congress Control Number: 2020947584

Additional copies of this publication are available from the National Academies Press, 500 Fifth Street, NW, Keck 360, Washington, DC 20001; (800) 624-6242 or (202) 334-3313; http://www.nap.edu.

Printed in the United States of America

Suggested citation: National Academies of Sciences, Engineering, and Medicine. 2020. *A framework for assessing mortality and morbidity after large-scale disasters*. Washington, DC: The National Academies Press. https://doi.org/10.17226/25863.

The National Academies of

SCIENCES · ENGINEERING · MEDICINE

The **National Academy of Sciences** was established in 1863 by an Act of Congress, signed by President Lincoln, as a private, nongovernmental institution to advise the nation on issues related to science and technology. Members are elected by their peers for outstanding contributions to research. Dr. Marcia McNutt is president.

The **National Academy of Engineering** was established in 1964 under the charter of the National Academy of Sciences to bring the practices of engineering to advising the nation. Members are elected by their peers for extraordinary contributions to engineering. Dr. John L. Anderson is president.

The **National Academy of Medicine** (formerly the Institute of Medicine) was established in 1970 under the charter of the National Academy of Sciences to advise the nation on medical and health issues. Members are elected by their peers for distinguished contributions to medicine and health. Dr. Victor J. Dzau is president.

The three Academies work together as the **National Academies of Sciences, Engineering, and Medicine** to provide independent, objective analysis and advice to the nation and conduct other activities to solve complex problems and inform public policy decisions. The National Academies also encourage education and research, recognize outstanding contributions to knowledge, and increase public understanding in matters of science, engineering, and medicine.

Learn more about the National Academies of Sciences, Engineering, and Medicine at **www.nationalacademies.org**.

The National Academies of
SCIENCES · ENGINEERING · MEDICINE

Consensus Study Reports published by the National Academies of Sciences, Engineering, and Medicine document the evidence-based consensus on the study's statement of task by an authoring committee of experts. Reports typically include findings, conclusions, and recommendations based on information gathered by the committee and the committee's deliberations. Each report has been subjected to a rigorous and independent peer-review process and it represents the position of the National Academies on the statement of task.

Proceedings published by the National Academies of Sciences, Engineering, and Medicine chronicle the presentations and discussions at a workshop, symposium, or other event convened by the National Academies. The statements and opinions contained in proceedings are those of the participants and are not endorsed by other participants, the planning committee, or the National Academies.

For information about other products and activities of the National Academies, please visit www.nationalacademies.org/about/whatwedo.

COMMITTEE ON BEST PRACTICES FOR ASSESSING MORTALITY AND SIGNIFICANT MORBIDITY FOLLOWING LARGE-SCALE DISASTERS

ELLEN J. MacKENZIE (*Chair*), Bloomberg Distinguished Professor and Dean, Johns Hopkins Bloomberg School of Public Health
SUE ANNE BELL, Assistant Professor, University of Michigan School of Nursing
H. RUSSELL BERNARD, Research Professor and Director, Arizona State University
ARAM DOBALIAN, Professor and Director, Division of Health Systems Management and Policy, The University of Memphis
MARCELLA F. FIERRO, Chief Medical Examiner (retired), Commonwealth of Virginia; Consultant Forensic Pathologist, Fierro Forensics
ELIZABETH FRANKENBERG, Director, Carolina Population Center, University of North Carolina
JOHN L. HICK, Faculty Emergency Physician, Hennepin Healthcare; Professor of Emergency Medicine, University of Minnesota
ALI S. KHAN, Dean, College of Public Health, University of Nebraska Medical Center
MAUREEN LICHTVELD, Professor and Chair, Department of Environmental Health Sciences, Tulane University School of Public Health & Tropical Medicine
CHARLES ROTHWELL, Director (retired), National Center for Health Statistics
RICHARD SERINO, Distinguished Senior Fellow, Harvard T.H. Chan School of Public Health
MICHAEL A. STOTO, Professor, Health Systems Administration and Population Health, Georgetown University
W. CRAIG VANDERWAGEN, Founder and General Manager, East West Protection, LLC
DANIEL WALL, Emergency Manager, City of Ventura
MATTHEW WYNIA, Director, Center for Bioethics and Humanities, University of Colorado

Study Staff

SCOTT H. WOLLEK, Study Director (*from August 2019*)
MICHELLE MANCHER, Study Director (*until August 2019*)
DANIEL L. CORK, Senior Program Officer

OLIVIA C. YOST, Program Officer
MARIAM SHELTON, Research Associate (*until December 2019*)
MICHAEL BERRIOS, Research Associate
ANDREW M. POPE, Senior Director, Board on Health Sciences Policy

Consultant

ANNA NICHOLSON, Doxastic, Inc.

Reviewers

This Consensus Study Report was reviewed in draft form by individuals chosen for their diverse perspectives and technical expertise. The purpose of this independent review is to provide candid and critical comments that will assist the National Academies of Sciences, Engineering, and Medicine in making each published report as sound as possible and to ensure that it meets the institutional standards for quality, objectivity, evidence, and responsiveness to the study charge. The review comments and draft manuscript remain confidential to protect the integrity of the deliberative process.

We thank the following individuals for their review of this report:

JAMES FICKE, The Johns Hopkins Hospital
NICHOLAS P. JEWELL, London School of Hygiene & Tropical Medicine
ROGER J. LEWIS, Harbor-UCLA Medical Center
NICOLE LURIE, Harvard Medical School
PABLO A. MARQUET, Pontificia Universidad Católica de Chile
SAMANTHA MONTANO, Massachusetts Maritime Academy
DAN MORGAN, National Transportation Safety Board
JOSEPH O. PREWITT DIAZ, American Red Cross International Services
WILLIAM ROUSE, Georgetown University
KIMBERLY SHOAF, The University of Utah
TENER VEENEMA, Johns Hopkins Bloomberg School of Public Health

ROBERT WALLACE, The University of Iowa
MARY C. WATERS, Harvard University
VICTOR WEEDN, The George Washington University

Although the reviewers listed above provided many constructive comments and suggestions, they were not asked to endorse the conclusions or recommendations of this report nor did they see the final draft before its release. The review of this report was overseen by **ALFRED O. BERG,** University of Washington School of Medicine, and **CHARLES E. PHELPS,** University of Rochester. They were responsible for making certain that an independent examination of this report was carried out in accordance with the standards of the National Academies and that all review comments were carefully considered. Responsibility for the final content rests entirely with the authoring committee and the National Academies.

Contents

Preface

From the moment of impact through the years it takes for communities to recover and rebuild, disasters have complex and far-reaching health impacts, extending beyond an assessment of mortality only. Exacerbating the toll of lives lost are serious morbidities, including not only direct physical injuries, but also trauma and stress-induced mental health effects, disaster-induced interrupted treatment aggravating underlying conditions, and, in some instances, exposures to environmental contaminants. Disadvantaged and underserved communities are in most cases disproportionately impacted by disasters; hence, any comprehensive disaster impact assessment must also take into account the social determinants of health.

Congress mandated this study in 2018 as part of the Disaster Recovery Reform Act, following the publication of significant discrepancies regarding the numbers of deaths caused by Hurricane Maria in Puerto Rico in September 2017, which brought to the forefront pointed questions about how estimates of total disaster-related mortality ought to be derived. Yet, the assessment of disaster-related health impacts is a complicated and multifaceted endeavor, requiring the coordination of diverse stakeholders within a nationwide patchwork of systems responsible for recording and reporting health and mortality data. Over the course of the committee's deliberations, we sought to pinpoint the most important challenges that undercut the ability of practitioners to gather, report, and use mortality and morbidity data to save lives and protect health. It became clear that responsibilities and practices across multiple stakeholders were fragmented and inconsistent, making it difficult if not impossible to compare and learn across disasters. Thus, while it may be possible to answer the narrow question "What is the best way to calculate the total mortality from a particular disaster in a given population over a given time frame?," any functional system for regularly assessing disaster-related mortality and serious morbidity will require sustained efforts to integrate disparate systems, harmonize and standardize definitions and practices, and cultivate the commitment of stakeholders to assess, report, and make data accessible and usable as a fundamental component of the disaster management enterprise. To realize this transformation, the committee strove to develop recommendations that are actionable and that provide a practical roadmap to overcome persistent barriers to achieving real, sustainable change that bolsters community resilience.

The committee's deliberations occurred during an unprecedented time; just as our term of appointment was about to wrap up, a novel infectious disease grew into a pandemic with enormous impacts on health and society. The original charge to the committee did not focus heavily on disasters related to infectious diseases, but this exclusion was reconsidered as the coronavirus disease 2019 (COVID-19) pandemic gathered momentum worldwide in early 2020. Following the Stafford Disaster Relief and Emergency Assistance Act declaration for all states in March 2020 and the escalating spread of severe acute respiratory syndrome coronavirus 2 (SARS-CoV-2) within the United States, many of the challenges already identified by the committee became starkly evident in real time, as early attempts to assess COVID-19-related mortality and morbidity were scientifically challenging and fraught with methodological, logistical, philosophical, and even political controversy. In May 2020 the study sponsor, the Federal Emergency Management Agency, approved the committee's request to include considerations related to the COVID-19 pandemic in the final report. The committee's intent for this inclusion is to provide practical context for the core recommendations set forth in the report, not to adjudicate the relative merits of current estimates of pandemic-related mortality or to comprehensively assess the impacts of the COVID-19 pandemic. We also did not want consideration of issues related to data on pandemics to become the focus of the report, which has much broader implications for disasters of all types. Therefore, at several places in the report we offer examples drawn from the ongoing pandemic that highlight administrative, logistical, and methodological challenges in assessing mortality and morbidity common to large-scale disasters of any provenance, and to illustrate how the committee's framework could be applied in practice to help overcome those barriers.

While the report focuses on the approaches and systems needed to accurately estimate disaster-related mortality and morbidity, the value of these data extends far beyond these estimates. For practitioners and policy makers, an integrated, holistic data system should inform targeted investments in response and recovery to strengthen community resilience between disasters. For individuals and communities, these data hold deep emotional significance and they can help survivors and their loved ones in a community in memorializing what has been lost. For society and at a global level, these data can even be used to prevent some disasters by helping to shape decisions in the context of the changing global climate as to where and how people live and whether to rebuild or retreat from geographic areas subject to frequent flooding, high temperatures, or wildland fires.

An area of critical significance, which the committee was not able to cover in great depth due to the narrowness of the Statement of Task, is the role of social determinants in disaster-related morbidity and mortality and how these factors relate to community resilience. It is well established that disasters affect populations inequitably: disparities in socioeconomic factors and other environmental, geographic, political, and biological dimensions heighten vulnerabilities and amplify the risks of death and morbidities for certain groups during and after a disaster. It is the committee's perspective that these issues are of fundamental importance. We strongly advocate for further study about how social determinants of health affect disaster-related health consequences, as well as how mortality and morbidity data can be contextualized and enriched by multidimensional data to develop and use more effective strategies to protect vulnerable groups and promote community resilience.

Lastly, although the committee's recommendations are targeted at the assessment of mortality and morbidity related to "large-scale" disasters (see the definition in Chapter 1), our plan of action, presented in Chapter 5, is intended to be read and adopted more broadly to develop stronger, more nimble systems that are primed and ready to respond to events of any magnitude or origin. This report is being released at a time of great uncertainty, with much remaining unknown about the health impacts of the as-yet unrelenting COVID-19 pandemic, and the next disaster that could occur at any time. It is the committee's hope that our recommendations will strengthen the nation's resolve and ability to save lives and protect health in the wake of this disaster and the next—whenever or wherever it strikes.

Ellen J. MacKenzie, *Chair*
Committee on Best Practices for Assessing Mortality and Significant Morbidity Following Large-Scale Disasters

Summary[1]

In the wake of a large-scale disaster, from the initial devastation through the long tail of recovery, protecting the health and well-being of the affected individuals and communities is paramount. Accurate and timely information about mortality and significant morbidity related to the disaster are critical to supporting situational awareness for the disaster management enterprise and driving public health action to save lives and prevent further health impacts. Conversely, failure to capture mortality and morbidity data accurately and consistently undercuts the nation's capacity to protect its population. Information about disaster-related mortality and morbidity adds value at all phases of the disaster management cycle. As a disaster unfolds, these data are crucial in guiding response and recovery priorities, ensuring a common operating picture and real-time situational awareness across stakeholders, and protecting vulnerable populations and settings at heightened risk. Public health messaging shaped by accurate morbidity and mortality data is critical for communicating vital information to the public, protecting them from ongoing and future hazards, and prompting protective actions from policy makers and other leaders. During the interim between disasters, these data provide the foundation for evaluation, prevention, mitigation, and preparedness activities designed to reduce morbidity and mortality when future events arise. In some instances, these data might also inform actions that can even prevent future disasters, such as through prompting actions to mitigate the risk of climate-related disasters. In sum,

[1] This Summary does not include references. Citations for the discussion presented in this Summary appear in subsequent chapters.

accurate assessment of mortality and morbidity from disasters is not merely an academic or historical exercise: the timely and accurate counting and attribution of deaths and morbidities can improve disaster response and lead to a more accurate assessment of the extent, types, and causes of morbidity and mortality in disasters and drive changes in policy, practice, and behavior that will prevent suffering and save lives.

Extracting the maximum value from these data depends on having standard practices and systems in place for collecting and reporting accurate information, analyzing it appropriately, and translating the data into action to protect disaster-affected communities. However, it is challenging to coordinate these efforts effectively and uniformly across the disaster management enterprise, which comprises a vast and intricate network of federal and state, local, tribal, and territorial (SLTT) systems as well as a plethora of stakeholders ranging from emergency management, health care, government agencies, the general public, policy makers, and the public and private sectors. The practices and systems currently in place are inadequately robust, coordinated, or reliable to leverage mortality and morbidity data to their fullest potential. Instead, these systems and stakeholders are often splintered, siloed, and unable to rapidly share information with each other. As a result, the same incident can generate dramatically different estimates of mortality and morbidity depending on the policies and practices of the home jurisdiction. Data that are not captured uniformly across jurisdictions, federal and SLTT agencies, and professions are less conducive to comparative analysis and may exclude valuable information about deaths and morbidities that are indirectly or partially attributable to a disaster. In other cases, available data about mortality and morbidity are squandered because they are not or cannot be acted on to add value to disaster management or because existing systems are not deriving the optimal value from the data to guide action. Additionally, the consistent and accurate collection of disaster-related mortality and morbidity data is often not prioritized because the stakeholders involved may not be aware of its importance. Multiple approaches exist to assess disaster-related mortality and morbidity. Also of critical importance is the reality that stakeholders may have certain vested interests to selectively use data to depict the estimated impacts of a disaster in a certain manner. Whether explicit or inadvertent, this can lead to controversy and confusion. Avoiding these problems requires improving processes for vital statistics, public health, emergency management and emergency response data systems; integrating these data sources with other sources of health data, including indicators of the social determinants of health (especially where morbidity data are concerned); and, perhaps most important, standardizing the way these data collection processes are implemented in SLTT agencies throughout the United States.

The entire disaster management enterprise would benefit from changes in practices and policies to strengthen the systems and structures involved in the consistent assessment of mortality and morbidity data during and following large-scale disasters. The increasing frequency and severity of disasters worldwide underscore the need for improvement and standardization of these systems and for stakeholders to be more flexible, coordinated, and adept to meet the core mission of protecting the health and well-being of people impacted by disasters and bolstering community resilience.

BACKGROUND AND RECOMMENDATIONS

While it is impossible to know definitively the full impact of a large-scale disaster on the people directly and indirectly affected, this report attempts to highlight how the administrative, organizational, logistical, and analytical components associated with each of the major estimation approaches can be improved to produce more accurate and complete reflections of the disaster's true effect. As such, the committee's recommendations for improving the function and value of the nation's systems and practices for assessing mortality and morbidity following large-scale disasters span the organizational, operational, analytical, and professional domains. To structure the process of developing their recommendations, the committee established a set of guiding precepts that synthesize the ethos and key characteristics of their vision for a highly effective system (see Box S-1).

BOX S-1
Guiding System Precepts—Abridged

A highly effective system for assessing morbidity and mortality of major disasters would:

- Collect and use data for community health protection as an essential component across all phases of disaster management.
- Incorporate both individual counts and population estimates to better understand a disaster's true effect.
- Leverage morbidity data and mortality data to support response, recovery, mitigation, and preparedness.
- Build on and use existing systems, capacities, and methodologies.
- Commit to the continuous improvement of systems over time.
- Adopt an enterprise approach to activate stakeholders and systems in times of crisis and during the inter-disaster period.
- Support the resilience and strengths of historically disadvantaged populations by using data to understand, mitigate, and eliminate inequalities in disaster impacts.

Organizational Leadership and an Enterprise Approach

Successfully implementing the recommendations set forth in this report will hinge on strong organizational leadership to foster mutual commitment across stakeholders to achieve a coordinated, enterprise-wide approach—aligning the programs and priorities of multiple stakeholders under a shared mission of improving the assessment of mortality and morbidity following large-scale disasters. The full spectrum of systemic changes needed to achieve this improvement across multiple—and often siloed—stakeholders and systems will not be realized unless these agencies, entities, and their leadership rise to meet this collective mission. Leadership at the federal and SLTT levels must buy-in as champions to drive lasting changes across multiple systems and overcome fragmentation. Throughout the disaster management cycle, cross-agency responsibilities will need to be adapted to meet this mission for domestic action.

No federal entity or standardized system is singularly responsible for coordination or oversight of the practices for collection, reporting, and dissemination of disaster-related mortality and morbidity data at the national level in the United States. Rather, these responsibilities are primarily the domain of states, territories, and even counties, creating a patchwork of data systems, standards, and processes. Furthermore, the systems and incentive structures currently in place are inadequate to facilitate collaboration among those entities. But in the face of a disaster, these entities must be nimble enough to flex and adapt beyond their day-to-day functions to contribute their unique tools and capacities to a shared enterprise. The leadership of federal agencies is critical in championing for and investing in the necessary systems improvements as well as setting national standards, but federal leadership will not be enough in view of the underlying structures of public health systems in the United States. SLTT entities will need to promote the value and facilitate the operationalization of these activities in tandem with federal efforts.

Uniform Philosophy for Attribution

Across professions and jurisdictions, multiple terms are used to denote a death or injury as related to a disaster and, if so denoted, the degree to which it is related. These different terms are often conflated, which can lead to misunderstandings and mischaracterization of the estimated impact of a disaster. It also undercuts the ability to appropriately compare assessments of disaster-related mortality and morbidity over time and across disasters. As discussed in Chapter 2, there is widespread variation in what is being assessed and the context in which it is being assessed. The current terminology and case definitions used to describe disaster-related mortality and morbidity do not adequately capture the differences in assessment methods used or the totality and temporality of disaster-related deaths and morbidity. The lack of a uniform framework for assessing disaster-related health impacts undermines the quality and usability of these data to inform disaster management, and it leads to confusion about or even misrepresentations of the impacts of disasters. The committee recommends the immediate adoption of a consistent framework, which includes approaches for assessment and case definitions, as well as a comprehensive understanding of how these approaches and definitions should be applied to the assessment of mortality and morbidity following large-scale disasters (see Recommendations 2-1 and 2-2).

Framework for Assessing Disaster-Related Mortalities and Morbidities

To contribute to improving the quality and utility of these data, the committee developed a framework to serve as an initial guide for (1) describing the two primary approaches for developing quantitative indicators of total mortality or morbidity and (2) parsing out individual case definitions that can be used to uniformly characterize the degree to which an individual death or morbidity is attributed to a disaster. First, quantitative indicators of an event's impact can be generated using two basic approaches: counts of affected individuals or population estimates. One approach is not always better than the other and both produce estimates of a disaster's impact at a distinct point of time, within a specific context, and based on particular assumptions. Each approach also encompasses a variety of methodologies and tools, each of which has its own unique timelines, challenges, and targets.

Estimating total mortality or morbidity by using counts of affected individuals uses data from record keeping systems such as death registration systems or case counts reported to public health agencies. While individual counting methods produce very precise estimates of mortality and morbidity (generally reported to the exact number), the accuracy of this approach is contingent on (1) a complete count of bodies or ill or injured individuals, and (2) accurate attribution of mortality or morbidity to the disaster using consistent case definitions. Because these preconditions are not always met, the committee recommends the adoption of the definitions provided in Box S-2 (see Recommendation 2-1 for the complete recommendation text) as a starting point.

The second basic approach to estimating mortality and morbidity is to use statistical methods, such as survey, sampling, or excess mortality methods. These methods typically generate more comprehensive data than the individual counting approach—because they inherently include both direct and indirect deaths, injuries, or illness—and produce results that are generalizable to the population level. They will typically also include confidence intervals to indicate the exact level of imprecision in the estimations.

BOX S-2
Uniform Case Definitions for Attributing Individual Deaths to a Disaster
(See Recommendation 2-1)

- Direct death: A death directly attributable to the forces of the disaster or a direct consequence of these forces.
- Indirect death: A death not from a direct impact but due to unsafe or unhealthy conditions around the time of the disaster, including while preparing for, responding to, and during recovery from the disaster.
- Partially attributable death: A death that cannot be definitively tied to the disaster but where the disaster more likely than not has played a contributing role in the death.

Approaches for Assessment: Counts and Estimates

These two general approaches (individual counts from administrative records and population estimates based on statistical approaches) both provide essential information in the face of a disaster. Each approach has its own strengths, weaknesses, appropriate uses, and methodologies and each approach makes assumptions and is subject to bias. These approaches are similar in that they pertain to a time period and to a geographical area, and estimates from both can be refined over time. Estimates based on individual counts of deaths recorded in administrative systems are valuable for understanding the immediate impact of disasters, but their accuracy depends on the completeness with which individual cases are recorded and reported. The individual counting methods within this approach often fail to capture certain types of disaster-related deaths including individuals who would not have died *but for* the disaster (e.g., carbon monoxide poisoning from a poorly placed generator or a fatal heart attack during disaster cleanup). More about methods and considerations for conducting individual counts can be found in Chapter 3. Comparatively, population-based estimation methods are crucial for capturing a full understanding of the impacts of a disaster on health and mortality. These methods may incorporate less precise information on cause of death, and in some applications (e.g., estimates of "excess" deaths) cannot distinguish which individuals would have survived in the absence of the disaster from those who would have died during the period regardless. A review of methodologies and tools associated with population estimates can be found in Chapter 4. The complex nature of disasters and the multiple pathways through which they affect human health make it difficult to quantify the impact of a specific disaster on human health with precision. Together, however, the two approaches can provide both timely information and a far more comprehensive picture of the health and mortality impacts of a disaster (see Recommendation 2-2).

Recommendation 2-1: Adopt and Support the Use of a Uniform Framework for Assessing Disaster-Related Mortality and Morbidity

The Department of Health and Human Services and the Department of Homeland Security, including the Office of the Assistant Secretary for Preparedness and Response, the Centers for Disease Control and Prevention, the Centers for Medicare & Medicaid Services, and the Federal Emergency Management Agency, should adopt and support the use of a uniform framework for assessing disaster-related mortality and morbidity before, during, and after a disaster by state, local, tribal, and territorial (SLTT) entities; public health agencies; and death investigation and registration systems. To implement this uniform framework nationally, the National Center for Health Statistics in conjunction with state and local vital records offices, medical examiners and coroners, medical certifiers, and all relevant professional associations should jointly adopt and apply this framework to practice, including the routine use of uniform case definitions and data collection, recording, and reporting practices. Additionally, all Stafford Disaster Relief and Emergency Assistance Act declarations should require affected states and regions to comply with the reporting requirements for individual count and population estimation approaches as described in the framework. Timely guidance should be disseminated to SLTT entities regarding the proper certification of individual deaths with provision for direct, indirect, and partially attributable deaths following a large-scale disaster.

The following terminology and approaches for defining mortality and morbidity following large-scale disasters should be adopted immediately:

- **Total reported mortality and morbidity estimation using individual counts:** Individual counts are point-in-time estimates of disaster-related mortality and morbidity derived from reported cases.
  - o *Direct death or morbidity*: A death or morbidity directly attributable to the forces of the disaster or a direct consequence of these forces.
  - o *Indirect death or morbidity*: A death or morbidity not from a direct impact but due to unsafe or unhealthy conditions around the time of the disaster, including while preparing for, while responding to, and during recovery from the disaster.
  - o *Partially attributable death or morbidity*: A death or morbidity that cannot be tied definitively to the disaster but

where the disaster more likely than not has played a contributing role in the death.
    - *Unrelated death or morbidity*: A death or morbidity that is unassociated with or cannot be attributed to the forces of a disaster.
- **Total mortality and morbidity derived from population estimates:** Population estimates are point-in-time estimates of the impact of a disaster at a population level derived using various statistical methods and tools, including sampling.

<u>Recommendation 2-2: Report Both Individual Counts and Population Estimates</u>

Both individual counts and population estimates should be used as accepted standards for reporting by state, local, tribal, and territorial entities and supported by the federal agencies as indicators of mortality and morbidity to determine the impact of disasters over time. State and federal reporting of total mortality and morbidity estimates following disasters should use both individual counts of direct and indirect deaths and population estimates of mortality and morbidity as these data become available following a disaster. Individual count data should be referred to as *reported cases* or *reported deaths* and should not be referred to as reflecting *total mortality* or a *death toll*. Total mortality estimates should be derived from population estimation methods, which provide a more complete assessment of overall impacts of large-scale disasters.

Sometimes, the availability of different estimates for assessing mortality and morbidity can create confusion, and at worst, the impression that impact of the disaster is being minimized or exaggerated by certain stakeholders via the selective use of data. This was a major public concern following Hurricanes Katrina and Maria, and more recently during the coronavirus disease 2019 (COVID-19) pandemic. When this happens, it is important to realize that the variation in estimates may reflect different, but appropriate, methods and targets. For example: Does the count include deaths that are indirectly or partially attributed to the disaster? Over what time period and in what geographic area are deaths or morbidities being estimated?

However, while there are legitimate reasons for analysts to use different approaches and methods for assessing the impact of a disaster, a certain approach or method may be more appropriate than others in specific instances. This report describes the efforts needed to select the most appropriate approaches, methods, and tools according to the context.

Differences in estimates of mortality and morbidity often reflect the great variation in the public health and emergency response data systems at the state and local levels in the United States. What is required for an individual death to count as being caused by a hurricane, for example, depends on the clarity and specificity of case definitions used within a jurisdiction and on the professional judgments of those making determinations. Whether an individual with respiratory illness is included in the COVID-19 case count depends on whether a test was available and reported. This variability provides an opportunity for intentional or inadvertent selective use of data to minimize or exaggerate the number of cases based on stakeholder interests. This report describes how this problem can be addressed by improving processes for vital statistics, public health, and emergency response data systems and standardizing the way they are implemented and the data are reported by SLTT agencies throughout the United States.

Operationalize Uniform Systems, Tools, and Practices for Assessing Individual-Level Mortality

In addition to widespread inconsistency in the practices and case definitions used to attribute deaths to a disaster, the quality and value of those data are threatened by variability in how deaths are registered and reported across the United States. Mortality data are currently collected and reported through a byzantine process that spans a disjointed network of federal and SLTT-level systems for death investigation and registration. No federal or nationally standardized system exists for death investigations; instead, these are carried out through a patchwork of different medicolegal death investigation systems that are governed at the SLTT level and thus vary by jurisdiction. For example, states may use a coroner system, medical examiner (ME) system, or a combination of both for certifying deaths—and there are notable differences in levels of training, appointment processes, and political standing for coroners and medical examiners, each of which can impact the quality of death investigations. In some states, these systems are centralized at the state level and in others these systems are decentralized at the county or district level. After a death is certified within the medicolegal death investigation system, it is registered at a state-level vital records office to create a death record. It is then shared with the National Center for Health Statistics (NCHS) via the National Vital Statistics System (NVSS). As described in Chapters 3 and 4, this heterogeneity across systems and lack of uniform standards for attributing mortality and morbidity to a disaster across different systems impedes meaningful analysis and undermines the value of these data in improving disaster management.

The committee identified multiple gaps in death investigation and registration systems that limit the accuracy and comparability of the individual-level data collected. For instance, different SLTT systems use incongruent definitions for what counts as a disaster-related death. Medical certifiers of death play a crucial role on the front lines of this process, as they are responsible for assessing whether and the degree to which a death is attributable to the disaster and then inputting that information such that the appropriate information flows up through state-level death registration system and NCHS. Despite their essential role, training for medical certifiers is inconsistent and often inadequate. Because of the variation in the types of medicolegal death investigation systems that exist throughout the United States, the qualifications of these certifiers vary from being a registered voter with a high school diploma and free of a felony conviction in some coroner systems to forensic pathologists with 4–6 years of postgraduate medical training and board certification working in medical examiner systems as autopsy physicians and public health officers (see Chapter 3 for discussion of variation in the medicolegal death investigation system). Additionally, the current medicolegal death investigation and registration systems were not designed to capture information in a way that facilitates interoperability and timely data sharing within and across SLTT and federal levels. This adds to the administrative burden on medical examiners and coroners (ME/Cs) who are often required to enter data on a death into multiple systems. Electronic registration and coding of causes and contributors of death can streamline the process of death registration, but not all ME/C jurisdictions have electronic case management systems nor do all states have fully electronic death registration systems (see Recommendations 3-1 and 3-2).

The committee also identified opportunities to address these gaps through a series of immediate and future priorities for investment to promote the adoption of standard and uniform practices for collecting, recording, and reporting these data. For example, all jurisdictions would benefit from collecting a set of standard baseline data points about a death (e.g., geocoding of place of death and place of residence; practices for describing contributing factors of death). The NVSS is well positioned to drive many of the necessary systemic changes to improve vertical coordination across stakeholders and the interoperability of electronic systems between themselves, medical certifiers, and state vital records offices. Additional federal-level requirements could help ensure that these baseline data are collected uniformly and accurately by medical certifiers, so the information can be coded and entered into the national database.[2] This will also require supporting those states without electronic death registration systems to put them in place.

[2] This does not warrant changes to death certificates, which are legal documents governed at the state level.

Recommendation 3-1: Strengthen Existing Systems to Improve Individual-Level Mortality Data Quality

The Centers for Disease Control and Prevention (CDC), through the National Center for Health Statistics (NCHS), should lead an enterprise-wide initiative to strengthen existing death registration systems to improve the quality of disaster-related mortality data at state, local, tribal, and territorial levels. These efforts should prioritize the standardization of methods for data reporting and recording and to improve the capacity of death investigation and registration systems to capture more detail on contributing causes of death following disasters.

The following immediate actions should be undertaken:

- NCHS should fund and support the transition of the remaining states and territories with paper-based death registration systems to electronic death registration systems (EDRSs) and lead, in collaboration with state vital records offices, the integration of best practices for capturing and coding disaster-related death data into state-based EDRSs.
- NCHS should directly fund improvements in and the standardization of medical examiner and coroner (ME/C) death e-filing systems and require interoperability with these systems and state EDRSs. Similarly, NCHS and state registrars should require that EDRSs adopt the following standard improvements:
    - Automatic filing of death information with state EDRSs via ME/C e-filing systems to reduce the administrative burden on medical examiners and coroners;
    - Automated and uniform alert flags, prompts, drop-down options, and decision-making support for use by medical certifiers when entering data into a death record in both a routine and just-in-time capacity;
    - Offline data entry and other continuity mechanisms; and
    - Geocoding of deaths based on both place of residence and location of death.

The following long-term actions should be prioritized:

- NCHS should fund and adopt, where appropriate, artificial intelligence technologies to improve the throughput of its automated medical coding systems so as to improve the throughput of ME/C deaths to a level equivalent to that of other natural causes of death.
- State vital records offices and ME/C offices, with the support of CDC, should develop continuity plans to sustain the functions of these offices during emergencies.

Recommendation 3-2: Standardize Data Collection and Reporting of Individual-Level Reported Disaster-Related Mortality

The National Center for Health Statistics (NCHS), working with the states, should update the Model State Vital Statistics Act to drive uniformity of data collection and recording with respect to disaster-related mortality. To promote uniformity in definitions and practices for collecting and recording disaster-related mortality data and enhance the quality and comparability of these data, NCHS should revise the Model State Vital Statistics Act to provide clear guidance and data standards to state vital records offices and medical certifiers. These changes should include the use of automated flags, prompts, and drop-down options to collect data on the relationship of a death to a recent disaster and provide decision-making support for medical certifiers.

Standards for Defining and Collecting Morbidity Data

Morbidity is a complex concept that covers a range of health outcomes from the physical to psychological, including cardiovascular, gastrointestinal, and respiratory diseases; physical injuries; and mental health outcomes. Collecting data about disaster-related morbidities presents its own set of challenges beyond those described for mortality data, given the broad definition of disaster-related morbidities, variation across disaster types, and logistical challenges associated with mining morbidity data from across broad network of unique federal, SLTT, and health care systems. Capturing disaster-related morbidity data is further complicated by several inextricably linked factors: for example, disasters can exacerbate pre-existing conditions and create additional health complications (e.g., the closing of dialysis centers in a disaster will create morbidity among people with kidney disease requiring dialysis); co-morbidities can predispose certain at-risk individuals to additional diseases in the post-disaster environment (e.g., individuals with diabetes are at additional risk for cardiac disease); and multiple social determinants of health (SDOH) can profoundly impact both mortality and morbidity in disasters. The appendixes to this report provide several case examples that explore these complications. Appendix D describes the impact of SDOH on disaster-related morbidity and mortality through two case examples. Appendix C provides a focused case study of the challenges in assessing mortality and morbidity during the early stages of the COVID-19 public health emergency. Both provide additional support for the report's core recommendations.[3]

---

[3] The Federal Emergency Management Agency, the study's sponsor, provided permission for the inclusion of COVID-19 considerations in the report.

When acted on appropriately, morbidity data can help to reduce mortality (i.e., by preventing morbidities from becoming mortalities) and can be used to shape public health actions, including community health education, and medical preparedness (see Chapter 2 for additional uses of morbidity data). For end users in the field of disaster management, in particular, estimates of morbidity resulting from a disaster may actually be of more value than mortality data in informing life-saving recovery, mitigation, and preparedness activities; enhancing real-time response; and providing information on health care utilization. Therefore, exclusive focus on mortality data, the traditional outcome of interest, at the expense of morbidity data is tantamount to focusing only on the most severe cases.

Currently, there is no consensus on which morbidities or indicators should be consistently tracked in common types of disasters (e.g., floods, hurricanes, blizzards, tornadoes, pandemics/epidemics) to provide actionable information to end users such as public health and emergency planners, health care systems, and SLTT and federal agencies. As with all data, different types provide different opportunities for use. The collection of significant morbidity data, defined for the purposes of this report as serious morbidities with high risk of immediate hospitalization and death, could provide critical data on population needs regarding access to health care resources. However, exclusively focusing on significant morbidities would likely fail to capture population trends for less immediately critical but far more prevalent and costly morbidities related to the social determinants of health, such as respiratory impacts, mental health outcomes, and exacerbation of existing co-morbidities (see Appendix D). Defining what data to prioritize for collection is a critical first step to building the capability to collect and use these data. Therefore, investment in an ongoing process is needed to develop, validate, and disseminate national standards for data collection of key morbidities caused or exacerbated by specific types of disasters (see Recommendation 3-3).

Recommendation 3-3: Develop a Set of Standards for Morbidity Data Collection

The Centers for Disease Control and Prevention, in collaboration with the Centers for Medicare & Medicaid Services, the Council of State and Territorial Epidemiologists, and the National Association of County & City Health Officials should establish and promulgate national standards for the collection of disaster-related morbidities before, during, and after disasters. These activities should include investment in research to identify common morbidities that occur as a result of or are exacerbated by the conditions of specific types of disasters (e.g., floods, hurricanes, blizzards, radiation events, pandemics, etc.) and across multiple disaster types. This should include the identification of minimum timelines for data collection, the development and validation of morbidity data systems for use by the disaster management enterprise, and pilot testing and implementation of approaches to collect these data in a standardized manner.

Analytical Methods for Population Estimates

As indicated in the guiding precepts (see Box S-1), in assessing the impacts of disasters, the committee recognizes the importance of both counting individuals who die and estimating the morbidity and mortality impacts of disasters on the entire population at risk using statistical methods. Accurate counts of individual deaths can provide timely information on the scale of an event and is critical for assigning individual-level benefits, but individual counts rarely provide an adequate picture of a disaster's impact on the mortality and morbidity of the population as a whole. For a number of reasons (described in detail in Chapter 3 and explored in regard to the COVID-19 case study in Appendix C), individual counting methods typically underestimate the total impact of a disaster on a population. Statistical estimation methods, by contrast, generate a more complete picture of the total impact of the disaster, but do not always yield an allocation of individual cases into mutually exclusive categories of death or illness resulting from the disaster versus from other causes. Survey and sampling methods and excess death methods are the primary methods encompassed by the population estimation approach. See Chapter 2 for a discussion of both individual count and population estimate approaches as they relate to the value and use of mortality and morbidity data and Chapter 4 for a discussion of population-level methods of estimation.

Given the variation in ways for attributing the cause of any death and morbidity, there can be more than one appropriate approach to answering the question: "How many total deaths and significant morbidities were caused by this disaster?" However, while there is no single standard method for generating mortality or morbidity estimates using population estimation, methodological best practices can be specified. A national research program is vital to further develop and validate these best practices and to indicate appropriate circumstances for the use of specific methods (see Recommendation 4-1). As in all areas of research, these practices should be characterized by clarity in the specification of study objectives and definition of terms, transparency in the statement of assumptions and the sourcing of data used in the study, and great caution in advancing any particular measure or method as a most perfect solution.

Developing an effective data and information structure for studying disaster impacts on mortality and morbidity should be a cornerstone of the nation's operational disaster response function. Because the analytical sophistication and high-quality fieldwork necessary to develop and implement data infrastructure nationally is generally beyond the capabilities and time availability of most SLTT health departments, the responsibility of building and sustaining the capacity of the nation's existing research and survey infrastructure to support the collection of survey data on the health effects of disasters rests at the federal level (see Recommendations 4-1 and 4-2).

> <u>Recommendation 4-1: Fund and Conduct Research on Analytical Methods for Population Estimates</u>
>
> **The Centers for Disease Control and Prevention, the National Institutes of Health, and the National Science Foundation should establish a national research program to advance analytical methods for conducting population-level estimates of mortality and morbidity related to disasters.** This national research program should include the development and refinement of minimum standard methods and protocols for conducting population-level mortality and morbidity assessments as well as the creation and testing of tools for use by researchers, states, and localities to enhance their capabilities to carry out and use these analyses.
>
> - Academic departments and institutes, which can be more flexible in initiating and conducting studies, should be included in these research efforts.
> - Because many of the estimates in the literature result from "one-off" efforts that do not build on or seek comparability with previous disasters, an initial step in this research should be a careful comparison of different estimates from the same emergency to gain an understanding of how methodological choices and assumptions affect the estimates.

> <u>Recommendation 4-2: Enhance Capacity to Collect and Analyze Population Estimates for Mortality and Morbidity</u>
>
> **The Department of Health and Human Services, together with state, local, tribal, and territorial (SLTT) agencies, should proactively develop partnerships to enhance the capacity to collect and analyze population-level disaster-related morbidity and mortality information.** This includes the identification of appropriate mortality and morbidity datasets and sampling frames that might be brought to bear and the pre-negotiation of data-sharing agreements to ensure access to these data when needed.
>
> The following immediate actions should be undertaken:
>
> - The Secretary of Health and Human Services should push forward the collection of survey data on disaster-exposed and

comparison populations to provide population-representative data on how disasters and their contributing stressors affect morbidity and to build the evidence base on differences in mortality and morbidity impacts across types of disasters.

- The federal statistical system, including the Centers for Disease Control and Prevention (CDC), the Substance Abuse and Mental Health Services Administration, and others should harness existing survey infrastructure and develop standard, Institutional Review Board (IRB)-approved sampling frames and methods for dealing with methodological challenges, such as population migration, for use by researchers conducting population estimates following large-scale disasters.
- The stakeholders listed above should address issues with informed consent procedures under the Common Rule, respondent burden issues under the Paperwork Reduction Act, and privacy under the Health Insurance Portability and Accountability Act Privacy Rule in advance and ensure that alternative arrangements are in place to protect privacy and confidentiality.
- SLTT agencies and academic research centers with the capability of conducting population estimates of disaster impact should formalize working relationships, data-sharing agreements, and IRB approvals in advance of a disaster to reduce delays in access to health data needed to conduct population estimates following a disaster and develop baseline assessments during the inter-disaster period.
- CDC and the Federal Emergency Management Agency should integrate frontline public health practitioners (e.g., epidemiologists and others) in the disaster response teams to help gather data and begin detailed analyses of mortality and morbidity data early in the disaster.

Access to and Use of Mortality and Morbidity Data

To maximize value, data on disaster-related mortality and morbidity should be available to all stakeholders and be provided in a manner that is actionable for informing response, recovery, and mitigation activities at all stages of the disaster management cycle. Ensuring equitable access to timely and actionable data is of particular importance in disaster-impacted localities that may have limited capacity to carry out their own data collection and analysis. Strategies to broaden access and improve the utility of these data are described in Chapters 3 and 4. For example, federal agencies (e.g., NCHS, Federal Emergency Management Agency, Office of the Assistant Secretary for Preparedness and Response, CDC) have the responsibility to actively support partners at the SLTT levels by providing them with actionable, location-specific information from the federal database, including baseline comparison mortality data and up-to-date data on disaster deaths (see Recommendation 4-3). Access to data does not equate to the actionability of data. For data to be actionable, the stakeholder requires the tools, capacity, and expertise to analyze these data and act appropriately. Therefore, investment in the development and deployment of ready-to-use tools that are tailored for use by SLTT stakeholders is critical to ensuring action (see Recommendation 4-3). Leveraging federal data and expertise to address limitations of federal mortality and morbidity data, such as routine mortality and morbidity surveillance, continuous quality improvement of data collection and integration systems, and retrospective geocoding of death registry entries in certain disaster-impacted areas would also enhance the accuracy and actionability of these data (see Recommendation 4-3).

Recommendation 4-3: Facilitate Access to and Use of Actionable Mortality and Morbidity Data by State, Local, Tribal, and Territorial (SLTT) Entities

- **The Department of Health and Human Services (HHS) should work with the Centers for Disease Control and Prevention, the Federal Emergency Management Agency (FEMA), the Office of the Assistant Secretary for Preparedness and Response (ASPR), and other federal agencies to facilitate access to essential mortality and morbidity data to SLTT entities and academic research institutions throughout the disaster cycle. These data should be provided proactively and in a manner that is actionable for situational awareness and disaster response at state and local levels.**
- **Additionally, state and federal agencies should fund the development and testing of analytical tools and work collaboratively with local entities to use mortality and morbidity data in meaningful ways.**
- The following immediate actions should be undertaken to ensure SLTT access to and use of mortality and morbidity data:
    - The National Center for Health Statistics (NCHS) should code and automatically provide, with the assistance of FEMA and ASPR, location-specific, baseline mortality data and up-to-date data on disaster deaths following a declared disaster and upon request, as well as offer ready-to-use tools within a set time frame following disasters to states and localities.

- o NCHS should make available to researchers and SLTT investigators the mortality data from the National Death Index.
- o NCHS and state vital records offices should retrospectively geocode death registry entries in select areas that were previously affected by large-scale disasters to provide sample data for modeling future impact and other research.
- o ASPR and CDC should provide state and local officials with guidance on standard practices for assessing mortality and morbidity and facilitate the analysis of these data by state and local health and emergency management officials.
- o CDC in collaboration with FEMA and ASPR should fund and conduct research to establish standard practices for analyzing disaster-related causes of death and its contributing causes, including guidance on standard timelines for data analysis (e.g., 30 days) and geographic parameters for defining a disaster's geographic scope.
- o CDC and the Centers for Medicare & Medicaid Services (CMS) should use existing systems to pilot the collection of relevant morbidity data following disasters to serve as an inter-disaster baseline.
- o CMS, in collaboration with electronic health record companies and health systems, should pilot and evaluate the inclusion of disaster-related *International Classification of Diseases, Tenth Revision* codes in electronic health records.
- o HHS should use both existing and novel data sources to improve mortality and morbidity data acquisition and reporting, including the use of surveys, artificial intelligence, machine learning, and other big data methods.

Professional Training and Support

A broad range of stakeholders across professions and jurisdictions is involved in capturing, recording, analyzing, and using disaster-related mortality and morbidity data. Major barriers identified by the committee include the ongoing siloing of death investigation and registration systems from the disaster management enterprise, disparate levels of professional training and expertise across medical certifiers, and poor continuing education regarding attribution and recording of disaster-related deaths. Cumulatively, these shortcomings hinder the ability of the nation to procure accurate and complete individual counts of reported deaths following a disaster. Supporting medical certifiers will require federal resources for ongoing guidance, education, and training to enable their accurate input of data into death records and to appreciate the importance of their part in the enterprise. Additionally, structural changes in medicolegal death investigation systems may be warranted (e.g., transition to systems staffed with MEs and promulgation of standardized education and continuing training requirements) to ensure that this critically important system is staffed by professionals with medically oriented training and professional backgrounds. This will ensure that these professionals are equipped to perform essential system functions and support the consistent and unbiased assessment of individual deaths following disasters. Federal agencies and ME/C professional organizations are essential to engaging and supporting this workforce and making the essential changes (see Recommendations 3-4 and 3-5).

Recommendation 3-4: Strengthen the Capacity of the Medicolegal Death Investigation System to Assess Disaster-Related Mortality

The Centers for Disease Control and Prevention (CDC), in collaboration with state agencies and professional associations, should strengthen the value, capacity, and capability of the medicolegal death investigation system to improve investigation, training, data development and collection, and case management.

The following immediate actions should be undertaken:

- CDC should fund and re-launch the Medical Examiner and Coroner Information Sharing Program to provide guidance and support to medical examiners, coroners, and other medical certifiers.
- The National Association of Medical Examiners, the International Association of Coroners & Medical Examiners, the American Board of Medicolegal Death Investigators, and state-based medical examiner and coroner professional organizations should support the proposed framework for collecting and recording uniform mortality and morbidity data, encourage the use of existing CDC tools and guidance by all professionals, and provide continuing education courses for their members that reflect this guidance.
- CDC, through the National Center for Health Statistics, along with appropriate licensing bodies should provide standardized training and materials designed for medical certifiers (physicians, nurse practitioners, physician assistants, and others as applicable by state) who encounter natural deaths and are responsible for entering death information into the death record.
- Death investigation systems should develop relationships with state or university-based demographers and epidemiologists to

formalize proactive data collection and sharing agreements for natural disasters that are typical for the state as well as mass mortality and morbidity due to disease.

- To promote more accurate death certification, the above agencies should incentivize and support the conversion of coroner systems to regionalized medical examiner systems staffed by forensic pathologists and medicolegal death investigators professionally trained to identify and classify disaster-related deaths per the framework described in Recommendation 2-1.

Recommendation 3-5: Strengthen the Role of the Medicolegal Death Investigation and State Death Registration Systems in the Disaster Management Enterprise

State, local, tribal, and territorial public health and emergency management departments should integrate the professionals and agencies from the medicolegal death investigation and death registration systems in all aspects of preparedness and planning. This should involve the consideration of moving mortality management out of Emergency Support Function #8 (ESF8) and creating a separate ESF dedicated to mortality management. This new function could complement ESF8 and ensure focused attention on assessing mortality during and after disasters, while those charged with ESF8 responsibilities are focused on providing services to survivors. This new function could include the involvement of medical examiners, coroners, and other relevant professionals in planning drills for mortality management; effective, efficient, and unbiased data collection during disasters; training for family assistance centers; and standards for after-action reports and other mortality data-reporting activities.

MEETING THE MISSION

In its review of the current landscape of practices, systems, and tools for assessing mortality and significant morbidity following large-scale disasters, the committee identified several persistent, systemic challenges as well as potential best practices that could be brought to scale. Chapter 5 offers a set of crosscutting recommendations intended to serve as a blueprint for moving forward. Box S-3 provides a high-level synthesis of these recommendations stratified into immediate actions and future priorities.

BOX S-3
Recommended Immediate Actions and Future Priorities

Recommended immediate actions needed to address current gaps in policy, practice, and infrastructure for mortality and morbidity assessment include

1. Adoption and use of a uniform framework for collecting, recording, and reporting mortality and morbidity data (Recommendations 2-1 and 2-2).
2. Investment in improvements to data systems and tools for collecting, recording, and reporting individual count data at a state, local, tribal, and territorial (SLTT) level (Recommendations 3-1 and 3-2).
3. Update of the Model State Vital Statistics Act and Regulations to facilitate more robust and uniform mortality data collection across the nation (Recommendation 3-2).
4. Creation of a process to develop, validate, and promulgate national standards for reporting on a core set of morbidity impacts specific to the common types of major disasters (Recommendation 3-3).
5. Investment in and development of the capacity to collect and analyze the data necessary for population estimates of mortality and morbidity (Recommendation 4-2).
6. Implementation of new tools and approaches to share and use mortality and morbidity data (Recommendation 4-3).
7. Consideration of a separate Emergency Support Function dedicated to mortality management (Recommendation 3-5).

Recommended future priorities to strengthen the nation's ability to prepare for and respond to disasters and emergencies of all types via the enhanced assessment of individual counts and population estimates of mortality and morbidity include

1. Integration of new technologies, as these become available, into existing electronic data systems and tools (Recommendation 3-1).
2. Investment in research to advance the science of mortality and morbidity assessment (Recommendations 3-1, 4-1, and 4-2).
3. Development and dissemination of resources for training professionals in the medicolegal death investigation system and for inclusion in SLTT disaster management (Recommendations 3-4 and 3-5).

1

Introduction

In the hours, days, weeks, and months following a disaster, coming to terms with the event's impact on human life is critical for affected communities, responders, and those watching the aftermath unfold from afar. Assessments of disaster-related mortality and morbidity ascribe a quantitative value to a traumatic event, and these assessments hold deep emotional, societal, financial, and logistical value. These data can assist a community in memorializing what has been lost; inform and justify the scale of a response; determine access to resources; and strengthen mitigation and response practices to save lives in the future. Furthermore, as climate change alters the frequency and severity of many natural disasters and the map of global vulnerability shifts and expands, these data can provide an accounting of the financial and societal costs of failure to prevent or mitigate the effects of climate change. These data are imperative for long-range planning related to large-scale infrastructure projects and even for addressing questions of where to build and whether to rebuild in the context of our changing world. Accurately quantifying mortality and morbidity caused by disasters is foundational to protecting the public's health and well-being in myriad ways. However, the practices, systems, and stakeholders that exist across the nation to support these essential efforts are less coordinated, robust, and reliable than they should be. These systematic inadequacies—both simple and complex—hamper the nation's capability to respond more effectively in moments of crisis and limit the ability to proactively and economically mitigate the effects of the next disaster. This report describes the importance of accurately assessing mortality and morbidity data and the diverse uses of these data. In addition to reviewing the current landscape of practices and methods used in the field and highlighting existing barriers and challenges, the report provides stakeholders with a blueprint for action to enhance the collection, reporting, and use of accurate information on the mortality and morbidity of major disasters.

STUDY BACKGROUND AND SCOPE

Following the October 2018 passage of the Federal Aviation Administration Reauthorization Act, which contained the Disaster Recovery Reform Act, the Federal Emergency Management Agency (FEMA) tasked the National Academies of Sciences, Engineering, and Medicine (the National Academies) to carry out a consensus study of best practices for conducting mortality and morbidity assessments following large-scale disasters. The Statement of Task (see Box 1-1) developed by FEMA charged the consensus study committee with reviewing and describing the current state of the field of assessing disaster-related mortality and morbidity. This includes examining current practices and methods for collecting, recording, sharing, and using data across state, local, tribal, and territorial (SLTT) stakeholders and evaluating best practices and areas for future resource investment.

The Statement of Task directs the committee to focus on *large-scale* disasters[1]—natural or manmade—as defined in the Robert T. Stafford Disaster Relief and Emergency Assistance Act (Stafford Act) (see Box 1-2). The Statement of Task also makes clear that in-depth exploration or recommendations that are directly related to syndromic surveillance, long-term surveillance of health impacts related to disasters, or the surveillance of emergency responders are outside the scope of the committee's work.

The concepts of mortality and morbidity are used heavily throughout the report. The term "mortality" is widely used to mean a death or deaths that occur regardless of cause. The term "morbidity" generally means a disease(s) or injury(ies) of varying degree of severity. At the end of this chapter, there is a section titled Terminology Choices and Key Concepts, where more context is provided for the various terms and concepts used throughout this report. These include an explanation of the term "significant morbidity," per the language used in the Statement of Task, as well as a discussion of the vocabulary used for the attribution of both mortality and morbidity to a disaster, among others.

---

[1] The Stafford Act declaration in response to the ongoing coronavirus pandemic resulted in the inclusion of the pandemic in the committee's deliberation and report. See Appendix C for a paper developed independently by two committee members on the assessment of coronavirus mortality.

BOX 1-1
Statement of Task for the Committee on Best Practices for Assessing Mortality and Significant Morbidity Following Large-Scale Disasters

An ad hoc committee will conduct a review and assessment of the current state of the field and best practices in assessing and quantifying mortality and significant morbidity following large-scale disasters, with a specific focus on disasters declared under the Robert T. Stafford Disaster Relief and Emergency Assistance Act (Stafford Act). The purpose of this study is to describe the current landscape of mortality and significant morbidity data collection and information-sharing processes used by state, local, tribal, and territorial (SLTT) public health agencies and to propose areas for future resource investment to enhance these practices. In identifying and evaluating best practices and resources, the committee will focus on those applicable to SLTT public health preparedness and response practitioners.

Specifically, the committee will:

- Describe the importance of mortality and significant morbidity data after disaster impact, their use, and the organizations that capture these data or could benefit from use of the data.
- Describe the current architecture, methodologies, and information systems currently in use or available to SLTT public health agencies for the sharing and reporting of these data, highlighting the diversity of processes and identifying potential best practices. In doing so the committee may consider current guidance for attributing deaths directly and indirectly to a specific disaster, the role of information technology systems, including limitations, and continuity mechanisms to ensure continued data collection in a post-impact environment.
- Identify current challenges to collecting, recording, and reporting mortality and significant morbidity data after disasters, including, as feasible, challenges related to lack of standardization for data collection and disaster attribution, coordination, and training. This shall include an analysis of timing for attribution of death to a specific incident (e.g., acute, delayed) and potential impacts on individuals and organizations.
- Identify best practices for collecting, recording, and reporting mortality and significant morbidity data after disasters, and recommend priority areas of emphasis and allocation of resources to enhance SLTT mortality and significant morbidity data collection and reporting after disasters, considering feasibility, sustainability, and impact to SLTT and health care organizations.
- Review analytic approaches and statistical methods for disaster-related mortality and significant morbidity and identify best practices for conducting prospective tracking and retrospective studies.

This study is intended to focus on non-infectious-disease-related disasters (e.g., hurricanes, earthquakes, etc.) as defined in the Stafford Act. Syndromic surveillance, long-term surveillance, and surveillance of responders are outside the scope of this study.

BOX 1-2
Overview of the Stafford Act

The Stafford Act of 1988 gives authority to the President to declare a major disaster or emergency and to authorize the distribution of federal aid and support to affected areas and individuals. Declared disasters and emergencies each receive different types and amounts of federal assistance, with an emergency involving a more limited scope of assistance (Liu, 2008). Between 2000 and 2009 the Stafford Act was triggered, on average, approximately 57 times per year (CRS, 2017). It is used most frequently in response to large-scale local and regional disasters (e.g., Midwest flooding in 2019, California wildfires in 2017, Hurricane Katrina in 2005) and terrorist incidents (e.g., September 11, 2011, attacks and Oklahoma City bombing in 1995).

> "Major disaster" means any natural catastrophe (including any hurricane, tornado, storm, high water, wind-driven water, tidal wave, tsunami, earthquake, volcanic eruption, landslide, mudslide, snowstorm, or drought), or, regardless of cause, any fire, flood, or explosion, in any part of the United States, which in the determination of the President causes damage of sufficient severity and magnitude to warrant major disaster assistance under this Act to supplement the efforts and available resources of States, local governments, and disaster relief organizations in alleviating the damage, loss, hardship, or suffering caused thereby.

> "Emergency" means any occasion or instance for which, in the determination of the President, Federal assistance is needed to supplement State and local efforts and capabilities to save lives and to protect property and public health and safety, or to lessen or avert the threat of a catastrophe in any part of the United States.

SOURCE: Robert T. Stafford Disaster Relief and Emergency Assistance Act, Public Law 707, 100th Congress (November 23, 1988).

Inclusion of COVID-19

Despite the original request for the committee to focus its deliberations on disasters other than infectious disease-related disasters, the emergence of the coronavirus disease 2019 (COVID-19) pandemic and subsequent issuance of a Stafford Act declaration in March 2020 for all states ultimately led to the selective inclusion of COVID-19 in the report. In the weeks following the emergence and initial spread of COVID-19, before transmission was widespread domestically, the committee did not consider the outbreak to be within the scope of the report. However, as the number of cases increased within the borders of the United States, it became clear that the administrative, logistical, and methodological challenges illustrated in the early attempts of assessing COVID-19-related mortality and morbidity mirrored many of the same issues found in other large-scale disasters. Following the Stafford Act declaration, the committee requested confirmation from the study sponsor that discussions of COVID-19 could be included in the report. FEMA provided its approval for the inclusion in May 2020. The committee chose to include a few illustrative examples throughout the report from the COVID-19 pandemic regarding mortality and morbidity assessment to highlight overlapping logistical and methodological barriers with other large-scale disasters. In short, the committee believes that experiences from COVID-19 illustrate the same need for coordination across stakeholders and consistent policies and systems to accurately identify and report cases as in other natural disasters. The pandemic also provides clear and timely examples of the uses of different methods for assessing morbidity and mortality, which help to illustrate their comparative strengths and weaknesses for different purposes.

At the same time, the widespread transmission of COVID-19 in the United States occurred toward the end of the committee's deliberation period and the committee did not have sufficient opportunity to consider the full implications of COVID-19 (a pandemic that remained very active and evolving even at the time of the report's final editing) and also did not wish for the contentious issues surrounding COVID-19 to overtake the core messages of the report. As a result, the committee has included in Appendix C a separate thought piece, which was independently authored by two committee members, on early experiences of assessing COVID-19 mortality and morbidity. This paper provides additional real-time context and support for the report's core recommendations by highlighting overlapping methodological, administrative, and logistical challenges with other disasters and unique features of the pandemic—and a more focused analysis of morbidity and mortality estimation challenges in this public health emergency than what is provided in the main body of the report.

Inclusion of Social Determinants of Health

An in-depth focus on the socio-environmental dimensions of health and how these factors function to heighten vulnerabilities to disasters (e.g., association between secondary exposures, such as contaminated water supplies post-disaster; pre-existing economic disparities; and exacerbation of gastrointestinal illnesses) (CDC, 2005; Furey et al., 2007; Marinova-Petkova et al., 2019; Nigro et al., 2011; Yee et al., 2007) was determined to be outside the scope of this study. For this reason, this report does not provide a detailed analysis of these issues or dedicated recommendations on strategies for integrating social determinants of health information into mortality and morbidity data systems or how these data, once collected, could inform the actions of the disaster management enterprise. The committee, however, feels strongly that the lack of such in-depth discussion is purely a reflection of the limited scope of the study's charge and not a reflection of the fundamental importance of these issues. In particular, while research documenting stark disparities in the impacts of disasters on underserved and historically disadvantaged communities is relatively robust, dedicated research on how to mitigate or eliminate these disparities is sparse and much needed. For instance, there would be tremendous value in strengthening the knowledge base regarding the role of community resilience in mitigating disaster-related impacts including mortality and morbidity. Considerations related to the intersection of the social determinants of health and mortality and morbidity assessment will be highlighted at various points throughout the report as a reminder of the critical importance of these issues (see especially Chapter 2). Additionally, a short supplemental paper drafted by staff, which includes two case studies on the contributory roles of the social determinants of health on community vulnerabilities to adverse health outcomes following disasters, has been included at the end of this report (see Appendix D).

Report Approach and Methodology

This report explores a broad range of issues relevant to the assessment of mortality and morbidity following large-scale disasters, with a specific focus on those disasters defined by the Stafford Act. To address the study's Statement of Task (see Box 1-1), the National Academies appointed a 15-member committee with a broad range of academic and professional expertise, including public health policy, planning, and ethics; epidemiological and statistical research methods and analysis; and SLTT disaster response and fatality management. The committee deliberated from May 2019 to June 2020 and during this time the committee held five in-person meetings.

Committee's Approach

Regarding the committee's approach, this study was brought before the committee due the extreme discrepancies in mortality estimates following Hurricane Maria in Puerto Rico in 2017. While this tragedy emotionally underpinned the committee's deliberations, the committee chose not to endorse a specific methodological approach or a particular singular way of assigning a "death toll" for all disasters. Instead, the committee interpreted the Statement of Task as asking, "What are the appropriate methods for tackling the problem of estimation and attribution?" and "How can these data be used to save lives and prevent suffering?" As such, the committee approached this study as an opportunity to provide stakeholders with an actionable roadmap that addresses persistent administrative, methodological, logistical, and organizational barriers to the effective assessment of disaster-related mortality and morbidity. Early in the deliberative process, it became evident that overcoming these barriers and achieving lasting change across multiple systems is reliant on the coordinated commitment of multiple entities. The committee's call for an enterprise approach to overcome persistent fragmentation in stakeholder responsibilities and systems ultimately forms the foundation for the report's final chapter, which lays out the recommendations as components of a broader plan. These recommendations seek to (1) provide a strong framework for conceptualizing mortality and morbidity assessment; (2) guide the appropriate selection and use of various estimation approaches; (3) strengthen data collection and reporting systems to enhance the quality and comparability of data; and (4) provide SLTT stakeholders with the actionable data, tools, resources, and training needed to use mortality and morbidity data to save lives.

Additionally, to further enhance the applicability of the report for all hazards, the committee sought to emphasize the similarity of challenges across disasters of all types and scales in the collection, recording, and use of mortality and morbidity data. Therefore, while the report's recommendations are focused directly on major disasters as defined in the Stafford Act and are referred to in this report as "large-scale disasters," the report's conclusions and recommendations can be read and adopted more broadly. Chapter 5 includes further discussion on the broader applicability of the committee's recommendations.

Report Methodology

The work of the committee was informed by several different mechanisms and activities—six public sessions, two webinars, two site visits, two public comment sessions, electronic public comments, and a literature review. The committee hosted multiple types of open-to-the-public, information-gathering sessions. In August 2019, the committee convened a 2-day, in-person public workshop that brought together stakeholders to discuss their experiences and perspectives on assessing disaster-related mortality and morbidity as well as related policy and practice considerations. This workshop included a public comment session. The third committee meeting held in October 2019 included four additional open sessions and were hosted during site visits in Butte County and Sacramento, California. During these October 2019 sessions, the committee engaged with city officials in the city of Paradise, representatives of the county public health office in Butte County, and the medical examiner of Sacramento County (see Appendix B for the public workshop and meeting agendas). In addition to these in-person events, the committee hosted two public webinars in February 2020, which featured researchers who use a variety of statistical approaches to develop population estimates in their respective fields. Public comments were formally solicited during the first and second in-person meetings of the committee in May and June 2019, respectively, and written comments from the public were accepted electronically for the entirety of the deliberative process. These public information-gathering sessions and the deliberations of the committee were supplemented by peer-reviewed and grey literature.

At the onset of deliberations, the committee worked in collaboration with the National Academies Research Center to develop and carry out a comprehensive review of the literature to support its work and provide additional evidence to inform the report's conclusions and recommendations. This primary review concentrated on journals in a series of databases, including Embase, Medline, PAIS, ProQuest, PubMed, PsycInfo, Scopus, SocINDEX, and Worldcat, among others, and concentrated on articles published between 1980 and 2019. The committee chose to focus its efforts on research related to disasters in the United States but did not automatically eliminate literature involving international disasters (e.g., 2004 Indian Ocean tsunami). A more detailed accounting of the search parameters for the primary literature review can be found in Appendix A. The intent of the committee's review of the literature on population estimation methods (see Chapter 4) was not to review every possible method and select a universal standard, but to explore the most relevant—and rigorous—methods that have been used, identify the benefits, shortcomings, and requirements for these methods, and, ultimately, develop a research agenda. The articles identified were reviewed for relevance to the Statement of Task and were made available to the committee, staff, and science writer. In addition to the primary comprehensive literature review, the committee drew from two supplemental papers drafted by members of the committee and staff (see Appendixes C and D) to provide additional supporting material for the report.

Guiding Precepts for an Effective Data System for Assessing Mortality and Morbidity

After reviewing the current landscape of practices for assessing mortality and morbidity following large-scale disasters, the committee established a set of guiding precepts to aid in developing its recommendations. The precepts describe the key qualities and philosophies of a responsive system for the collection and use of mortality and morbidity data that enables proactive decision making by stakeholders. These precepts, which follow, and their implications are incorporated throughout the report.

Collect and use data for community health protection as an essential component across all phases of disaster management

The fundamental responsibilities of emergency management and public health—at every level and capacity—are to protect human health, support recovery, and prevent similar consequences from occurring in the future. High-quality mortality and morbidity data can improve preparedness, mitigation, response, and recovery capabilities if they are widely accessible, appropriately analyzed, and used effectively. Efforts to improve the timeliness and accuracy of mortality and morbidity data should be underpinned by the broader ethos of saving lives, protecting health, and preparing for future disasters.

Incorporate both individual counts and population estimates to better understand a disaster's true effect

The two primary approaches for assessing disaster-related mortality and morbidity, individual counts and population estimates, have important and complementary values. The committee seeks to balance the two approaches in contributing to a comprehensive picture of a disaster's true effect. These estimation approaches have different uses, advantages, and drawbacks, but both are critical for accurately and comprehensively assessing and describing a disaster's impact on human health and for developing and improving approaches to limit the future consequences of disasters.

Leverage morbidity data and mortality data to support response, recovery, mitigation, and preparedness

Focusing exclusively on disaster-related mortality—the traditional outcome of interest—is shortsighted. Using morbidity data—both during the crisis and in the inter-disaster period—to evaluate and guide disaster management efforts provides greater opportunities for reducing future mortality outcomes and increasing the resilience of the community.

Build on and use existing systems, capacities, and methodologies

Efforts to drive systems-level improvements benefit from using existing capabilities and capacities as well as identifying shared goals and existing resources to support stakeholders across fields and disciplines. Failure to strengthen the broader system for collecting, recording, and reporting mortality and morbidity data weakens the ability of the nation to respond effectively to changing health threats. Changes that occur only in siloes or at certain levels will be insufficient to optimize the use of mortality and morbidity data.

Commit to the continuous improvement of systems over time

Access to valuable individual counts and population estimates of morbidity and mortality is foundational to understanding a disaster's impact. The specific data needs, appropriate tools, effective practices, and key stakeholders evolve over time, and thus systems need to respond by evolving in parallel. Adopting a systems-level learning approach can provide a foundation for continuously improving the integrity and interpretation of mortality and morbidity data, thus enabling greater protection of human life.

Adopt an enterprise approach to activate stakeholders and systems in times of crisis and during the inter-disaster period

Effectively collecting and using mortality and morbidity data requires collaboration across the disparate institutions and organizations that are directly and indirectly involved in disaster response, recovery, mitigation, and preparedness. An enterprise approach across the disaster management enterprise would unite stakeholders under common goals and mitigate the complexity of operationalizing improved practices and methods.

Support the resilience and strength of historically disadvantaged populations by using data to understand, mitigate, and eliminate inequalities in disaster impacts

Mortality and morbidity data can offer valuable contextual information about population-specific vulnerabilities and provide evidence for targeted mitigation and preparedness efforts to protect and improve the resilience of these populations.

VALUE AND MEANINGFUL USE OF MORTALITY AND MORBIDITY DATA IN DISASTER MANAGEMENT

The overarching aims of quantifying mortality and morbidity following a disaster are to facilitate actions that save lives, to protect health, and to prepare for the future (CDC, 2016). To achieve these aims, accurate data must be effectively communicated to a broad range of stakeholders that spans emergency management, government agencies, health systems, the general public, policy makers and political leadership, and other public- and private-sector stakeholders (see Chapter 2). The value of these data shifts across stakeholders, across the disaster management cycle, and over time (see Figure 1-1). Value is also determined by the type and quality of the data collected, how and when data are captured, and how these data are analyzed. Although mortality and morbidity data hold value for a variety of reasons, the primary focus of this report is how these data can be used to improve future health outcomes in large-scale disasters.

Two strands of work emerge following a disaster: one is driven by the need for immediate information on mortality, morbidity, and other relevant contextual data to facilitate response and recovery efforts, while the other seeks to better understand what happened during the response and recovery and how mitigation and prevention efforts can be informed and improved with better data. Quantifying the public health impacts of

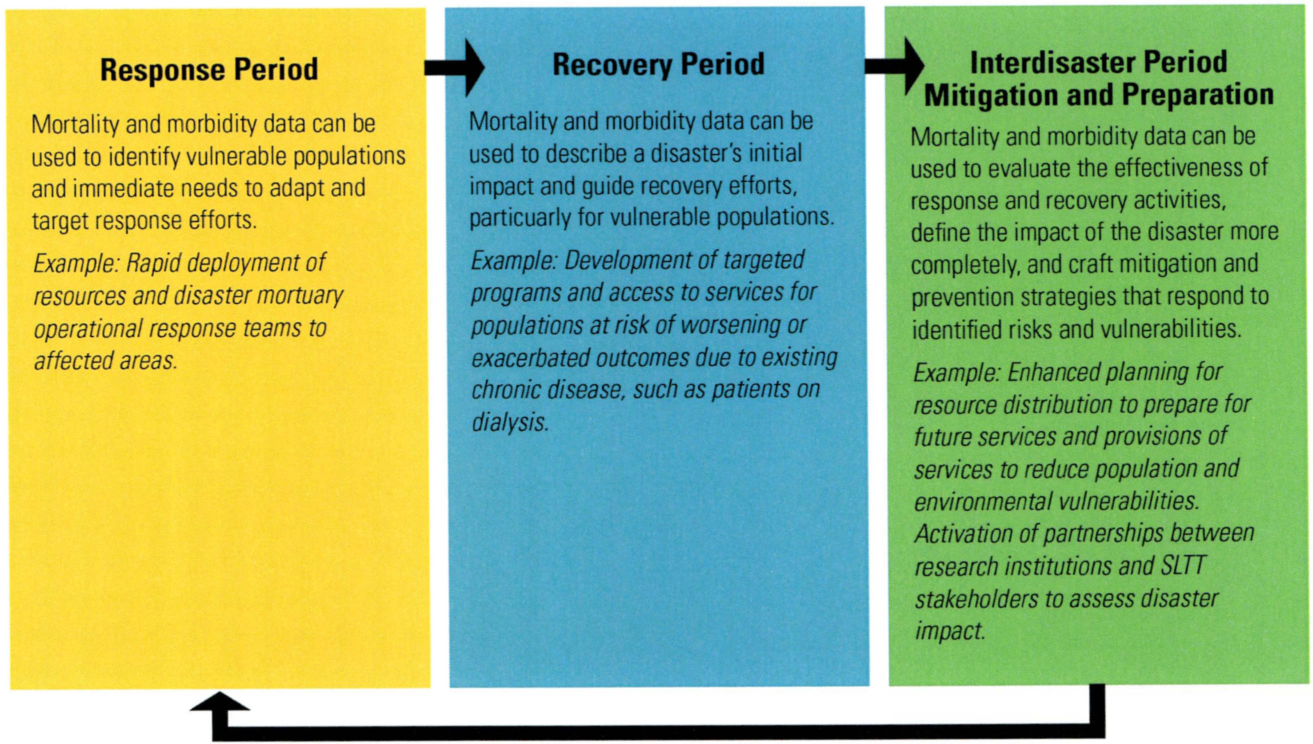

FIGURE 1-1 Changing uses of mortality and morbidity data over a disaster lifecycle.

disasters is important not only for informing immediate response efforts, but also for offering insights into the effectiveness of policies and interventions to strengthen future response and recovery efforts (Khan et al., 2014). Understanding the potential impact of a threat is essential for preparation, planning, mitigation, and response.

Modeling based on morbidity and mortality data can also help elucidate a particular future or past threat and provide an estimate of the likely impact the threat will have or had on a given population. When compared to baseline data, these analyses can help determine whether there is sufficient local-level capacity to manage that threat and whether federal resources may be required. These different approaches—individual counts and population estimates—used for estimating disaster-related mortality and morbidity as well as the practical uses for these data and relevant barriers will be discussed in greater detail in Chapters 3 and 4.

CURRENT ISSUES IN MORTALITY AND MORBIDITY ASSESSMENT

Despite the importance of mortality and morbidity data in protecting human life, the nation lacks the capacity to assess disaster-related mortality and morbidity in a standardized way across states, tribal nations, territories, and localities. Additional challenges that hinder the collection, reporting, and recording of accurate mortality and morbidity data include (1) an inconsistent adoption of uniform definitions for disaster-related mortality, (2) a lack of standards for defining and quantifying disaster-related morbidity, and (3) a lack of capacity and support for the medicolegal system to accurately collect and record the data. Furthermore, the valuable data that are already being collected about disaster-related mortality and morbidity are not being used effectively; the organizations that collect and use these data function in professional silos with insufficient capacity and inadequate tools to effectively analyze and use the data. These challenges and others identified by the committee will be discussed in subsequent chapters.

What Counts as a Disaster-Related Death or Morbidity?

A major barrier to accurately assessing the mortality and morbidity associated with a disaster is the lack of consensus concerning the key concepts and definitions across the extensive network of systems and stakeholders involved in collecting, reporting, and using mortality and morbidity data. Most fundamentally, there is no agreement about what counts as a disaster-related death or morbidity, there are no standard practices or uniformly adopted case definitions for attributing different degrees of disaster-relatedness to a death, and there are no established standards or data systems for attributing and collecting data on disaster-related morbidities. This enterprise-wide lack of uniformity and consistency in standards and practices for assessing mortality and morbidity undermines the accuracy of the data that are collected and squanders valuable data that are not collected at all. It also undercuts the ability to gain insights from comparing the impacts of a disaster—or of similar disasters—across settings and over time.

Disaster-Related Death

According to the Centers for Disease Control and Prevention (CDC), disaster-related mortality is routinely underestimated nationwide.[2] A primary reason is that critical information indicating that a death is associated with a disaster is often omitted from a decedent's official death record. In many cases, reports of the total deaths due to a disaster are based exclusively on counts of individual death records. If those death records lack detail about association to a recent disaster, the estimates will predictably underestimate the true toll. Chapter 3 describes current practices for collecting and recording data in the death record. Relying only on counts of individual death records has further disadvantages as well. For instance, this approach routinely excludes individuals who died of myocardial infarction, stroke, diabetic ketoacidosis, inability to obtain dialysis, disaster-related infections, and many other physical and mental health conditions that might not have arisen in the absence of the disaster. Such deaths are every bit as real and every bit as important as direct deaths counted by examining death certificates; however, these deaths are most effectively captured and described by using population-based estimation methods (see Chapter 4). Obvious mismatches between mortality as presented by individual counts versus population estimates can ignite controversy and confusion—as was most recently seen following Hurricane Maria in Puerto Rico in 2017 (see Box 1-3)—in addition to perpetuating inaccurate perceptions of a disaster's true effect.

Disaster-Related Morbidities

Morbidity is an exceptionally complex and broad term that encompasses a vast range of short- and long-term health outcomes from the physical to psychological, including cardiovascular, gastrointestinal, and respiratory diseases; physical injuries; and mental health outcomes. Mortality is easier, comparatively, to define. Disaster-related morbidity is no

[2] "Brief History of Centers for Disease Control and Prevention Disaster-Related Mortality Activities." Paper provided to the committee at the August 29, 2019, workshop in Washington, DC. Available by request from the Public Access Records Office by emailing PARO@nas.edu.

BOX 1-3
Variation in Hurricane Maria Mortality Counts and Estimates

From September 19–21, 2017, Hurricane Maria hit Puerto Rico as a Category 4 hurricane, triggering a humanitarian crisis on the island from which it is still recovering. Having been battered by Category 5 Hurricane Irma only 2 weeks prior, the island suffered significant damage to its already strained infrastructure, with widespread power outages and heavy debris hampering rescue and recovery efforts. Following the hurricane, only 5 percent of the island's power grid was operational, and less than half of the population had access to potable water (Bacon, 2017).

It was in this environment that officials in Puerto Rico initially reported 64 fatalities as a result of Hurricane Maria (Kishore et al., 2018). The Puerto Rican government contracted The George Washington University in collaboration with the University of Puerto Rico Graduate School of Public Health to conduct a broader analysis of deaths caused by the disaster. The report, which was released on August 28, 2018, estimated roughly 2,975 excess deaths could be attributed to Hurricane Maria, compared with a similar period in previous years (Milken Institute School of Public Health, 2018). A separate evaluation independently conducted by researchers at Harvard University that was based on community surveys and published online on May 29, 2018, in the *New England Journal of Medicine* estimated that as many as 4,645 (95% confidence interval, 793 to 8,498 deaths) excess deaths occurred (Kishore et al., 2018).

Hurricane Maria serves as an example of challenges in measuring the true effect of a major disaster and the value that population estimation methods can provide in the absence of robust individual counts. Additionally, this disaster highlights several of the logistical, political, administrative, and analytical challenges to assessing the true mortality and morbidity associated with an event that will be addressed later in this report.

less broad than all-cause morbidity and includes infectious diseases exacerbated by extreme socio-environmental conditions, such as population displacement, overcrowding, lack of access to clean water (Kouadio et al., 2012), chronic diseases brought on by stress or aggravated by disaster conditions (Miller and Arquilla, 2008), and chronic conditions that become acute (Mokdad et al., 2005). In addition to physical morbidities, intense exposure to stressors is associated with mental health sequelae such as suicide attempts and substance abuse (McFarlane and Williams, 2012). The relationship between disasters and morbidities of all types has increasingly become a research subject of interest, particularly as our understanding of the causal links among the social determinants of health, disasters, and morbidities has developed (see Appendix D).

Collecting data about disaster-related morbidities, specifically, presents its own set of challenges, given the broad scope of morbidities that can be tied, to some degree, to a disaster and the conditions it creates; the influence of pre-existing and co-morbid conditions; variation in the landscape of morbidities across disaster types; and the logistical challenges associated with mining morbidity data from across a broad network of unique federal, SLTT, and health care systems. As with disaster-related mortalities, there is no established standard for what counts as a disaster-related morbidity or what data or indicators should be consistently tracked across common types of disasters (e.g., hurricanes, blizzards, tornadoes, pandemics/epidemics) to provide actionable information to end users such as public health and emergency planners, health care systems, and SLTT and federal agencies. As with all data, different data types provide different opportunities for use. The COVID-19 pandemic has demonstrated how the availability of multiple methods for assessing mortality and morbidity can create confusion and make these numbers susceptible to manipulation or the appearance thereof.

Defining which morbidity data are of value to the disaster management enterprise and developing standards for the data systems that generate these data are critical first steps to building the capability to collect and use these data effectively (see Chapters 3 and 4). A discussion of how the committee chose to define significant morbidity as it relates to a disaster can be found later in this chapter.

Federal Efforts and Guidance to Improve the Assessment of Mortality and Morbidity

Wide variation persists in what counts as a disaster-related death across counties, states, and the federal government (see Table 3-2 for federal and state criteria for attributing deaths to COVID-19). Some federal and professional guidance exists for medical certifiers certifying individual deaths attributable to a disaster, but this guidance has not been consistently adopted across jurisdictions to harmonize the variation in case definitions and inconsistencies in data collection and reporting practices. Along with the lack of a universal, methodologically sound framework for understanding disaster-related mortality and morbidity, these factors (and others) limit the ability to intervene to reduce the health impacts of future disasters (Combs et al., 1999). Furthermore, the variability in the ways that disaster-related mortality and morbidity are reported in different jurisdictions can even obfuscate the impact of an event that has already happened.

Over the past few decades, CDC and partners have worked to improve data collection and reporting practices at state and local levels by developing standard case definitions and tools to support stakeholders—primarily medicolegal death investigation professionals (see Chapter 3)—in the attribution of disaster-related mortality. In 1999, CDC published uniform disaster mortality case definitions for attributing direct and indirect deaths to a disaster[3] (Combs et al., 1999) (see Box 1-4). These have been used to categorize deaths after the fact in retrospective studies of large-scale disasters (Brunkard et al., 2008; CDC, 2004, 2006; Ragan et al., 2008). To bolster national awareness about the importance of attributing deaths to a disaster, CDC has also developed guidance to support professionals working in the medicolegal system in completing death certificates with accurate information. This guidance includes *A Reference Guide for Certification of Deaths in the Event of a Natural, Human-Induced, or Chemical/Radiological Disaster* (NCHS, 2017) and instructions for completing the cause of death section on a death certificate. The guide is based on CDC's uniform disaster mortality case definitions and offers a flow chart for making determinations about attribution; it also includes examples of common causes of direct disaster-related death and common circumstances leading to indirect disaster-related deaths. To address challenges in gathering death-scene data, CDC's *Death Scene Investigation After Natural Disaster or Other Weather-Related Events* toolkit supports investigators by providing a common framework for collecting and documenting consistent disaster-related death-scene information (CDC, 2017). Additional tools piloted and supported by CDC are discussed in Chapter 3.

Despite these federal efforts, the adoption of these uniform case definitions, data recording practices, and reporting methods remains inconsistent among SLTT-level stakeholders, who are primarily responsible for collecting and recording disaster-related mortality and morbidity data. A multitude of different terms, interpretations of policy, and professional practices for recording attribution across SLTT medicolegal systems are used to categorize and describe the degree of association between an individual- or population-level health outcome and exposure to a disaster. Fatality management templates and protocols to support uniform standards and practices for medical examiners, coroners, and other medical certifiers have been developed by various states and by professional associations (e.g., the National Association of Medical Examiners), but adherence to these standards is voluntary. Furthermore, many of the templates and protocols do not provide specific guidance about which data points for disaster-related mortality are important to collect or about how they should be recorded within information systems to benefit emergency management and public health. These inconsistencies in data recording make it difficult to compare data across localities and states and also limit the effective use of these data (see Chapter 3).

[3] "Brief History of Centers for Disease Control and Prevention Disaster-Related Mortality Activities." Paper provided to the committee at the August 29, 2019, workshop in Washington, DC. Available by request from the Public Access Records Office by emailing PARO@nas.edu.

BOX 1-4
Uniform Case Definitions for Attributing Direct and Indirect Deaths to a Disaster

A *directly related death* is defined as a death directly attributable to the forces of the disaster or by the direct consequences of these forces, such as structural collapse, flying debris, or radiation exposure. A key question for the medical examiner and coroner (ME/C) or other certifier to ask is: Was the death caused by the actual environmental forces of the disaster such as wind, rain, flood, earthquake, or blast wave, or by the direct consequences of these forces such as structural collapse, chemical spill, or flying debris? If so, this is a directly related death that was caused by natural or human-induced forces.

An *indirectly related death* occurs when the unsafe or unhealthy conditions present during any phase of the disaster (i.e., pre-event or preparations, during the actual occurrence, or post-event during cleanup after a disaster) contribute to a death. Key questions for ME/C or other certifier to ask are: (1) Did unsafe or unhealthy conditions from the environmental forces of the disaster contribute to the death? These conditions could be the loss or disruption of usual services (e.g., utilities, transportation, or health care). If so, this is an indirectly related death. (2) Did the forces, whether natural or human-induced disaster, lead to temporary or permanent displacement, property damage, or other personal loss or stress that contributed to the death? These indirect circumstances involve personal loss or lifestyle disruption. If so, this is also an indirectly related death.

SOURCE: NCHS, 2017.

Public Health Emergency Preparedness and Response Cooperative Agreement Requirements for Mortality and Morbidity Data

CDC's Public Health Emergency Preparedness (PHEP) cooperative agreement outlines the responsibility of SLTT public health agencies to aggregate and analyze mortality and morbidity data after any disaster as an essential public health capability. All 50 states, 4 major metropolitan areas, and 8 territories are recipients of the PHEP cooperative agreement. The CDC tools mentioned above have now been included in the updated CDC Public Health Emergency Preparedness and Response Capabilities of the PHEP cooperative agreement (CDC, 2018, 2020). Despite commitment from certain federal and SLTT agencies and the requirements of the PHEP agreement, CDC guidance and standards have not yet been widely adopted in practice nationwide (Noe, 2019).

Stakeholders

The responsibilities for collecting, recording, and reporting mortality and morbidity data are distributed across many different stakeholders and entities—some of which have competing interests and conflicting policies—at the local, state, regional, and federal levels. Different agencies and organizations are accountable for different components of this complex process and have responsibility for different pieces of data following large-scale disasters (see Box 1-5 for a list of the stakeholders involved). Three critical federal players are CDC, FEMA, and the Office of the Assistant Secretary for Preparedness and Response in the Department of Health and Human Services. Other important stakeholders are hospital and health

BOX 1-5
Stakeholder Involvement

Federal
Assistant Secretary for Preparedness and Response
Census Bureau
Centers for Disease Control and Prevention
Centers for Medicare & Medicaid Services
Department of Defense
Department of Homeland Security
Department of Veterans Affairs
Federal Emergency Management Agency
Federal Interagency Council on Statistical Policy
Government Accountability Office
National Center for Health Statistics
National Institutes of Health
National Weather Service/National Oceanic and Atmospheric Administration
Office of Management and Budget

State, Tribal, and Territorial
Association of State and Territorial Health Officials
Council of State and Territorial Epidemiologists
Medical examiners and coroners (state-specific)
State health departments
State vital records offices

County and Localities
County health departments
Medical examiners and coroners
National Association of County & City Health Officials
School systems
Vital records

systems, health care providers, nursing homes, social support cultural centers, care systems for end-stage renal disease, epidemiologists, morgues and medical examiners, state and local governments, and communities. The major users of mortality and morbidity data are widely dispersed across the general public, political leadership, the private sector, and the public sector. However, these stakeholders' responsibilities are commonly siloed, and the integration of disaster epidemiology into disaster management and policy making remains limited (Malilay et al., 2014). For example, despite the critical importance of the medicolegal system in collecting essential data for disaster management, this group of stakeholders is rarely engaged in emergency management and public health planning for disasters.

Other
Academic schools of public health
American Academy of Forensic Sciences
American Board of Medicolegal Death Investigators
American Public Health Association
American Statistical Association
Association of Schools and Programs of Public Health
Community-based organizations and research partners
Emergency medical services
Environmental health groups
Faith-based organizations
International Association of Coroners & Medical Examiners
International Association of Emergency Managers
Health and other insurance companies
Health information exchanges
Health information systems
Homeless shelters and outreach organizations
Hospitals and health systems
Law enforcement (criminologists, forensics)
National Association for Public Health Statistics and Information Systems
National Association of Medical Examiners
Nongovernmental organizations
Nursing home and home-health trade organizations
Organizations that support institutionalized and incarcerated populations
Organizations that support people with disabilities and lived experience populations
Organizations that support undocumented immigrants
Public health institutes
Red Cross
Social media (Facebook, Twitter, Google)

TERMINOLOGY CHOICES AND KEY CONCEPTS

From the outset, it is important to clarify the terminology choices made by the committee and explain how these distinctions support improved assessment of mortality and morbidity following large-scale disasters. The concepts will be discussed in greater detail in future chapters.

Terminology for Estimating Impact

Multiple terms have been used to denote the presence and degree of a relationship between a death or injury and a disaster (e.g., key affected populations, excess deaths from violent causes, disaster-attributed mortality, incident morbidity). These terms are often conflated, resulting in misunderstandings about estimated impacts and poor comparability of mortality and morbidity assessments over time and across disasters. Additional challenges relate to characterizing *what* is being assessed and the *context* in which it is being assessed. These issues lead to further confusion over how to measure total mortality and morbidity and how these data can be best used by policy makers and other stakeholders.

Throughout the report, the committee has adopted a set of uniform terms to describe quantitative indicators of disaster impact and the methods and data used to develop them. Chapter 2 provides more detail on these terms and the committee's rationale, but a brief summary is provided here to facilitate the reader's entry into the report. First, the terms *individual count* (i.e., estimates derived from individual death records) and *population estimate* (i.e., estimates derived from population-based estimation methods) are used throughout the report to refer to the two main approaches for estimating a disaster's impact on mortality and morbidity. These two approaches can be used to describe essential information about mortality and morbidity and encompass distinct methodologies and tools. Additional terms used in the report include

- *Direct mortality and morbidity*: those killed or injured directly by the disaster;
- *Indirect mortality and morbidity*: those killed or injured indirectly as a result of the disaster; and
- *Partially attributable mortality and morbidity*: those killed or injured in part or possibly as a result of the disaster.

These terms were selected for use in the report based on several foundational concepts explored further in Chapter 2. First and most significantly, disasters are complex events with multifactorial health consequences, and there can be more than one appropriate approach to answering the question "How many deaths and severe morbidities were caused by this disaster?"

No single, standardized methodological approach to assessing disaster-related mortality and morbidity can be applied universally to generate a singular estimate that sufficiently describes a disaster's impact. However, while there is no standard method for generating mortality or morbidity estimates, best practices among the available methodologies can now be specified for both individual counts and population estimates, as can the appropriate circumstances for their uses. Gaining a comprehensive understanding of a disaster's impact on human health requires more than one method of assessment.

The second foundational concept is that quantitative assessments of disaster impact represent an estimation of impact at a distinct point of time, within a specific context, and based on particular assumptions. Estimates of total mortality and morbidity—both individual counts and population estimates—are not static and can change over time as additional data are gathered or updated, as additional mortality or morbidity occurs, or as the assumptions for characterizing the estimate evolve.

The third concept is that each approach is valuable and imprecise in different ways and has different appropriate uses. Individual counts rely on administrative data, such as death records, to estimate the number of reported deaths in a certain geographical area at a defined point in time and are valuable for an initial understanding of the immediate impact of disasters or causes of death (e.g., carbon monoxide poisonings from improper generator use in the home). However, this method can be undermined by inaccuracies in the ways that data are recorded and reported; individual counts also fail to count certain individuals, such as those who die of natural causes during a disaster but would not have died *but for* the disaster (see Chapter 3). Population-based estimation methods are crucial for capturing a full understanding of the impacts of a disaster on health and mortality and for illustrating population-level trends and associations (e.g., an increase in myocardial infarctions following Hurricane Sandy in New Jersey) (Swerdel et al., 2014). These methods may incorporate less precise information on cause of death and in some applications (e.g., estimates of "excess" deaths) cannot distinguish which individuals would have survived in the absence of the disaster from those who would have died during the period regardless (see Chapter 4). The complex nature of disasters and the multiple pathways through which they affect human health make it difficult to quantify the impact of a specific disaster on human health with precision. Together, however, the two approaches can provide both timely information and a far more comprehensive picture of the health and mortality impacts of a disaster.

Finally, and especially in pandemics, is the matter of temporality. Disasters such as hurricanes or wildfires occur over a period of days or weeks (although recovery can take months or years). Attributed mortality and morbidity counts and estimates change over time for two reasons: some long-term consequences take time to occur, and all data systems have lags that vary over time. In pandemics both of these factors apply, but there is an additional dynamic: the continued infection of new cases, which reflects efforts to control the pandemic through social distancing and other methods. For instance, for the reasons discussed above, COVID-19 deaths are sometimes seen as more reliable than case counts. But deaths lag hospitalizations, the onset of symptoms, and the time of infection by 3 to 4 weeks. The daily number of deaths, therefore, is a seriously lagging indicator of the efficacy of control efforts, and thus a poor guide for deciding whether, say, social distancing measures can be relaxed.

Defining Significant Morbidity

The qualification of *significant* morbidity, rather than all degrees and types of disaster-related morbidity, was specifically noted in the committee's Statement of Task, but the term was not explicitly defined by the study sponsor. Further discussions with FEMA during the committee's first meeting provided some clarity concerning this term and, per FEMA's guidance, limited the committee's deliberations to very serious morbidities, both physical and mental. Because no standard practices or systems to collect disaster-related morbidity data exist at a national level (see Chapter 4), no standard definition for describing what counts as significant disaster-related morbidity exists in the literature. However, this term has been used previously to describe a serious risk of immediate hospitalization or risk to life due to the restriction of critical bodily functions for specific diseases and conditions, such as end-stage liver disease (Brown et al., 2016) and chronic obstructive pulmonary disease (Cushen et al., 2017). The term *significant* is highly subjective, and significant morbidity could realistically encompass a wide range of physical and mental injuries that are deemed significant in different ways by different stakeholders. In the absence of a widely accepted scientific or operational definition for significant morbidity and based on the guidance of the sponsor, this report will approach significant morbidity from the context described above—injuries or illnesses that place an individual at high risk of hospitalization or imminent death, such as acute cardiovascular events or the worsening of a chronic condition such as kidney disease.

While this report will focus on practices for assessing significant morbidity as it is described above, readers should approach the report with the understanding that the recommendations are applicable to the assessment of morbidity at all levels. Throughout the report text, the committee will use the term *morbidity* to refer to significant morbidity per the above context unless otherwise stated. A discussion of the many uses for disaster-related morbidity data can be found in Chapter 2; a discussion of challenges and opportunities for improving the assessment of disaster-related morbidity can be found in Chapters 3 and 4.

Finally, the inherent complexity of morbidity, the variation of morbidities across disasters, and the current lack of standards and infrastructure for systematically assessing morbidity following disasters indicates that what counts as significant morbidity is likely less important than the question of what should be counted. It is beyond the committee's capacity to develop an evidence-based set of standards and indicators to frame the future collection of morbidity data, as considerable investment in research will need to occur to develop the body of research to support such a job. However, the committee stresses that the identification of key morbidities across common disaster types could add value to early efforts to capture disaster-related morbidity data in a systematic manner by SLTT and federal stakeholders. See Chapter 3 for a discussion of potential key morbidities that could be targeted by data collection efforts and how these individual counts could be used by SLTT entities and Chapter 4 for information about survey methods for collecting these data and analytical approaches for developing population estimates of morbidity.

ORGANIZATION OF THIS REPORT

This report seeks to provide federal and SLTT stakeholders with actionable guidance for improving the assessment of mortality and significant morbidity of disasters. Although the committee's charge focused primarily on major disasters as defined by the Stafford Act, the report's recommendations are largely applicable to other disasters and emergencies. Each chapter includes highlighted conclusions that provide evidence for the report's recommendations, which are laid out in the final chapter of the report. In Chapter 2 the committee explores the importance of and various uses for mortality and morbidity data. The chapter also lays out the committee's framework approaches for conceptualizing disaster-related mortality and morbidity estimates and describes a recommended set of standard definitions. Chapter 3 provides an overview of the diversity in the nation's death investigation systems and explores the current landscape of individual-level mortality and morbidity data collection, recording, and use across this network. In that chapter the committee also identifies barriers to the collection, reporting, and use of individual counts and provides a set of best practices for the implementation of individual counting methods for assessing mortality and morbidity from disasters. Chapter 4 reviews analytical methods used to develop population estimates of mortality and morbidity from disasters and provides recommendations on operational practices. Chapter 5 provides a summary of the report's major conclusions and recommendations and sets forth a suggested plan of action for use by relevant stakeholders. Several appendixes with supplemental material selected by the committee can be found at the end of the report. Appendix A includes the committee's preliminary literature review search strategy and Appendix B contains a record of all of the public sessions hosted by the committee over the course of its deliberations. Appendix C includes a companion piece developed independently by two members of the committee about the assessment of mortality and morbidity from the COVID-19 pandemic. Appendix D contains two supplemental case studies on how the social determinants of health can affect the assessment of mortality and morbidity. Appendix E contains the committee and staff biographies.

REFERENCES

Bacon, J. 2017. *Why Puerto Rico faces a monumental recovery effort.* USA Today. https://www.usatoday.com/story/news/nation/2017/09/26/why-puerto-rico-faces-monumental-recovery-effort/703515001 (accessed June 22, 2020).

Brown, C. L., B. G. Hammill, L. G. Qualls, L. H. Curtis, and A. J. Muir. 2016. Significant morbidity and mortality among hospitalized end-stage liver disease patients in Medicare. *Journal of Pain and Symptom Management* 52(3):412–419.

Brunkard, J., G. Namulanda, and R. Ratard. 2008. Hurricane Katrina deaths, Louisiana, 2005. *Disaster Medicine and Public Health Preparedness* 2(4):215–223.

CDC (Centers for Disease Control and Prevention). 2004. Preliminary medical examiner reports of mortality associated with Hurricane Charley—Florida, 2004. *Morbidity and Mortality Weekly Report* 53(36):835–837.

CDC. 2005. *Vibrio* illnesses after Hurricane Katrina—multiple states, August–September 2005. *Morbidity and Mortality Weekly Report* 54(37):928–931.

CDC. 2006. Mortality associated with Hurricane Katrina—Florida and Alabama, August–October 2005. *Morbidity and Mortality Weekly Report* 55(9):239–242.

CDC. 2016. *A primer for understanding the principles and practices of disaster surveillance in the United States.* Atlanta, GA: Centers for Disease Control and Prevention.

CDC. 2017. *Death scene investigation after natural disaster or other weather-related events.* Atlanta, GA: Centers for Disease Control and Prevention. https://www.cdc.gov/nceh/hsb/disaster/docs/DisasterDeathSceneToolkit-P.pdf (accessed June 26, 2020).

CDC. 2018. *Public health emergency preparedness and response capabilities.* https://www.cdc.gov/cpr/readiness/capabilities-change.htm (accessed June 26, 2020).

CDC. 2020. *Public Health Emergency Preparedness (PHEP) cooperative agreement.* https://www.cdc.gov/cpr/readiness/phep.htm#:~:text=Eight%20U.S.%20territories%20and%20freely,%2C%20and%20Republic%20of%20Palau (accessed June 4, 2020).

Combs, D. L., L. E. Quenemoen, R. G. Parrish, and J. H. Davis. 1999. Assessing disaster-attributed mortality: Development and application of a definition and classification matrix. *International Journal of Epidemiology* 28(6):1124–1129.

CRS (Congressional Research Service). 2017. *Stafford Act declarations 1953–2016: Trends, analyses, and implications for Congress.* CRS report no. R42702. https://crsreports.congress.gov/product/pdf/R/R42702 (accessed June 25, 2020).

Cushen, B., R. Morgan, and R. Summer. 2017. Chronic obstructive pulmonary disease. In S. R. Quah (ed.), *International encyclopedia of public health, 2nd ed.* Cambridge, MA: Academic Press. Pp. 28–35.

Furey, J. S., H. Fredrickson, C. Foote, and M. Richmond. 2007. Post-Katrina fecal contamination in Violet Marsh near New Orleans. *International Journal of Environmental Research and Public Health* 4(2):84–92.

Khan, Y., B. Schwartz, and I. Johnson. 2014. Surveillance and epidemiology in natural disasters: A novel framework and assessment of reliability. *PLOS Currents* doi: 10.1371/currents.dis.6773eb9d5e64b733ab490f78de346003.

Kishore, N., D. Marqués, A. Mahmud, M. V. Kiang, I. Rodriguez, A. Fuller, P. Ebner, C. Sorensen, F. Racy, J. Lemery, L. Maas, J. Leaning, R. A. Irizarry, S. Balsari, and C. O. Buckee. 2018. Mortality in Puerto Rico after Hurricane Maria. *New England Journal of Medicine* 379(2):162–170.

Kouadio, I. K., S. Aljunid, T. Kamigaki, K. Hammad, and H. Oshitani. 2012. Infectious diseases following natural disasters: Prevention and control measures. *Expert Review of Anti-Infective Therapy* 10(1):95–104.

Liu, E. C. 2008. *Would an influenza pandemic qualify as a major disaster under the Stafford Act?* Congressional Research Service report to Congress. https://digital.library.unt.edu/ark:/67531/metadc627007/m1/1/high_res_d/RL34724_2008Oct20.pdf (accessed June 25, 2020).

Malilay, J., M. Heumann, D. Perrotta, A. F. Wolkin, A. H. Schnall, M. N. Podgornik, M. A. Cruz, J. A. Horney, D. Zane, R. Roisman, J. R. Greenspan, D. Thoroughman, H. A. Anderson, E. V. Wells, and E. F. Simms. 2014. The role of applied epidemiology methods in the disaster management cycle. *American Journal of Public Health* 104(11):2092–2102.

Marinova-Petkova, A., I. Guendel, J. P. Strysko, L. L. Ekpo, R. Galloway, J. Yoder, A. Kahler, A. Artus, A. R. Hoffmaster, W. A. Bower, H. Walke, B. R. Ellis, T. Hunte-Ceasar, E. M. Ellis, and I. J. Schafer. 2019. First reported human cases of leptospirosis in the United States Virgin Islands in the aftermath of Hurricanes Irma and Maria, September–November 2017. *Open Forum Infectious Diseases* 6(7):ofz261.

McFarlane, A. C., and R. Williams. 2012. Mental health services required after disasters: Learning from the lasting effects of disasters. *Depression Research and Treatment* 970194.

Milken Institute School of Public Health. 2018. *Ascertainment of the estimated excess mortality from Hurricane María in Puerto Rico*. Washington, DC: The George Washington University. https://publichealth.gwu.edu/sites/default/files/downloads/projects/PRstudy/Acertainment%20of%20the%20Estimated%20Excess%20Mortality%20from%20Hurricane%20Maria%20in%20Puerto%20Rico.pdf (accessed June 26, 2020).

Miller, A. C., and B. Arquilla. 2008. Chronic diseases and natural hazards: Impact of disasters on diabetic, renal, and cardiac patients. *Prehospital and Disaster Medicine* 23(2):185–194.

Mokdad, A. H., G. A. Mensah, S. F. Posner, E. Reed, E. J. Simoes, M. M. Engelgau, and Chronic Diseases and Vulnerable Populations in Natural Disasters Working Group. 2005. When chronic conditions become acute: Prevention and control of chronic diseases and adverse health outcomes during natural disasters. *Preventing Chronic Disease* 2(Spec No):A04.

NCHS (National Center for Health Statistics). 2017. *A reference guide for certification of deaths in the event of a natural, human-induced, or chemical/radiological disaster*. Hyattsville, MD: National Center for Health Statistics. https://www.cdc.gov/nchs/data/nvss/vsrg/vsrg01.pdf (accessed June 26, 2020).

Nigro, O. D., A. Hou, G. Vithanage, R. S. Fujioka, and G. F. Steward. 2011. Temporal and spatial variability in culturable pathogenic *Vibrio* spp. in Lake Pontchartrain, Louisiana, following Hurricanes Katrina and Rita. *Applied and Environmental Biology* 77(15):5384–5393.

Noe, R. 2019. *Session 3: Current capabilities in assessing and using morbidity and mortality data in real-time during a large-scale disaster.* Presentation at the August 29, 2019, public meeting of the National Academies of Sciences, Engineering, and Medicine's Committee on Best Practices for Assessing Mortality and Significant Morbidity Following Large-Scale Disasters, Washington, DC.

Ragan, P., J. Schulte, S. J. Nelson, and K. T. Jones. 2008. Mortality surveillance: 2004 to 2005 Florida hurricane-related deaths. *The American Journal of Forensic Medicine and Pathology* 29(2):148–153.

Swerdel, J. N., T. M. Janevic, N. M. Cosgrove, J. B. Kostis, and the Myocardial Infarction Data Acquisition System Study Group. 2014. The effect of Hurricane Sandy on cardiovascular events in New Jersey. *Journal of the American Heart Association* 3(6):e001354.

Yee, E. L., H. Palacio, R. L. Atmar, U. Shah, C. Kilborn, M. Faul, T. E. Gavagan, R. D. Feigin, J. Versalovic, F. H. Neill, A. L. Panlilio, M. Miller, J. Spahr, and R. I. Glass. 2007. Widespread outbreak of norovirus gastroenteritis among evacuees of Hurricane Katrina residing in a large "megashelter" in Houston, Texas: Lessons learned for prevention. *Clinical Infectious Diseases* 44(8):1032–1039.

2

Value and Use of Mortality and Morbidity Data

The act of quantifying mortality and morbidity following a traumatic event, such as a large-scale disaster, holds deep emotional, societal, financial, and logistical value and serves a multitude of different uses for different stakeholders. Accurately quantifying disaster-related mortality and morbidity is a complex and challenging endeavor. The meaningful use of morbidity and mortality data is often undermined by the fact that no uniform framework or standard vocabulary for conceptualizing disaster-related mortality and morbidity data is in use across all jurisdictions, federal and state, local, tribal, and territorial (SLTT) agencies, and professional domains. Data are captured inconsistently, and data that are collected are not being used to their fullest potential due to the siloing of agencies and systems. The first part of this chapter lays out a potential framework for conceptualizing disaster-related mortality and morbidity and introduces updated case definitions developed by the committee. The second part of the chapter discusses the value and meaningful use of mortality and morbidity data by various stakeholders across the disaster lifecycle and provides examples of how these data are currently used or could be used. Chapters 3 and 4 will focus on the analytical and operational challenges and practices related to the collection, reporting, and recording of individual counts and population estimates of mortality and morbidity.

CONCEPTUALIZING ALL-CAUSE MORTALITY AND MORBIDITY

Significant confusion and disagreement persist across systems and stakeholders regarding what counts as a disaster-related death or morbidity, which profoundly affects the ability to use mortality and morbidity data in meaningful ways. Resolving this discordance and moving toward consistently applied standards and harmonized practices will require more than merely developing simple case definitions, however. It will require taking a broader understanding of disaster-related mortality and morbidity data that considers the context, timing, and methods by which data are collected and recorded as well as considering the methods used to assess and use the data to protect the health of the public. Although a framework with common definitions can be helpful in catalyzing and supporting the adoption of this more comprehensive type of approach, no uniform framework is widely used in current practice.

A framework to guide the assessment of mortality and morbidity would provide a methodological structure for more accurately and completely categorizing and reporting those outcomes in a consistent manner. Ideally, such a framework would strike a balance between uniformity and flexibility, would be applicable to all disasters (e.g., small- or large-scale, human-induced or naturally occurring), and would include case definitions that are designed to capture all mortality and morbidity related to the event while also excluding cases that are unrelated (Combs et al., 1999). A uniform approach for quantitatively describing a disaster's health impacts would also enable analyses of the effectiveness of disaster management activities across different disasters. A uniform approach could also support:

- More consistent assessment of the human impact of disasters across all jurisdictions;
- Delivery of adequate resources for recovery;
- Forecasting of needs for similar incidents in the future;
- Identification of behavioral contributors to disaster-related mortality and morbidity to inform interventions to modify future behavior;
- Exploration of population impacts to promote health and offer relevant services and support for prevention and recovery; and
- Identification of vulnerable populations and their specific needs to improve services and reduce additional morbidity, injury, and death.

To address the need for a uniform approach for conceptualizing and assessing mortality and mortality data following large-scale disasters, the committee developed a framework that can be adopted across all systems and jurisdictions (see Table 2-1). This framework incorporates the two primary methodological approaches for estimating disaster-related mortality and morbidity and builds on a body of literature of analytical prospective and retrospective methodologies (Kishore et al., 2018; Santos-Burgoa et al., 2018; Stephens et al., 2007).

TABLE 2-1 Proposed Framework of Approaches for Defining Mortality and Morbidity Following Large-Scale Disasters

Term	Description	Example
Total reported mortality and morbidity estimation using individual counts: Individual counts are point-in-time estimates of disaster-related mortality and morbidity derived from reported cases.		
Term	Description	Example
Direct	A death or morbidity directly attributable to the forces of the disaster or a direct consequence of these forces.	Deaths from structural collapse, flying debris, radiation exposure, drowning during the event; delayed deaths directly related to initial impact (e.g., head injury leading to coma with eventual death from aspiration pneumonia)
Indirect	A death or morbidity not from a direct impact but due to unsafe or unhealthy conditions around the time of the disaster, including while preparing for, responding to, and during recovery from the disaster.	Deaths due to loss of medical or transport services (e.g., death due to lack of access to dialysis); exposure to hazards such as chemicals; deaths related to disaster response, such as carbon monoxide poisoning from improper use of generators; deaths or illness due to diarrheal disease among shelter residents
Partially attributable	A death or morbidity that cannot be definitively tied to the disaster but where the disaster more likely than not has played a contributing role in the death.	Death due to drug overdose in a patient who had been abstinent and re-started drug use during or immediately after the disaster; death from myocardial infarction or stroke during a disaster in a patient with pre-existing cardiovascular disease; death due to suicide following or during a disaster in a patient with pre-existing mental illness
Total mortality and morbidity derived from population estimates: Population estimates are point-in-time estimates of the impact of a disaster at a population level derived using various statistical methods and tools, including sampling. **Examples:** Increase in all-cause mortality in the 4 weeks after a hurricane derived from excess mortality data; increase in myocardial infarctions in the 6 months following a disaster derived from claims data; estimation of population infection rates using serological prevalence studies; increase in asthma exacerbation episodes in the wake of a large wildfire using data from electronic health records.		

This proposed framework builds on and provides standard meaning to the disaster mortality definitions promoted by the Centers for Disease Control and Prevention and works in tandem with designations for natural and unnatural deaths used by medical examiners and coroners. It is important to note that the case definitions proposed by the committee are aligned with—and not intended to replace—the language already being used in the medical examiner and coroner community to categorize different manners and causes of death. Most states offer five options for coding the manner of death: natural, homicide, suicide, accidental, and undetermined (NAME, 2002). The manner of death is *how* that injury or illness led to the death, while the cause of death refers to the specific illness or injury that led to death (Washoe County Regional Medical Examiner's Office, 2020). Natural deaths are those that have internal physiological causes. The term unnatural death is used by medical examiners and coroners to categorize a death that did not occur due to natural causes (IOM, 2003). As discussed below, the committee's case definition for a direct death will capture only unnatural disaster-related deaths, while the case definitions for indirect deaths and partially attributable deaths can capture both natural and unnatural deaths. Another potential advantage of using the committee's uniform case definitions and framework is that it offers medical certifiers of individual cases of mortality (e.g., doctors, nurse practitioners) greater autonomy in categorizing a death as being indirectly related or partially attributable to a disaster without triggering a mandatory review by the

BOX 2-1
Additional Stakeholder Considerations for Mortality and Morbidity Estimation

It is critically important to be aware that stakeholders may have certain vested interests in reducing or increasing the estimated impacts of a disaster. The committee's intent in moving away from focusing on a single, largely unchanging "death toll" to using morbidity and mortality data to more fully describe the human impact of a disaster over time—including recognizing the potential legitimacy of multiple approaches for assessing mortality and morbidity—is to help avoid confusion or the impression that data are being manipulated for stakeholder-specific purposes. For example, stakeholders with interests in reducing or increasing the estimated impacts of a disaster could potentially—either explicitly or inadvertently—apply different approaches to present different versions of a disaster's impact. This was a major public concern following Hurricanes Katrina and Maria and, more recently, during the COVID-19 pandemic (see Appendix C). Competing stakeholder interests surround these data, the manipulation of which can pose major policy and public health safety risks, but it is important to realize that variation in estimates might reflect different, but appropriate, methods and targets. Still, while there are legitimate reasons for stakeholders to use different methods for assessing the impact of a disaster, some methods will be more appropriate than others for specific purposes (see Chapters 3 and 4 for methodological best practices for individual counts and population estimation approaches). Risks of inappropriate uses of methods and data can be mitigated if key stakeholders commit to exclusively using and promoting the universal adoption of (1) a methods-based framework for attributing mortality and morbidity to a disaster, (2) standard methods for analyzing the data, and (3) standard operations and practices for data collection, reporting, and use across all jurisdictions and stakeholders.

medical examiner. Chapter 3 provides more detail about the roles of these stakeholders in mortality data collection and reporting.

Most significantly, this framework shifts the paradigm for defining a disaster's health impacts from a singular death toll toward a more inclusive understanding of the complex impact of a disaster on human life. In a major disaster, for example, the total mortality estimate can remain dynamic for years, as individuals succumb to injuries or health conditions that occurred as a result of their exposure to the disaster. Even the number of deaths that can be directly attributed to the force of the disaster (i.e., direct deaths) can change over time, because people injured in the event may eventually die of those same injuries or morbidities years later. Insufficient research exists to define a clear minimum timeline by which disaster-related mortality and morbidity should be tracked; however, setting such guidelines for the capture of data is critical (see Recommendations 3-2 and 3-3 on standards for collection of mortality and morbidity data). Box 2-1 provides an overview of some additional stakeholder considerations that provide further rationale

Mortality and morbidity estimates also determine how a disaster is presented in the media. Media coverage of a disaster tends to be very selective and may either over-represent or inadequately account for the severity and number of deaths or morbidities (Tzvetkova, 2017). Estimates made based on media reports during the immediate aftermath of a disaster may not be subsequently updated for completeness or validated (Green et al., 2019). It is important to resist political and media pressures to publicize early case-based mortality counts before they are verified. Establishing clearly defined criteria for case definitions within a standardized approach can allow those providing information to the media to say that (1) this is what has been reported so far, (2) the process of counting and estimating is ongoing, and (3) more information will be provided in the future.

Clear communication of disaster-related mortality and morbidity data to the public is essential; an example would be the statements, "According to current reports, the disaster has caused X number of deaths directly and it has contributed to another X number of deaths as of X date." Data-informed public messaging also helps to avert the spread of rumors and misinformation, given that enormous pressure to provide mortality counts can build in the first hours after a disaster's impact. Certain states have sought to prevent the spread of rumors immediately following a disaster. For example, Florida's statewide reporting system centralizes the counting of all deaths at the state level, with individual counties not tasked with counting and reporting their deaths independently. This approach allows initial counts of disaster-related deaths to be communicated to the public by a single source with access to all mortality data from across the state, in addition to ensuring consistency and timeliness of data. The Federal Emergency Management Agency also provides a website to dispel commonly held misconceptions surrounding its activities related to morbidity and mortality estimates (FEMA, 2020).

for the use of a uniform approach to assessing disaster-related mortality and morbidity.

Methodological Approaches for Assessing Total Disaster-Related Mortality and Morbidity

Disasters are complex events with such multifactorial health consequences that no single number can sufficiently describe a disaster's health impact. This precludes the possibility of any universal methodological approach that can be used across all disasters to generate an estimation of mortalities or morbidities related to that disaster. This complexity also gives rise to a persistent challenge in the assessment of mortality and morbidity, which is the widespread conflation of the outputs of two different but complementary methodological approaches for estimating disaster-related mortality and morbidity: (1) individual counts, which are numbers derived from individual administrative case reports, and (2) population estimates, which are based on statistical approaches. The committee's proposed framework includes both of these essential methodological approaches. Both approaches provide essential information in the face of a disaster, but they differ in their assumptions, data requirements, strengths, weaknesses, and appropriate uses (see Table 2-2). They are similar in that they pertain to a defined point in time and to a geographical area, and both can be refined over time as the situation evolves or as new data become available. When applied appropriately, the two approaches can help answer different questions, elucidate different sets of risk factors, and uncover different potential points of intervention. Therefore, both individual counts and population estimates contribute to a comprehensive picture of a disaster's health impacts, which can be used to inform response and recovery and to prepare for future events.

Individual counts are estimates that are based on counts of deaths recorded in administrative systems and are valuable for understanding the immediate impact of disasters. However, the accuracy of this approach depends on the completeness with which individual cases are recorded and reported. Depending on the strength and precision of the data collection system to capture information about each bit of data accurately and consistently, individual count methods often fail to capture certain types of disaster-related deaths (e.g., individuals who die of natural causes during a disaster and would not have died *but for* the disaster). However, individual counting methods, if deployed successfully, can provide an early estimate of the number of reported individual deaths, injuries, and cases of illness that are considered to be directly or indirectly caused by the disaster or partially attributable to it. Operational considerations for the collection, recording, reporting, and use of individual counts can be found in Chapter 3.

TABLE 2-2 Strengths, Weaknesses, and Uses for Individual Counts and Population Estimate Approaches

Strengths	Weaknesses	Uses
Individual Counts		
• Can offer a more rapid assessment of the immediate impact of the disaster at a defined point in time. • Allow for more specific details on the degree of attribution of the mortality—direct, indirect, and possible or partially related—to the disaster.	• Accuracy depends on the strength and precision of the data system to capture complete data on reported cases; therefore, more likely to underestimate impact. • Often fail to capture cases that lack evidence for inclusion in the count (e.g., partially attributable mortalities); therefore, more likely to underestimate impact.	• Rapidly identify affected population needs and allocation of resources. • Provide rapid updates on impact to the public. • Provide specificity to causes of death and morbidity so that interventions may be deployed. • Allow development of early public health messaging.
Population Estimates		
• Can provide a more comprehensive understanding of the impacts of a disaster on the health of the population. • Are able to capture a broader range of disaster-related deaths and morbidity, including indirect effects and partially attributable effects.	• Often substantial lag time in performing these analyses compared with individual counts. • Cannot always distinguish which individuals would have survived in the absence of the disaster from those who would have died during the period regardless. • Often require complex statistical modeling and assumptions.	• Offer critical in-depth analyses following the disaster to inform disaster mitigation and preparedness practices. • Identify population-level trends. • Provide more complete estimate of total impact across a population.

SOURCE: Adapted from Appendix C.

Unlike individual counts, population estimates of total disaster-related mortality and morbidity are derived by estimating the number of mortalities and morbidities using statistical means, such as representative and complex sampling, survey-based methods or using a variety of excess mortality and morbidity methods (e.g., comparing deaths or illness rates in the disaster-affected population to rates observed in the same population during the previous year or during a relevant time period). Population-based estimation methods are crucial for capturing a full understanding of the impacts of a disaster on health and mortality. These methods are often reported in ways that convey the appearance of less precision (i.e., they provide a point estimate with confidence intervals) compared with reports of individual counting methods (which provide a single number, but no confidence intervals, thereby implying greater certainty around the estimate) and in some applications (e.g., estimates of excess deaths) they cannot distinguish individuals who would have survived in the absence of the disaster from those who would have died during the period regardless. Chapter 4 will explore the landscape of population estimation methods and identify potential best practices for conducting and using these analyses.

It is critical to recognize that individual counts are not always superior to population estimates based on samples or vice versa. For some audiences, the term "count" might imply greater precision than the term "estimate," but this assumption is incorrect and both approaches can produce valuable estimates of the true effect of a disaster, which are useful for different purposes. Importantly, both are estimates in the sense that they are ways of gauging total impact that are inherently incomplete and subject to variability over time and according to the specific methods used. Therefore, focusing solely on individual counts limits the scope of an investigation. A more effective strategy is to apply both approaches to assessing mortality and morbidity, which makes the assessment more valuable in terms of understanding the complex nuances of the disaster's impact and the population's vulnerabilities.

Multifactorial Problem

Another concept critical to understanding disaster-related mortality and morbidity is that all quantitative assessments developed using either approach represent a description of the disaster's impact at a specific point in time based on a unique set of conditions and assumptions. These estimates can change over time as more data are gathered, additional mortality and morbidity occur, new assumptions are developed, and updated analyses are performed. Regardless of the methodological approach applied, the assessment of mortality and morbidity is a complex multifactorial problem that is influenced by time, resources, capability, and the health of the affected population. It is impossible to definitively know the true impact of a disaster on human life. Instead, this report attempts to highlight how the administrative, organizational, logistical, and analytical components associated with each of these approaches can be improved to make counts and estimates more accurate and complete reflections of the disaster's true effect.

As a data recording and reporting system matures and is able to more accurately count individual deaths, it will capture progressively more of the deaths that are included in the population-based estimates. This will consequently lessen the disparity between the population estimates of mortality and the number of individual deaths reported, for example. Still, certain categories of indirect and partially attributable mortality and morbidity may always be more difficult to detect in practice at the individual level (e.g., heart attack, stroke) and will tend to be better captured through population estimation methods.

> *Conclusion 2-1: Current terminology and case definitions used to describe disaster-related mortality and morbidity fail to capture the differences in assessment methods used and the totality and temporality of disaster-related deaths and significant morbidity. The lack of a uniform framework for assessing disaster-related health impacts undermines the quality and usability of these data in informing disaster management.*

Accuracy of Individual Counts and Degree of Attribution

The precision of estimates of disaster-related mortality and morbidity made using individual counts depends on the accuracy of decisions that are made about the strength of association of an individual outcome to a disaster. In the case of mortality, medical examiners, coroners, or other medical certifiers[1] must consider for each individual death (1) the type of death, (2) the degree to which the death can be attributed to a disaster, and (3) the temporality of the death—"the timescale over which the death is expected and can be attributed to a disaster in the context of different types of disasters" (Green et al., 2019, p. 452). Given the multidimensionality of these judgments, the different parameters that the responsible parties use to assess the degree of attribution drive variation in the types and quantities of outcomes that are collected and recorded. See Chapter 3 for a discussion of the variation in data collection and recording practices throughout the medicolegal system. Multiple terms have been used to denote the presence and degree of a relationship between a death or injury and a disaster. These are often conflated, resulting in misunderstandings about disasters' impacts and also poor comparability between mortality and morbidity assessments over time and across disasters. Another fundamental disadvantage of the individual counting approach is the risk of failing to count difficult-to-capture cases, such as natural deaths that would not have occurred but for the disaster.

To improve consistency and provide guidance for attributing mortality and morbidity to a disaster using an individual-count approach, the committee developed a set of terms for use throughout the report: namely, an individual reported disaster-related mortality or morbidity can be categorized

---

[1] Medical certifiers are medical professionals with the authority to record a cause of death and sign a death registration following a death, typically in a hospital or a health care setting. Medical certifiers are commonly physicians, nurse practitioners, or physician assistants, although this varies by state based on state law (see Chapter 3 for more information on medical certifiers and death registration).

as directly related, indirectly related, or partially attributable to a disaster. These terms are intended to be flexible enough yet also to be precise enough to support accurate and consistent decision making on whether a case is related to the disaster's impact or other consequences and, if so, to what extent (see Table 2-1). Consistent use of these three terms is also intended to facilitate more effective communication to the media and public about the different ways that an individual reported death or morbidity can be related to a disaster.

Direct Mortality and Morbidity

Direct deaths or morbidities are directly attributable to the disaster itself, such as deaths due to blunt force injury or drowning as a consequence of a disaster's physical force. In the language of cause of death reporting, a direct death is always an unnatural death (Green et al., 2019). Direct deaths tend to be the primary focus of data collection efforts, particularly in the medicolegal death investigation system, because these outcomes are generally the most straightforward to collect and record. However, exclusively capturing direct deaths and failing to account for direct morbidities or for indirect or partially attributable deaths underestimates the actual short- and long-term impacts of the disaster. Additionally, the attribution of individual direct deaths to a disaster does not have an obvious natural end point. As discussed above, a person who dies as a direct consequence of a disaster should always be considered a direct death or morbidity, even if the death occurs many years later. Box 2-2 provides an overview of data sources for individual counts of disaster-related deaths and morbidity.

Indirect Mortality and Morbidity

Indirect disaster-related mortality and morbidity data capture natural and unnatural deaths and morbidities that are associated with—but not directly caused by—the event. Essentially, the criteria for an indirect death require that the death would not have occurred "but for" the conditions present due to the disaster. Indirect deaths include outcomes due to unsafe or unhealthy conditions around the time of the disasters or during any phase of the disaster lifecycle that contribute to a death (Combs et al., 1999) (see Table 2-1). For example, carbon monoxide poisoning due to unsafe generator use during a power outage resulting from a hurricane, or deaths due to lack of access to essential medications or treatments, such as dialysis, should be recorded and reported as indirect deaths. Indirect mortality and morbidity data can offer a wealth of information about a disaster's impact and provide actionable evidence to inform disaster response and on how to prevent deaths during future events. However, accurately

BOX 2-2
Data Sources for Individual Counts of Disaster-Related Deaths

Data from death certificates are the primary source used to attribute individual deaths directly, indirectly, or partially to a disaster. Death certificate information can be accessed through death investigation reports by medicolegal death investigators, state medical examiners' and coroners' systems, physicians and other medical certifiers completing death certificates, and from the electronic death registration systems of state and federal vital statistics departments (Noe, 2018). Access to death certificate information may be delayed during recovery operations, but a number of alternative sources of mortality data exist, including funeral home records, emergency medical services scene transport records, hospital medical records, media reports and memorial websites, the Red Cross disaster-related mortality report form, and the Federal Emergency Management Agency's records of individual funeral benefits distributed (Horney, 2017).

capturing and recording indirect deaths can be hampered by subjectivity in determinations by medical examiners, coroners, or medical certifiers and often by incomplete evidence to support attribution at the time the death is certified. Strategies that could help prevent the loss of these valuable data on indirect mortality and morbidity include (1) establishing a common policy and philosophical approach for collecting and recording these data, (2) providing professional training to reduce variation in practice, and (3) developing improved tools and methods for capturing these data. In addition, providing a third category for individuals for whom their mortality or morbidity might be partially attributable to the disaster should help mitigate the risk of losing valuable data on these individuals' outcomes.

Partially Attributable Mortality and Morbidity

Partially attributable mortality and morbidity is an intentionally nebulous category compared to direct or indirect deaths or morbidities. It encompasses those deaths or morbidities that cannot be tied to the disaster with a high degree of certainty but where the death, injury, or illness was more likely than not to be at least partially related to the disaster. In other words, the death would be unlikely to have occurred "but for" the disaster, but it cannot be tied definitively to it. For instance, this category would include a person who dies because the disaster caused stress or exhaustion that exacerbated a pre-existing chronic condition (Green et al., 2019), such as a person with known heart disease who suffered a heart attack while in a shelter environment. At present there is no term commonly in use to define these types of deaths or morbidities, and because these deaths can be variably labeled as indirect, the lack of a common terminology generates inconsistency and possible bias across jurisdictions or individual certifiers. The committee aims to address this problem with the category of partially attributable deaths. Importantly, this category is not static, and partially attributable deaths or morbidities can be reclassified as indirect deaths or morbidities as more evidence of causation becomes available.

Population Estimation Methods

Population estimates quantify mortality and morbidity related to a disaster at a population level through statistical analyses and epidemiological approaches to assess the size and characteristics of the population affected. The analytical approaches used to develop population estimates include surveys using representative or complex sampling of affected populations as well as estimates derived by comparing observed deaths or morbidities during the disaster time to what was observed in a prior time frame or to a comparison population (Green et al., 2019; Kishore et al., 2018; Stephens et al., 2007). Population estimates often include a broader range of disaster-associated effects than are captured by individual counts, which frequently undercount the true number of cases, because population estimates inherently include indirect and partially attributable deaths and morbidities. Thus, for example, population estimates of disaster deaths will often be larger than the number of direct or indirect deaths captured through individual count methods, sometimes by very large margins (see Appendix C for examples). Population estimates have been developed by researchers following many previous disasters. For instance, modeling excess mortality is a statistical approach for conducting population estimates. Models of excess mortality developed following Hurricane Maria in 2017 in Puerto Rico demonstrate the value of comparing immediate all-cause mortality reported in a community during a disaster to a baseline number of deaths that would be expected in the same community from a disaster of that magnitude (Santos-Burgoa et al., 2018). Other analytical approaches, such as those used in other social science fields such as demography and anthropology can be applied to estimate the size of an affected population and develop excess mortality and morbidity estimates, particularly in situations where the affected population is hard to count. For example, mortality estimates following the 1985 Mexico City earthquake were made using a network scale-up method to determine the estimated victim count (Bernard et al., 1991). Sampling approaches and analyses of electronic medical records and related data are especially useful for understanding the long-term, non-fatal consequences of disasters, including mental health issues (see Chapter 4).

ATTRIBUTING MORBIDITY TO A DISASTER

While the cause of death may sometimes be difficult to determine, mortality itself is easier to define than morbidity. Morbidities related to disasters represent an exceptionally broad range of health outcomes that span physical injuries, chronic and infectious conditions, and psychological impacts in addition to having long-term impacts on communities, health systems, and economies. The physical and mental health effects of disasters can be immediate or delayed (Adeola and Picou, 2012) and can occur as a result of the direct forces of the disaster, such as an injury, or as a result of the conditions brought forth by the disaster. The latter includes such scenarios as the interruption of mental health services or the decline of health maintenance activities (e.g., blood pressure testing or access to prescription drugs), which exacerbate existing vulnerabilities and pre-existing co-morbidities to produce additional morbidity and mortality (Bourque et al., 2009; Schnall et al., 2011).[2] For example, research following Hurricane Katrina found that the interruption of health maintenance activities was an indicator for additional future morbidity since up to one-half of evacuees seeking shelter in the Astrodome and Red Cross facilities lacked access to their prescription medications (Brodie et al., 2006; Greenough et al., 2008). Common disaster-related morbidities include infectious diseases (Kouadio et al., 2012), chronic diseases exacerbated by disaster conditions (Miller and Arquilla, 2008; Mokdad et al., 2005), and mental health problems, including self-harm and substance abuse, caused or worsened by exposure to intense stressors (McFarlane and Williams, 2012) (see Table 2-3 for an overview of select research on disaster-related morbidities).

Further complexity is added by the fact that different disasters produce a different landscape of morbidities (Bourque et al., 2009). A major flood is not expected to produce an increase in burns and a wildfire should not generally lead to an increase in near-drownings. In disasters where large populations are temporarily displaced in close-quartered shelters, gastrointestinal and respiratory infections are likely to be prevalent (Schnall et al., 2011), while terrorist attacks are likely to result in physical and psychological trauma. Chronic diseases such as asthma, cardiovascular conditions, and diabetes and their associated co-morbidities represent a larger proportion of morbidities associated with disasters, particularly environmental disasters, in the United States (Schnall et al., 2011).

What should count as a disaster-related morbidity might also be shaped by the intended uses of the data—for example, to address hospital capacity issues, to assess short- or long-term disabilities versus specialty conditions,

[2] See Appendix D for an exploration of the causal links across social determinants of health and disaster-related morbidity and mortality through the lens of COVID-19.

TABLE 2-3 Selected Research on Physical and Psychological Morbidities Associated with Disaster Exposure

Morbidity Type	Disaster Type	Major Findings
Carbon monoxide poisoning (Bourque et al., 2009)	Hurricane	Number of cases, associated with improper use of generators, peaked within 3 days of hurricane landfall.
Asthma/other respiratory symptoms (Bourque et al., 2009)	Terrorism	Higher rates of lower-airway hyper-responsiveness among first responders to Ground Zero, possibly as a result of exposure to airborne contaminants from fires, dust, and equipment exhaust.
Water- and vector-borne diseases (Watson et al., 2007)	Flood, tsunami	Overcrowding and population displacement coupled with disruption or lack of regular sanitation services has led to increases in diseases such as measles, hepatitis, gastrointestinal diseases, and food poisoning, etc.
Depression (Goldmann and Galea, 2014)	Hurricane, terrorism	Depression is considered to be one of the most prevalent disaster-related mental disorders.
Substance use disorders and overdoses (Goldmann and Galea, 2014)	Terrorism	Increased rates of cigarette, alcohol, and marijuana use among New Yorkers following the September 11, 2001, terrorist attacks.
Heart attack (Nakagawa et al., 2009; Swerdel et al., 2014)	Hurricane, earthquake	Rates of heart attacks and other cardiovascular conditions elevated in the months and years following a disaster, compared with pre-disaster levels.

or to evaluate the impact on the health system more broadly during the response and recovery periods.

Despite the range of information that is possible to collect, the variation in morbidity across disasters, and the ongoing lack of a standard approach for collecting morbidity data, it is likely that a group of key morbidities could be distilled across common disasters (e.g., hurricanes, tornadoes, floods, wildfires, and extreme temperature events). This standard dataset could provide a starting point for the collection of more standardized data points and approaches for data collection and analysis (see Recommendation 3-3 and Conclusion 3-6). Potential morbidities on target for consistent data collection across a range of common disasters should move beyond the definition of "significant morbidity" and be inclusive of morbidities that are known to be associated with those common socioeconomic and environmental conditions prevalent following most disasters. These include morbidities associated with mass displacement, environmental exposure, extreme stress, and lasting infrastructure damage, among others. These data, even if imperfect and incomplete to start, could provide actionable information for disaster management policy and practice.

In particular it is well documented that socially disadvantaged and underserved communities suffer disproportionally from disasters and morbidities. More research is needed on how to best mitigate these disparities before, during, and after a disaster. To achieve this aim, research and decisive action are needed to develop a consensus around which morbidities and other appropriate indicators would be most useful to collect before, during, and after every disaster or specific types of disasters, and what analytical methods and systems should be developed or enhanced to facilitate the collection, analysis, and use of these data (Bourque et al., 2009). More discussion about gaps and potential opportunities for collecting, recording, and using morbidity data for individual counts can be found in Chapter 3. Further discussion of methods for population estimates can be found in Chapter 4.

OVERLOOKED VALUE OF MORBIDITY DATA

Assessing health outcomes is a critical component of improving rapid response and recovery following a disaster through the allocation of resources and targeted public health messaging and enhancing prevention and mitigation activities during the inter-disaster period (Schnall et al., 2011). The collection and use of morbidity data, however, is an often overlooked component of the disaster management enterprise, which tends to focus on mortality as an indicator of disaster-related health impacts. When acted on appropriately, morbidity data can help to reduce mortality (i.e., by preventing morbidities from becoming mortalities) and can be used to help shape public health messaging and medical preparedness. For end users in the field of disaster management, in particular, estimates of morbidity resulting from a disaster may actually be of more value than mortality data in informing life-saving mitigation and preparedness activities and in enhancing real-time response. Therefore, an exclusive focus on mortality data, the traditional outcome of interest, at the expense of morbidity data is tantamount to focusing only on the worst case and diverts responders' attention from efforts that could reduce human suffering and save additional lives.

A recent example of the power of morbidity data to prevent additional suffering is the testing and tracking of individual coronavirus disease 2019 (COVID-19) cases throughout the world. In Singapore and Hong Kong, among other places, surveillance data were used successfully in the early months of the pandemic to identify and isolate cases in order to prevent additional mortalities and avoid a drain on medical resources, especially in intensive care units (Purnell and Solomon, 2020). For hospitals, evidence-based models for quantifying expected morbidities following a disaster may be of much greater value than expected mortality models, because injuries and disease tend to consume a great deal of health system resources.

Evaluation of Health System Access, Capacity, and Cost

Morbidity data can be used to assess health system functions, costs, and access to care over time in order to support the shifting needs of patients with chronic conditions such as diabetes (Lee et al., 2016) during and after a disaster. For example, in the 6 years following Hurricane Katrina, Peters et al. (2014) noted a three-fold increase in the percentage of admissions to Tulane University Hospital for acute myocardial infarction (Peters et al., 2014). Another 2009 modeling study found that Hurricane Katrina also (1) had a significant effect on diabetes management, (2) had exacerbated existing racial/ethnic health disparities, and (3) had an estimated lifetime cost of $504 million for the affected adult population (Fonseca et al., 2009). This research indicates that not only do disaster-related morbidities put pressure on local and regional health care systems but that access to care and the costs of obtaining care are significant and represent variables that could be addressed proactively with better and earlier access to descriptive morbidity data combined with data on related sociodemographic factors. Overall, the disaster management enterprise remains underinvested in understanding morbidity and how using morbidity data can contribute to saving lives, protecting health, and improving health equity, as will be discussed in Chapters 3 and 4.

VALUE AND USE OF DATA ACROSS THE DISASTER LIFECYCLE

Morbidity and mortality data add value to all phases of the disaster lifecycle, from the immediate aftermath of an event through the recovery and inter-disaster periods. The value of these data and how they can be used optimally will shift over time. For instance, quantifying the health impacts of a disaster can help to determine the disaster's scale and inform resource deployment at the early stages. During later phases, the data can be used for predictive planning, risk mitigation, and other efforts to improve preparedness and strengthen public health systems to perform better during future disasters. Figure 1-1 in Chapter 1 provides a more detailed description of the use of mortality and morbidity data across the disaster lifecycle. The integration of applied epidemiology into disaster management can provide a reliable, actionable evidence base for decision makers and other stakeholders (Malilay et al., 2014). However, extracting the value of mortality and morbidity data is dependent on the right data being collected and having the right methods and systems in place to effectively analyze and use the data. This requires determining the types of data with the most value in ensuring people's well-being at each phase of the disaster management cycle.

In terms of their functional value, mortality and morbidity data enable the Federal Emergency Management Agency (FEMA), the Department of Health and Human Services (HHS), and other federal and SLTT agencies involved in a response to (CDC, 2016):

- quantify disaster health impacts and ongoing hazards;
- detect and track epidemiological trends;
- limit further health impacts;
- ensure a common operating picture;
- inform resource allocation;
- shape public messaging and control rumors;
- provide support to individuals and families;
- target interventions and other public health responses;
- monitor and evaluate the effectiveness of the response and recovery efforts; and
- evaluate the effectiveness of prevention and mitigation activities and inform preparedness planning.

Value and Use of Data During Response and Recovery Period

The response and recovery periods include the disaster impact and its immediate aftermath and includes emergency response efforts and efforts to restore infrastructure and services (DOI, 2020). The timing of optimal data use during the response and recovery periods depends on the type of disaster, its severity, and the areas and populations affected. However, the primary value of data during these periods is to track the evolution of the disaster in order to save lives and limit further deaths and health consequences. For example, the HHS emPOWER program draws on data from the Centers for Medicare & Medicaid Services (CMS) to create dynamic maps, tools, and resources to identify and provide support during disasters to CMS beneficiaries who live alone and are dependent on electricity for their health care needs (ASPR, 2020). The program has been deployed successfully during Hurricane Matthew in Florida (2016) and during the severe wildfires in Los Angeles, California (2017) (Finne, 2018).

Accurate real-time and historical mortality and morbidity data are critical for ensuring a common operating picture and real-time situational awareness as a disaster unfolds and recovery efforts begin. All stakeholders need reliable, accurate information with which to inform their decisions. Therefore, a lack of shared information and poor access to data among stakeholders can hinder response efforts. Although mortality and morbidity data present a significant opportunity to better target future planning, mitigation, and response efforts—particularly for vulnerable communities—the usability of these data is reliant on their consistent collection, reporting, and interpretation (see Chapter 3).

Targeting Response and Recovery Efforts and Resource Allocation

During the immediate response period, reliable real-time mortality and morbidity data can be used to assess and respond to the evolving current needs. For example, the data can guide the strategic allocation of resources in response to situational needs, which can help limit future morbidity and mortality. For example, the Assistant Secretary for Preparedness and Response's Emergency Support Function #8 (ESF8)—Public Health and Medical Services—offers federal support to strengthen SLTT-level disaster response capabilities. Under ESF8, the National Disaster Medical System can respond to spikes in mortality and morbidity to provide human resources in settings where health system capacity and infrastructure have been compromised by a disaster. Disaster medical assistance teams (DMATs) can help triage mass casualties and provide acute care, while disaster mortuary operational response team (DMORT) medical examiner and coroner services can provide standalone morgue operations and human remains identification services (ASPR, 2012). Spikes in mortality can provide real-time evidence for the need for support from DMATs and DMORTs. Rapid increases in initial mortality and morbidity counts could also indicate the need for specific types of health care services or resources. These initial raw data captured immediately following a disaster can also help responders predict and prepare for subsequent waves of mortality and morbidity that often occur during the following days, especially if health delivery systems and transportation infrastructure are incapacitated (Malilay et al., 2014).

In addition to the use of real-time data to address current needs, historical morbidity data can be used in the immediate aftermath of a disaster to model expected trajectories and outcomes and to identify vulnerable populations. These models can provide essential details for informing the planning and execution of the response that cannot be derived rapidly from other sources. For example, prospective models based on historical data could predict whether local-level capacity is capable of continuing to manage the current threat or if state or federal resources may be needed. These approaches would be particularly valuable for determining current or future access to basic resources such as food, clean water, and energy in vulnerable communities as well as for identifying and addressing critical gaps in service delivery (Malilay et al., 2014). For example, following Hurricane Maria in Puerto Rico, individuals requiring dialysis or diabetes medication were often unable to access them due to a lack of power and clean water and debris blocking access roads (Cordero, 2019).

Financial and Emotional Support for Survivors and Families

Mortality and morbidity data can also help alleviate the devastating impacts of disasters on individuals and families by guiding the provision of resources and support. Mortality data in particular have major financial implications for individuals and families seeking funeral assistance from FEMA, because one of the eligibility requirements for this support is documentation that the death occurred either directly or indirectly as a result of the disaster impact (NCHS, 2017).[3] If a death was not attributed as such by the medical examiner, coroner, or other medical certifier, then the death may be ruled ineligible for funeral assistance, or assistance may be delayed (Bowden, 2018). Data are also used to determine eligibility for other types of resources and support, to guide social and medical benefits and payouts in a standardized way, to streamline assistance programs, and to reduce public confusion about how to access support. For instance, FEMA can use data following a disaster to provide timely individual and public assistance to supplement SLTT resources, such as the crisis counseling program that

[3] Under the Other Needs Assistance provision of the Individuals and Households Program, FEMA provides financial assistance to help with the cost of uninsured expenses for a death or interment caused directly or indirectly by a presidentially declared emergency or major disaster (see 44 C.F.R. § 206.119(c)(4)). Applicants must submit an official death certificate clearly indicating that the death was attributed to the emergency or disaster, either directly or indirectly, or a signed statement from an SLTT government-licensed medical official (e.g., medical examiner or coroner) directly or indirectly attributing the death to the emergency or disaster (FEMA, 2019).

offers funds for mental health services to communities in disaster-affected areas as defined by the Robert T. Stafford Disaster Relief and Emergency Assistance Act (Stafford Act) (FEMA, 2016; State of Michigan, 2020).

Public Health Emergency Communication and Response

Effective public health messaging in a disaster-affected area is shaped by accurate and timely mortality and morbidity data. Timely and clear communication following a disaster keeps the public informed about the unfolding event, protects them from ongoing hazards, and dissuades individuals from taking risks due to a lack of awareness or haste. For example, historical and real-time mortality and morbidity data can be used to identify and communicate risks to the public such as carbon monoxide poisonings, unsafe drinking water sources, fallen electrical wires, or hazardous chemical and environmental exposures (Malilay et al., 2014). These data can also be used to inform the timing and frequency of communicating the existence of digital tools and resources that are available to individuals in their immediate area or in an unfamiliar area to which they have been evacuated. For example, the communication of accessible tools like RxOpen's real-time pharmacy information could enhance access to critical medications for these groups (RxOpen, 2020). For disaster survivors with chronic health conditions, limited access or a lack of access to essential medications and medical equipment can directly affect immediate and future health.

Value and Use of Data During the Inter-Disaster Period

The inter-disaster period encompasses mitigation and preparedness efforts that occur in the interim phase between the end of one disaster and the beginning of the next (Malilay et al., 2014). The core value of mortality and morbidity data during this period is to save lives and protect human health during the next disaster (Green et al., 2019). Such data can be used to identify vulnerabilities and exposure-related risk factors, to improve the allocation of resources on a regional level, and to proactively inform the design of interventions to reduce morbidity and mortality from future events (Malilay et al., 2014). In the case of human-caused disasters (such as terrorism, or climate change-related events), better data on health effects and interactions might not only mitigate disaster impacts but even help to prevent future disasters.

Building Health System Capacity

To support health systems in building response capacity, mortality and morbidity data can be used to predict demands on health care delivery systems, to guide resource and service usage patterns, to strengthen physical infrastructure, and to organize staff and systems to deploy during a future response (Malilay et al., 2014). Gaps in access to care and gaps along the continuum of care can also be identified to improve health systems during and between disasters. Data can be used to assess costs to the medical system at set intervals following a disaster and to perform cost-effectiveness analyses to compare the costs associated with a large-scale disaster response versus the costs of prevention, mitigation, and planning; this can help to prioritize resource allocation and investment in lower-cost planning activities (Malilay et al., 2014). Additionally, mortality data from previous disasters can inform the windows of coverage for FEMA assistance and other benefits for future disasters.

Improving Policy and Practice

Mortality and morbidity data can be used to muster appropriate levels of support for legislation and funding for programs, infrastructure, and resources. More accurate predictions of excess mortality from certain types of disasters could serve as powerful levers for policy change to prevent such disasters or mitigate their impacts. Furthermore, comparing actual morbidity and mortality data following a disaster to historical data for similar prior disasters can feed back into continuous improvement of preparedness policies and activities (Schnall et al., 2017). Mortality and morbidity data also can be used reflexively to evaluate and improve mortality and morbidity data collection practices. These efforts may include assessing the effectiveness of specific case definitions and data sources with respect to different health outcomes (Malilay et al., 2014) and developing institutional best practices for collecting, using, and sharing data (e.g., standardized practices for assessing morbidity and mortality).

Cultivating Community Resilience

Protecting the public by investing in community resilience[4] is a long-term public health goal, so data should be collected with sufficient granularity to be relevant at the community level. Data can be used to strengthen community resilience to future disasters in myriad ways. In addition to strengthening community-level health systems and emergency management infrastructure, data can be used to understand biopsychosocial and environmental conditions—including the proximal and distal influencers of disparities—that affect a community's susceptibility to disaster-related mortality

[4] Community resilience is multidimensional, spanning six types of community capital: natural/environmental, buildings and infrastructure, financial and economic capital, human and cultural capital, social capital, and political capital (NASEM, 2019).

and morbidity. Mortality and morbidity data are critical for understanding and mitigating the disproportionate impacts of disasters on vulnerable populations. These populations need to be identified during the inter-disaster period so that their access and functional needs can be supported through targeted interventions and messaging (Browning et al., 2006; Feehan and Salganik, 2016; Lowe et al., 2013; Mace et al., 2018; Wolkin et al., 2015).[5] For example, in discussions with community leaders, the committee learned that the response to the Camp Fire that struck Paradise, California, revealed that the city was reliant on the Butte County Health Department for access to public health data. When the county was unable to provide needed data during the disaster and recovery, Paradise officials were forced to look to the local hospital to provide data that could have been used to enhance preparedness and response capacities at the local and county levels. Furthermore, data on disaster-related mortality and morbidity are important for helping communities access resources and support services as well as for supporting fundraising and advocacy. In Florida, for example, the committee learned that data from the state's robust women, infants, and children program showed a significant disaster-related reduction in the number of certain program participants after a hurricane, which informed strategies to reengage with specific communities. Demonstrating the value of data collected during disasters can also help to improve transparency and build trust between emergency management and communities.

Mortality and morbidity data hold important value for monitoring a community's progress over time in the recovery period, which can last for years. Longitudinal morbidity data can be used to track long-term health sequelae of disasters, including mortality risk.[6] Some of these outcomes are shaped by age, gender, and other sociodemographic factors that have been established by longitudinal studies conducted after Hurricane Katrina (Adams et al., 2011; Adeola and Picou, 2012), Hurricane Maria (Santos-Burgoa et al., 2018), and the 2004 Indian Ocean tsunami (Frankenberg et al., 2014; Ho et al., 2017). Studying relative mortality over time also allows for charting the effects of cumulative stress and chronic disease as the survivors age (Ho et al., 2017). Going forward, standardizing the collection of longitudinal mortality and morbidity data would enable comparisons of

[5] Medically vulnerable groups include people who are hospitalized, people who have electricity grid–sensitive conditions (e.g., hypertension and diabetes) and people living with infectious diseases such as tuberculosis and AIDS (Bernard et al., 2010). Grid-sensitive conditions are especially common among people in nursing homes and people receiving home care (Banks, 2013; DeSalvo et al., 2014). Socially vulnerable groups include people in financially precarious situations who become homeless and unemployed, leading to indirect deaths by overdose or suicide, as well as local homeless populations.

[6] Longer-term physical health consequences are a particular concern when a disaster causes environmental hazards that can persist for years (e.g., oil spills or radiation) (Frankenberg et al., 2014).

specific communities at selected points in time after incidents in order to develop common 6-month, 1-year, 3-year, and 5-year datasets, for example.

Stress, posttraumatic stress disorder, depression, and anxiety are common mental health morbidities and co-morbidities after a disaster (Adams et al., 2014; Adhikari Baral and Bhagawati, 2019; Beaglehole et al., 2018; Buttke et al., 2012; Mulchandani et al., 2019; Norris et al., 2002). Using data to better understand the risk factors for these mental health sequelae could help to inform screening, prevention, and intervention efforts in communities affected by disasters (Adams et al., 2014).

Ongoing Public Health Communication

Another valuable use of mortality and morbidity data is in evaluating how effectively public health messaging is able to drive behavioral change and reduce risk across the disaster management cycle (Malilay et al., 2014). For instance, data on the health consequences of improper generator use could be used to shape messaging and policy in ways to mitigate similar mortality in subsequent disasters (Schnall et al., 2017).

Value of Multidimensional Mortality and Morbidity Data

As described throughout this chapter, mortality and morbidity data represent a wide variety of uses and values. These data, if accurate and complete, can be used to identify at-risk populations, among other uses, and respond with appropriate actions to support recovery, mitigate root vulnerabilities, and prepare to prevent future harm, which represents great value to the field of disaster management. Critically, mortality and morbidity data alone represent just one category of data and further contextualization of these data with other rich data points, such as race and ethnicity, socioeconomic status, among others, provides for a multidimensional understanding of those same mortality and morbidity data. The integration of these data represents real opportunities to identify the underlying causal pathways and sub-population inequities existing at the intersection of the social determinants of health (SDOH), disaster exposure, and disaster-related mortality and morbidity, which could in turn allow for the improved design and targeting of resources and programs to the sub-population in greatest need. The contextualization of morbidity and mortality using SDOH data adds additional value and evidence to foster a stronger and more responsive disaster management enterprise that prioritizes community resilience.

The contributory role of SDOH on vulnerability should not be deemphasized. For example, Thomas-Henkel and Schulman (2017, p. 1) write, "SDOH can account for up to 40% of individual health outcomes, particularly among low-income populations, [and] their providers are increasingly focused on strategies to address patients' unmet social needs (e.g. food insecurity, housing, transportation, etc.)." Co-morbidities are one significant consequence of these unmet social needs (Valderas et al., 2009), which add distinct complexity to the assessment and use of disaster-related mortality and morbidity data. Certain socio-environmental factors—population density, exposure to pollution, outdoor manual labor—are known to increase biological susceptibility to disease, and those impacts seep into individual treatment decisions and care of various medical conditions (McKibben, 2020). During and after a disaster, these influences are even more pronounced. Other SDOH, such as race and economic status, are known to be associated with persistent inequities in health and are critical to examine alongside disaster-related mortality and morbidity data to provide a foundation of evidence for promoting community resilience. Excluding an assessment of SDOH in the overall assessment of post-disaster mortality and morbidity significantly limits the opportunity to prevent disaster-related mortality and morbidity; an oversight that would have especially deleterious consequences for regions with large communities of disadvantaged and underserved populations and that are also susceptible to natural disasters, such as Puerto Rico, the U.S. Gulf Coast, and areas experiencing frequent wildfires (e.g., California).

RECOMMENDATIONS

Mortality and morbidity data related to large-scale disasters represent a poorly tapped resource for critical information to improve the nation's ability to respond to disasters and save lives. Fundamentally, the lack of a consistently used framework for attributing mortality and morbidity results in the inconsistent collection and reporting of data on the scope and causes of mortality and morbidity over time and across disasters. The committee's framework responds to this critical gap and is unique in that it balances the value of both individual count and population estimation methods for developing quantitative indicators of total mortality or morbidity and provides updated individual count case definitions to characterize the level of attribution for all deaths related to disasters of all types.

Recommendation 2-1: Adopt and Support the Use of a Uniform Framework for Assessing Disaster-Related Mortality and Morbidity

The Department of Health and Human Services and the Department of Homeland Security, including the Office of the Assistant Secretary for Preparedness and Response, the Centers for Disease Control and Prevention, the Centers for Medicare & Medicaid Services, and the Federal Emergency Management Agency, should adopt and support the use of a uniform framework for assessing disaster-related mortality and

morbidity before, during, and after a disaster by state, local, tribal, and territorial (SLTT) entities; public health agencies; and death investigation and registration systems. To implement this uniform framework nationally, the National Center for Health Statistics in conjunction with state and local vital records offices, medical examiners and coroners, medical certifiers, and all relevant professional associations should jointly adopt and apply this framework to practice, including the routine use of uniform case definitions and data collection, recording, and reporting practices. Additionally, all Stafford Disaster Relief and Emergency Assistance Act declarations should require affected states and regions to comply with the reporting requirements for individual count and population estimation approaches as described in the framework. Timely guidance should be disseminated to SLTT entities regarding the proper certification of individual deaths with provision for direct, indirect, and partially attributable deaths following a large-scale disaster.

The following terminology and approaches for defining mortality and morbidity following large-scale disasters should be adopted immediately:

- **Total reported mortality and morbidity estimation using individual counts:** Individual counts are point-in-time estimates of disaster-related mortality and morbidity derived from reported cases.
  - o *Direct death or morbidity*: A death or morbidity directly attributable to the forces of the disaster or a direct consequence of these forces.
  - o *Indirect death or morbidity*: A death or morbidity not from a direct impact but due to unsafe or unhealthy conditions around the time of the disaster, including while preparing for, while responding to, and during recovery from the disaster.
  - o *Partially attributable death or morbidity*: A death or morbidity that cannot be tied definitively to the disaster but where the disaster more likely than not has played a contributing role in the death.
  - o *Unrelated death or morbidity*: A death or morbidity that is unassociated with or cannot be attributed to the forces of a disaster.
- **Total mortality and morbidity derived from population estimates:** Population estimates are point-in-time estimates of the impact of a disaster at a population level derived using various statistical methods and tools, including sampling.

Recommendation 2-2: Report Both Individual Counts and Population Estimates

Both individual counts and population estimates should be used as accepted standards for reporting by state, local, tribal, and territorial entities and supported by the federal agencies as indicators of mortality and morbidity to determine the impact of disasters over time. State and federal reporting of total mortality and morbidity estimates following disasters should use both individual counts of direct and indirect deaths and population estimates of mortality and morbidity as these data become available following a disaster. Individual count data should be referred to as *reported cases* or *reported deaths* and should not be referred to as reflecting *total mortality* or a *death toll.* Total mortality estimates should be derived from population estimation methods, which provide a more complete assessment of overall impacts of large-scale disasters.

REFERENCES

Adams, V., S. R. Kaufman, T. van Hattum, and S. Moody. 2011. Aging disaster: Mortality, vulnerability, and long-term recovery among Katrina survivors. *Medical Anthropology* 30(3):247–270.

Adams, Z. W., J. A. Sumner, C. K. Danielson, J. L. McCauley, H. S. Resnick, K. Grös, L. A. Paul, K. E. Welsh, and K. J. Ruggiero. 2014. Prevalence and predictors of PTSD and depression among adolescent victims of the spring 2011 tornado outbreak. *Journal of Child Psychology and Psychiatry* 55(9):1047–1055.

Adeola, F. O., and J. S. Picou. 2012. Race, social capital, and the health impacts of Katrina: Evidence from the Louisiana and Mississippi Gulf Coast. *Human Ecology Review* 19(1):10–24.

Adhikari Baral, I., and K. C. Bhagawati. 2019. Post traumatic stress disorder and coping strategies among adult survivors of earthquake, Nepal. *BMC Psychiatry* 19(1):118.

ASPR (Assistant Secretary for Preparedness and Response). 2012. *Public health emergency—Emergency Support Function #8*. https://www.phe.gov/Preparedness/planning/mscc/handbook/chapter7/Pages/emergency.aspx (accessed June 2, 2020).

ASPR. 2020. *HHS emPOWER program fact sheet*. https://empowermap.hhs.gov/HHS%20emPOWER%20Program_Fact%20Sheet_FINAL_v9_508.pdf (accessed June 26, 2020).

Banks, L. 2013. Caring for elderly adults during disasters: Improving health outcomes and recovery. *Southern Medical Journal* 106(1):94–98.

Beaglehole, B., R. T. Mulder, C. M. Frampton, J. M. Boden, G. Newton-Howes, and C. J. Bell. 2018. Psychological distress and psychiatric disorder after natural disasters: Systematic review and meta-analysis. *British Journal of Psychiatry* 213(6):716–722.

Bernard, H. R., E. C. Johnsen, P. D. Killworth, and S. Robinson. 1991. Estimating the size of an average personal network and of an event subpopulation: Some empirical results. *Social Science Research* 20(2):109–121.

Bernard, H. R., T. Hallett, A. Iovita, E. C. Johnsen, R. Lyerla, C. McCarty, M. Mahy, M. J. Salganik, T. Saliuk, O. Scutelniciuc, G. A. Shelley, P. Sirinirund, S. Weir, and D. F. Stroup. 2010. Counting hard-to-count populations: The network scale-up method for public health. *Sexually Transmitted Infections* 86(Suppl 2):ii11–ii15.

Bourque, L., J. Siegel, M. Kano, and M. Wood. 2009. Morbidity and mortality associated with disasters. In H. Rodríquez, E. L. Quarantelli, and R. R. Dynes (eds.), *Handbook of disaster research*. New York: Springer. Pp. 97–112.

Bowden, J. 2018. FEMA has approved 3 percent of requests for Puerto Rico funeral aid. *The Hill*, September 11. https://thehill.com/homenews/administration/406169-fema-has-approved-just-3-percent-of-requests-for-puerto-rico-funeral (accessed June 26, 2020).

Brodie, M., E. Weltzien, D. Altman, R. J. Blendon, J. M. Benson. 2006. Experiences of Hurricane Katrina evacuees in Houston shelters: Implications for future planning. *American Journal of Public Health* 96(8):1402–1408. doi: 10.2105/AJPH.2005.084475.

Browning, C. R., S. L. Feinberg, D. Wallace, and K. A. Cagney. 2006. Neighborhood social processes, physical conditions, and disaster-related mortality: The case of the 1995 Chicago heat wave. *American Sociological Review* 71(4):661–678.

Buttke, D., S. Vagi, A. Schnall, T. Bayleyegn, M. Morrison, M. Allen, and A. Wolkin. 2012. Community assessment for public health emergency response (CASPER) one year following the Gulf Coast oil spill: Alabama and Mississippi, 2011. *Prehospital and Disaster Medicine* 27(6):496–502.

CDC (Centers for Disease Control and Prevention). 2016. *A primer for understanding the principles and practices of disaster surveillance in the United States, 1st ed.* Atlanta, GA: Centers for Disease Control and Prevention.

Combs, D. L., L. E. Quenemoen, R. G. Parrish, and J. H. Davis. 1999. Assessing disaster-attributed mortality: Development and application of a definition and classification matrix. *International Journal of Epidemiology* 28(6):1124–1129.

Cordero, J. 2019. *Session 1: Hurricane Maria in Puerto Rico*. Presentation at the August 29, 2019, public meeting of the National Academies of Sciences, Engineering, and Medicine's Committee on Best Practices for Assessing Mortality and Significant Morbidity Following Large-Scale Disasters, Washington, DC.

DeSalvo, K., N. Lurie, K. Finne, C. Worrall, A. Bogdanov, A. Dinkler, S. Babcock, and J. Kelman. 2014. Using Medicare data to identify individuals who are electricity dependent to improve disaster preparedness and response. *American Journal of Public Health* 104(7):1160–1164.

DOI (Department of the Interior). 2020. *Natural disaster response and recovery*. https://www.doi.gov/recovery (accessed August 1, 2020).

Feehan, D. M., and M. J. Salganik. 2016. Generalizing the network scale-up method: A new estimator for the size of hidden populations. *Sociological Methodology* 46(1):153–186.

FEMA (Federal Emergency Management Agency). 2016. *Crisis counseling assistance and training program guidance*. https://www.samhsa.gov/sites/default/files/images/fema-ccp-guidance.pdf (acccessed June 26, 2020).

FEMA. 2019. *Fact sheet—funeral assistance*. https://www.fema.gov/media-library-data/1565189678667-0fdafea4dbca363ed6380cf2ae453aa8/FACTSHEET_Funeral AssistanceFINA2019Compliant.pdf (accessed August 2, 2020).

FEMA. 2020. *Rumor control*. https://www.fema.gov/rumor-control (accessed June 10, 2020).

Finne, K. P. 2018. *HHS emPOWER program: Translating research into practice*. PowerPoint presentation. sites.nationalacademies.org/cs/groups/dbassesite/documents/webpage/dbasse_187829.pdf (accessed June 26, 2020).

Fonseca, V. A., H. Smith, N. Kuhadiya, S. M. Leger, C. L. Yau, K. Reynolds, L. Shi, R. H. McDuffie, T. Thethi, and J. John-Kalarickal. 2009. Impact of a natural disaster on diabetes: Exacerbation of disparities and long-term consequences. *Diabetes Care* 32(9):1632–1638.

Frankenberg, E., M. Laurito, and D. Thomas. 2014. The demography of disasters. In *International Encyclopedia of the Social and Behavioral Sciences (Area 3), 2nd ed.* Amsterdam, The Netherlands: North Holland. Pp. 1–22.

Goldmann, E., and S. Galea. 2014. Mental health consequences of disasters. *Annual Review of Public Health* 35(1):169–183. https://doi.org/10.1146/annurev-publhealth-032013-182435.

Green, H. K., O. Lysaght, D. D. Saulnier, K. Blanchard, A. Humphrey, B. Fakhruddin, and V. Murray. 2019. Challenges with disaster mortality data and measuring progress towards the implementation of the Sendai Framework. *International Journal of Disaster Risk Science* 10:449–461.

Greenough, P. G., M. D. Lappi, E. B. Hsu, S. Fink, Y.–H. Hsieh, A. Vu, C. Heaton, and T. D. Kirsch. 2008. Burden of disease and health status among Hurricane Katrina-displaced persons in shelters: A population-based cluster sample. *Annals of Emergency Medicine* 51(4):426–432.

Ho, J. Y., E. Frankenberg, C. Sumantri, and D. Thomas. 2017. Adult mortality five years after a natural disaster. *Population and Development Review* 43(3):467–490.

Horney, J. 2017. *Disaster epidemiology: Methods and applications*. London: Academic Press.

IOM (Institute of Medicine). 2003. *Medicolegal death investigation system: Workshop summary*. Washington, DC: The National Academies Press. https://doi.org/10.17226/10792.

Kishore, N., D. Marqués, A. Mahmud, M. V. Kiang, I. Rodriguez, A. Fuller, P. Ebner, C. Sorensen, F. Racy, J. Lemery, L. Maas, J. Leaning, R. A. Irizarry, S. Balsari, and C. O. Buckee. 2018. Mortality in Puerto Rico after Hurricane Maria. *New England Journal of Medicine* 379(2):162–170.

Kouadio, I. K., S. Aljunid, T. Kamigaki, K. Hammad, and H. Oshitani. 2012. Infectious diseases following natural disasters: Prevention and control measures. *Expert Review of Anti-infective Therapy* 10(1):95–104.

Lee, D. C., V. K. Gupta, B. G. Carr, S. Malik, B. Ferguson, S. P. Wall, S. W. Smith, and L. R. Goldfrank. 2016. Acute post-disaster medical needs of patients with diabetes: Emergency department use in New York City by diabetic adults after Hurricane Sandy. *BMJ Open Diabetes Research and Care* 4(1):e000248.

Lowe, D., K. L. Ebi, and B. Forsberg. 2013. Factors increasing vulnerability to health effects before, during and after floods. *International Journal of Environmental Research and Public Health* 10(12):7015–7067.

Mace, S. E., C. J. Doyle, K. Askew, S. Bradin, M. Baker, M. M. Joseph, and A. Sorrentino. 2018. Planning considerations for persons with access and functional needs in a disaster—Part 1: Overview and legal. *American Journal of Disaster Medicine* 13(2):69–83.

Malilay, J., M. Heumann, D. Perrotta, A. F. Wolkin, A. H. Schnall, M. N. Podgornik, M. A. Cruz, J. A. Horney, D. Zane, R. Roisman, J. R. Greenspan, D. Thoroughman, H. A. Anderson, E. V. Wells, and E. F. Simms. 2014. The role of applied epidemiology methods in the disaster management cycle. *American Journal of Public Health* 104(11):2092–2102.

McFarlane, A. C., and R. Williams. 2012. Mental health services required after disasters: Learning from the lasting effects of disasters. *Depression Research and Treatment* 2012:970194.

McKibben, B. 2020. Racism, police violence, and the climate are not separate issues. *The New Yorker*. https://www.newyorker.com/news/annals-of-a-warming-planet/racism-police-violence-and-the-climate-are-not-separate-issues (accessed September 1, 2020).

Miller, A. C., and B. Arquilla. 2008. Chronic diseases and natural hazards: Impact of disasters on diabetic, renal, and cardiac patients. *Prehospital and Disaster Medicine* 23(2):185–194.

Mokdad, A. H., G. A. Mensah, S. F. Posner, E. Reed, E. J. Simoes, M. M. Engelgau, and Chronic Diseases and Vulnerable Populations in Natural Disasters Working Group. 2005. When chronic conditions become acute: Prevention and control of chronic diseases and adverse health outcomes during natural disasters. *Preventing Chronic Disease* 2(Special Issue):A04.

Mulchandani, R., M. Smith, B. Armstrong, C. R. Beck, I. Oliver, and English National Study of Flooding and Health Study Group. 2019. Effect of insurance-related factors on the association between flooding and mental health outcomes. *International Journal of Environmental Research and Public Health* 16(7):1174.

Nakagawa, I., K. Nakamura, M. Oyama, O. Yamazaki, K. Ishigami, Y. Tsuchiya, and M. Yamamoto. 2009. Long-term effects of the Niigata-Chuetsu earthquake in Japan on acute myocardial infarction mortality: An analysis of death certificate data. *Heart* 95(24):2009–2013.

NAME (National Association of Medical Examiners). 2002. *A guide for manner of death classification, 1st ed.* https://name.memberclicks.net/assets/docs/4bd6187f-d329-4948-84dd-3d6fe6b48f4d.pdf (accessed August 1, 2020).

NASEM (National Academies of Sciences, Engineering, and Medicine). 2019. *Building and measuring community resilience: Actions for communities and the Gulf Research Program*. Washington, DC: The National Academies Press. https://doi.org/10.17226/25383.

NCHS (National Center for Health Statistics). 2017. *A reference guide for certification of deaths in the event of a natural, human-induced, or chemical/radiological disaster.* Hyattsville, MD: National Center for Health Statistics. https://www.cdc.gov/nchs/data/nvss/vsrg/vsrg01.pdf (accessed June 26, 2020).

Noe, R. 2018. Applications: Disaster-related mortality surveillance: Challenges and considerations for local and state health departments. In J. A. Horney (ed.), *Disaster epidemiology: Methods and applications*. London: Academic Press. Pp. 55–63.

Norris, F. H., M. J. Friedman, P. J. Watson, C. M. Byrne, E. Diaz, and K. Kaniasty. 2002. 60,000 disaster victims speak: Part I. An empirical review of the empirical literature, 1981–2001. *Psychiatry* 65(3):207–239.

Peters, M. N., J. C. Moscona, M. J. Katz, K. B. Deandrade, H. C. Quevedo, S. Tiwari, A. R. Burchett, T. A. Turnage, K. Y. Singh, E. N. Fomunung, S. Srivastav, P. Delafontaine, and A. M. Irimpen. 2014. Natural disasters and myocardial infarction: The six years after Hurricane Katrina. *Mayo Clinic Proceedings* 89(4):472–477.

Purnell, N., and F. Solomon. 2020. Coronavirus doesn't have to be so deadly. Just look at Hong Kong and Singapore. *The Wall Street Journal.* https://www.wsj.com/articles/coronavirus-doesnt-have-to-be-so-deadly-just-look-at-hong-kong-and-singapore-11590491418 (accessed October 28, 2020).

RxOpen. 2020. *Facilities map.* http://rxopen.org (accessed June 26, 2020).

Santos-Burgoa, C., J. Sandberg, E. Suárez, A. Goldman-Hawes, S. Zeger, A. Garcia-Meza, C. M. Pérez, N. Estrada-Merly, U. Cólon-Ramos, C. M. Nazario, E. Andrade, A. Roess, and L. Goldman. 2018. Differential and persistent risk of excess mortality from Hurricane Maria in Puerto Rico: A time-series analysis. *Lancet Planet Health* 2(11):e478–e488.

Schnall, A. H., A. F. Wolkin, R. Noe, L. B. Hausman, P. Wiersma, K. Soetebier, S. T. Cookson. 2011. Evaluation of a standardized morbidity surveillance form for use during disasters caused by natural hazards. *Prehospital and Disaster Medicine* 26(2):90–98.

Schnall, A., R. Law, A. Heinzerling, K. Sircar, S. Damon, F. Yip, J. Schier, T. Bayleyegn, and A. Wolkin. 2017. Characterization of carbon monoxide exposure during Hurricane Sandy and subsequent nor'easter. *Disaster Medicine and Public Health Preparedness* 11(5):562–567.

State of Michigan. 2020. *Michigan awarded two federal grants to strengthen behavioral health services during COVID-19 crisis.* https://www.michigan.gov/coronavirus/0,9753,7-406-98158-526521--,00.html (accessed June 26, 2020).

Stephens, K. U., Sr., D. Grew, K. Chin, P. Kadetz, P. G. Greenough, F. M. Burkle, Jr., S. L. Robinson, and E. R. Franklin. 2007. Excess mortality in the aftermath of Hurricane Katrina: A preliminary report. *Disaster Medicine and Public Health Preparedness* 1(1):15–20.

Swerdel, J. N., T. M. Janevic, N. M. Cosgrove, J. B. Kostis, and the Myocardial Infarction Data Acquisition System Study Group. 2014. The effect of Hurricane Sandy on cardiovascular events in New Jersey. *Journal of the American Heart Association* 3(6):e001354.

Thomas-Henkel, C., and M. Schulman. 2017. *Screening for social determinants of health in populations with complex needs: Implementation considerations*. Center for Health Care Strategies, Inc. https://www.chcs.org/media/SDOH-Complex-Care-Screening-Brief-102617.pdf (accessed September 1, 2020).

Tzvetkova, S. 2017. Not all deaths are equal: How many deaths make a natural disaster newsworthy? *Our World in Data*, July 19. https://ourworldindata.org/how-many-deaths-make-a-natural-disaster-newsworthy (accessed June 28, 2020).

Valderas, J., B. Starfield, B. Sibbald, C. Salisbury, and M. Roland. 2009. Defining comorbidity: Implications for understanding health and health services. *Annals of Family Medicine* 7(4):357–363. https://www.ncbi.nlm.nih.gov/pmc/articles/PMC2713155/pdf/0060357.pdf (accessed September 1, 2020).

Washoe County Regional Medical Examiner's Office. 2020. *What is the difference between manner and cause of death?* https://www.washoecounty.us/coroner/faq/difference_cause_and_manner_of_death.php (accessed August 1, 2020).

Watson, J., M. Gayer, and M. Connolly. 2007. Epidemics after natural disasters. *Emerging Infectious Diseases* 13(1):1–5. doi: 10.3201/eid1301.060779.

Wolkin, A., J. R. Patterson, S. Harris, E. Soler, S. Burrer, M. McGeehin, and S. Greene. 2015. Reducing public health risk during disasters: Identifying social vulnerabilities. *Journal of Homeland Security and Emergency Management* 12(4):809–822.

3

Operational Considerations for Individual Counts of Mortality and Morbidity

Disaster-related mortality and morbidity can be measured using two primary approaches—individual counts and population estimates—both of which contribute to the comprehensive assessment of a disaster's impact. This chapter discusses the many operational considerations related to individual counts in order to explore how these data can be collected and used in disaster management. Discussions of analytical approaches for conducting population estimates of disaster-related mortality and morbidity can be found in Chapter 4. This chapter begins by exploring the heterogeneity in death investigation and registration systems and how this, among other factors, affects the collection, reporting, and recording of individual mortality count data. The latter part of the chapter focuses on the current practices, tools, and systems for using individual mortality data and identifies potential best practices and opportunities for bringing these practices to scale. Because of the differences between disaster-related mortality and morbidity data for individual counts, the chapter handles these issues separately. Box 3-1 provides a brief overview of how mortality and morbidity can be attributed when there have been individual counts of mortality and morbidity as described in the framework in the prior chapter. Several examples of the assessment of coronavirus disease 2019 (COVID-19)-related mortality and morbidity are included in this chapter to highlight overlapping administrative and logistical challenges that persist regardless of disaster type.

The individual counting approach to estimating total reported mortality and morbidity is reliant on the capture of all relevant cases and the appropriate attribution and recording of each case. This process of capturing

BOX 3-1
Attribution of Mortality and Morbidity in Individual Counts: Overview of Proposed Framework

As described in detail in Chapter 2 (see Table 2-1), disaster-related mortality and morbidity can be estimated using two main approaches: individual counts or population estimates. Each approach offers an estimation of the disaster's impact, and each has unique benefits, uses, and shortcomings. The committee proposed a framework that balances the benefits and uses of each approach and conceptualized how causalities can be attributed when using individual counting methods.

In the framework, the committee describes three categories to describe the degree of attribution of a reported death or morbidity to a disaster—direct, indirect, and partially attributable. Direct mortality and morbidity are those reported cases that can be directly attributable to the forces of the disaster. An indirect mortality or morbidity is not due to the immediate forces of the disaster but is associated with unsafe or unhealthy conditions around the time of the disaster—including while preparing for and responding to the disaster and during recovery from the disaster. This includes deaths that would not have occurred *but for* the disaster. These two categories generally align with the Center for Disease Control and Prevention's definitions for direct and indirect disaster-related deaths, and many deaths—in particular direct deaths—are subject to certification by a medical examiner or coroner. However, the committee's framework differs in that it provides a third category of partially attributable morality or morbidity, which cannot be definitively tied to the disaster but where the disaster more likely than not has played an important role in that outcome.

and recording data on reported mortalities and morbidities involves a multitude of factors at the state or local level—policies and case definitions for individual attribution; the availability of evidence and guidance to support decision making, the structure of the state or local medicolegal death investigation system, the process of death registration, and the training and professional judgment of medical examiners, coroners, and other medical certifiers to perform this work accurately and consistently. No standard practices, policies, or systems exist for recording these data. Additionally, the range of known and unknown morbidities and their complex associations with the disaster exposure are vast, and the process of assessing morbidity is challenged further by a lack of understanding of how chronic conditions and their sequelae can be attributed directly or to some other degree in the context of a disaster. The additional consideration of how to capture indirect and partially attributable deaths adds further complexity. These categories of individual deaths are not likely to be referred to the medical examiner or coroner and are more likely to be recorded by other medical certifiers in clinical or residential settings, such as a hospital or nursing home, where evidence to connect the death to a disaster may not be considered or may be unavailable.

Additionally, as described in Chapter 2, there are other issues related to inequity and vulnerability, which further complicate the collection and use of reported mortality and morbidity data at an individual level. For example, not all individuals with a disaster-related morbidity will present themselves to health care providers, as the ability to access care is tied to broader social and environmental contexts. Likewise, these same underlying factors simultaneously heighten an individual's risk of harm (e.g., pollution exposure or overcrowded housing) (McKibben, 2020). These associations complicate the collection of complete mortality and morbidity data and limit their actionability. Although this report will not discuss the integration and use of social determinants of health data into mortality and morbidity data to enhance their actionability for use in disaster management, Appendix D provides two high-level case studies, which examine how social determinants of health relate to mortality and mortality during and following disasters.

THE INVESTIGATION AND REGISTRATION OF DEATHS IN THE UNITED STATES

In the United States, individual mortality data are collected through a process that spans multiple medical, legal, and administrative systems: the nationwide network of state, local, tribal, and territorial (SLTT) medicolegal death investigation systems combined with state- and federal-level death registration systems. Understanding the challenges related to estimating disaster-related mortality using individual counting approaches requires an understanding of the process of registering a death. This begins when the certification of a death is performed by a medical certifier. The next step is for the death to be recorded in state and national death registration systems, which allows for state and federal mortality data to be compiled, analyzed, and disseminated. This section provides an overview of how these systems function and communicate to generate the individual-level mortality data used for estimating total reported mortality. Examining the function of these systems is essential to understanding the structural and administrative barriers that hinder the process of developing accurate individual counts.

Medicolegal Death Investigation Systems

The medicolegal death investigation system is responsible for investigating deaths and certifying the cause and manner of death for unnatural or unexplained deaths. This includes deaths due to homicide, suicide, unintentional injuries, and drug overdoses, among others. Those deaths processed via the medicolegal death investigation system account for 20 percent of all deaths (IOM, 2003). The medicolegal death investigation system has critical importance beyond the legal system and represents a great value to public health and research. Data collected in the system can be used to inform epidemiological investigations, disease and injury prevention programs, and preparedness and response practices and planning. In the United States the medicolegal death investigation system consists of a patchwork of different types of systems at the state and local levels for investigating these deaths. No federal or standardized medicolegal death investigation system is in use across all states and territories. The United States has about 2,400 medical examiner and coroner (ME/C) jurisdictions nationwide (NSTC, 2016) (see descriptions of these professions below). Medicolegal death investigation systems may be centralized at the state level or decentralized at the county or district level and may involve a coroner system, a medical examiner system, or a combination of both (CDC, 2015) (see Figure 3-1). For instance, the state of Florida has a decentralized medical examiner system, where county medical examiners are responsible for reporting data to the state commission, which is responsible for setting policy. This is different from states such as Maryland, Rhode Island, and Virginia, which have statewide systems that report to the state's chief medical examiner, who is responsible for policy setting. In Texas, the structure of the medicolegal system varies by county; some counties are served by the medical examiner's office, while others assign coroner duties to a justice of the peace or sheriff.

Within this diverse patchwork of medicolegal death investigation systems, death investigations are performed by ME/Cs, who have vastly different levels of professional training and requirements for education and professional experiences, as set by state code. These qualifications vary from being a registered voter with a high school diploma and free of a felony conviction in some coroner systems to being a forensic pathologist with 4–6 years of postgraduate medical training and specialty board certification working in medical examiner systems as autopsy physicians and public health officers. Medical examiners are required to have a doctorate of medicine, and they have varying professional requirements, with some states requiring more specialized certifications than others. Medical examiners are typically pathologists or forensic pathologists or simply physicians of any medical specialty who serve at a county, district, or state level. Unlike medical examiners, coroners are elected or appointed into office and serve an individual county or locality. Coroners generally do not have a medical background, although they may receive some training in certain jurisdictions (IOM, 2003). Despite the essential skills and expertise that medical examiners bring to the medicolegal death investigation system, the number of professionals in the field is in decline and funding remains insufficient (IOM, 2003; NSTC, 2016).

Many studies have recommended the conversion of coroner-based systems to medical examiner systems where deaths are investigated by medical death investigators, autopsies are performed by forensic pathologists, and deaths are certified by physician medical examiners with expertise in

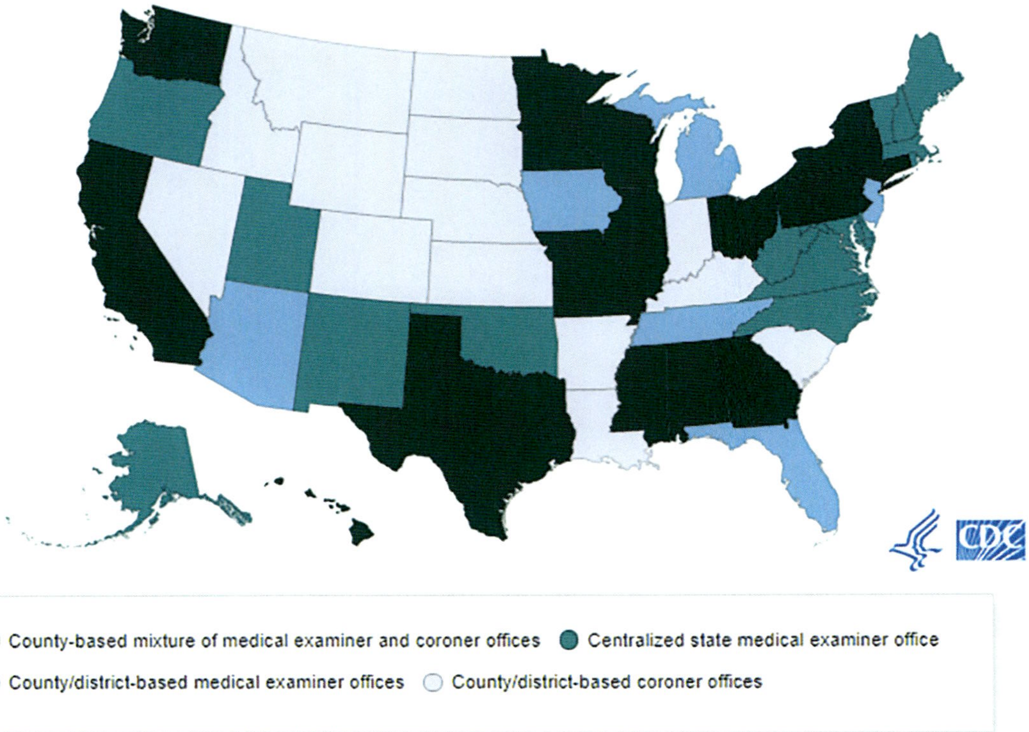

FIGURE 3-1 Variation in types of death investigation systems in the United States.
SOURCE: CDC, 2015.

identifying and documenting causes of death (IOM, 2003).[1] A 2009 report by the National Research Council, *Strengthening Forensic Science in the United States: A Path Forward*, recommended that Congress should authorize and appropriate incentive funds to establish regional medical examiner offices. Such a program would bring baseline standards for expertise and uniformity in the certification and coding of deaths, professional excellence in determining the causes of death, and economies of scale in staffing, facilities, electronic case management systems, and supplies.

Other Medical Certifiers

The medical certifier is responsible for determining the cause and manner of death, making an assessment of whether a death is related to a disaster, and recording primary data on the death. The type of medical certifier responsible in a particular situation depends on the circumstances of the death (see Box 3-2) and can be not only a medical examiner or coroner, but also another medical certifier such as a justice of the peace, sheriff, sheriff-coroner, hospital physician, pathologist, nurse practitioner, or other licensed health professional or responsible party depending on the state (Ruiz et al., 2018). In order to accurately collect data on individual-level deaths, death certifiers need to be supported with appropriate training, standards, and functional systems for recording the death within state and federal vital statistics systems (see later section on Training).

BOX 3-2
Medical Certifiers of Death in the United States

Certain classes of deaths are typically investigated by medical examiners or coroners prior to being recorded by vital statistics offices. These include

1. sudden unexpected deaths in adults and children;
2. unattended deaths, such as deaths that occur outside a health care system;
3. unnatural deaths, including accidental deaths, homicides, or suicides; and
4. deaths in custody.

Natural deaths, however, may be certified by physicians, nurse practitioners, physician assistants, pathologists, or registered hospice nurses, as allowed by state regulations.

---

[1] A cause of death is the specific illness or injury that led to death. The manner of death is *how* that injury or illness led to the death. Natural deaths have internal physiological causes; the term "unnatural death" is often used by medical examiners and coroners to categorize a death that did not occur due to natural causes (Snohomish County, 2020).

Death Registration Systems in the United States

After a death is certified by a ME/C or other medical certifier, it must be registered at the state-level vital records office, creating a death record. It is at this point that the medicolegal death investigation systems and the death registration systems meet. The state-level death registration system takes in data entered from multiple sources at the local and county levels, such as information from the case management systems used by ME/Cs and information from other medical certifiers and funeral homes, in order to create death records in state-based electronic death registration systems (EDRSs). ME/C case management systems, which collect and store data for ME/Cs and are separate from the state EDRS, receive information from death scene investigations, toxicology reports, and autopsy reports. Physicians and other medical certifiers of death input data directly into the state-based EDRS, while funeral home systems provide the EDRS with demographic information on deaths.

The state-level death registration system in turn shares death record information with the National Center for Health Statistics (NCHS) through the National Vital Statistics System (NVSS). NVSS compiles national statistics on disaster-related mortality from information provided on death records; if the medical certifier has not recorded a disaster name and coded the death as disaster-related, then the death may not be reported as such (Horney, 2017; NVSS, 2017) (see Box 3-3). Therefore, the state and federal vital statistics offices play critical roles in the collection, recording, and

BOX 3-3
Entry and Coding of Disaster-Related Death Information

In order for the National Vital Statistics System to code a death as associated with a disaster, the death record data entered by the medical examiner and coroner (in the case of unnatural or unexplained deaths) or by medical certifiers (in the case of natural deaths) must include descriptive information specific to the disaster. Under the current format of the death record, this could mean terms related to specific disasters, such as Hurricane Maria 2017, Camp Fire 2018, COVID-19 pandemic 2020, tornado, or flood. The inclusion of these descriptive details within the cause of death allows for these individuals' deaths to be assigned a disaster-related *International Classification of Diseases, Tenth Revision* code by the National Center for Health Statistics. Failure by the medical certifier to include these terms when a death is related to a known or suspected degree to a disaster prevents the coding of the death as disaster related and that death will not be reflected in federal or state counts of individual disaster deaths.

SOURCE: Horney, 2017.

reporting of mortality data and are foundational to the accurate and timely assessment of individual mortality counts following large-scale disasters.

Ideally, this interactive network of independent ME/C, state, and national electronic mortality data systems would be interoperable and would facilitate rapid data sharing (see Figure 3-2). However, not all ME/C jurisdictions are equipped with electronic case management systems, nor have all states transitioned to fully electronic death registration systems (e.g., American Samoa, Connecticut, Guam, North Carolina, Northern Mariana Islands, Rhode Island, Virgin Islands, and West Virginia have not) (NAPHSIS, 2020a). Additionally, because ME/C case management systems are not interoperable with state EDRSs, ME/Cs have to preform duplicate data entry in each system, which creates an administrative burden on already overworked professionals. In a crisis, this time burden is even more of an issue and could affect data quality if ME/Cs do not enter sufficient descriptive data about deaths into the EDRS. Furthermore, the way in which these systems output disaster information varies widely, from basic line list to electronic transfer. The development of a national network of ME/C case management systems, which would require investment by the Centers for Disease Control and Prevention (CDC) and states, would address the chronic issues related to poor interoperability and minimum standards for data quality and collection. Such a network could feature electronic and interoperable systems between ME/C case management, state EDRS, and NVSS; standard coding practices for disaster-related deaths; and mechanisms for rapidly sharing data with communities to facilitate recovery and promote preparedness for future disasters.

Data Sharing Within and Between States and Territories

The ability to share mortality data across stakeholders within a state or locality is critical for the inclusion of these data in the public health response to and surveillance of a disaster. However, sharing data is not always simple, and barriers to sharing data have been noted within localities with decentralized medical examiner or coroner systems, where the vital records office functions separately from the public health department, or where plans are not in place to provide alternative methods of data sharing (e.g., daily mortality reports or access to preliminary death record data) (Horney, 2017). Some mechanisms do currently exist to facilitate data sharing across states and territories. The State and Territorial Exchange of Vital Events system, operated by the National Association for Public Health Statistics and Information Systems, provides a platform for secure inter-jurisdictional exchange of mortality data between state-level electronic death registration systems and the national system (NAPHSIS, 2020b).

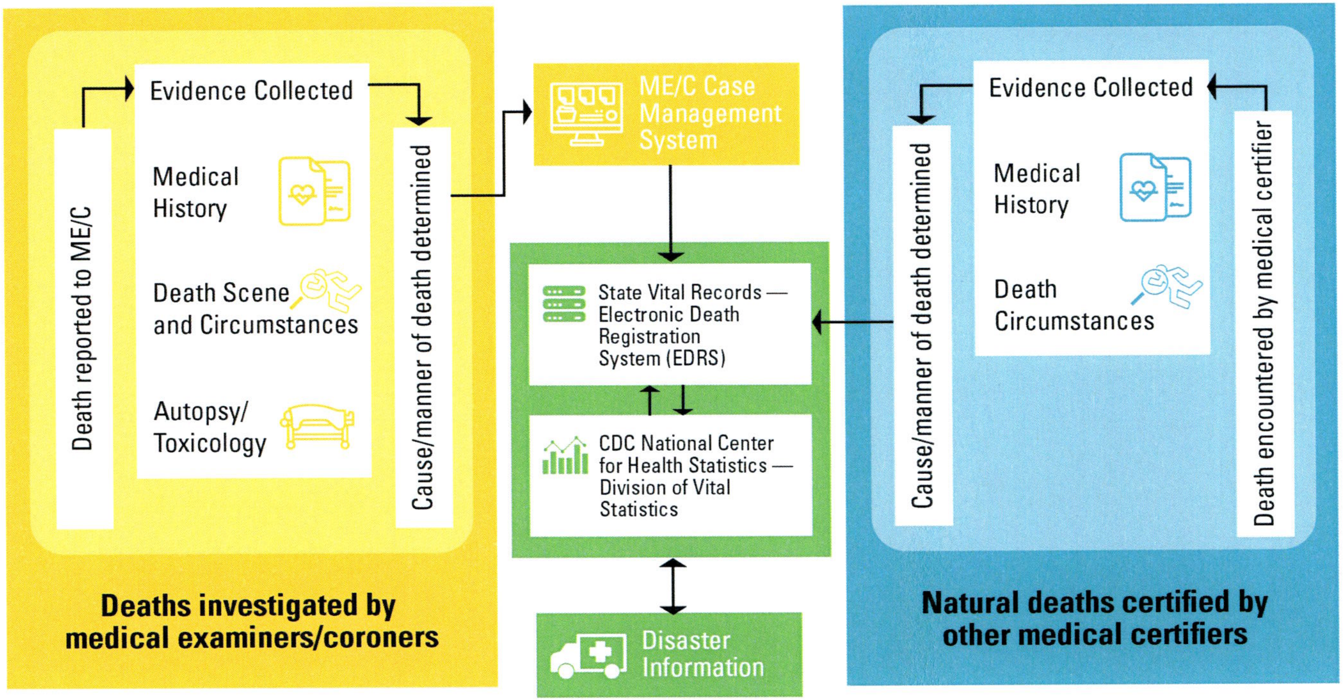

FIGURE 3-2 Simplified ideal process of certifying and registering a death in the United States.
NOTE: CDC = Centers for Disease Control and Prevention; ME/C = medical examiner and coroner.
SOURCE: Adapted from FEMA, 2019.

Death Certificates Versus Death Records

In the age of paper-based reporting, the death certificate was considered to be the primary source of individual-level mortality data. However, with the advent of electronic death registration systems, the information collected in the death registration system, which is called the death record, is actually the primary source of individual mortality data. A portion of this death record is used to create the death certificate, which is used for legal purposes, and the other portion is a statistical record containing detailed medical and demographic data. The death record is sent to the federal level for automated medical coding and editing by NVSS for the creation of statistical files for state and federal use. NCHS does issue a national standard death certificate that complies with the *International Classification of Diseases, Tenth Revision* (ICD-10) standards to facilitate uniform data collection and reporting for statistical analysis. States are required to collect standard vital statistics data that are captured in the death record, and states may and do add additional data items for their own registration or statistical needs, such as opioid overdoses, maternal mortality, and smoking. The death record of the EDRS is now the source of the state death certificate and the statistical information used in mortality attribution at the local, state, and federal levels.

CHALLENGES WITH UNIFORM ATTRIBUTION ACROSS THESE SYSTEMS

Today, SLTT medicolegal systems and the state and federal death registration systems function in conjunction with one another, but originally these systems developed independently due to their historically different purposes. Death investigation systems and vital statistics registration systems in the United States evolved as state-level functions. Understanding the impact of the heterogeneity of medicolegal death investigation and death registration systems and the many different stakeholder roles is foundational to understanding the challenges related to operationalizing the collection, reporting, and recording of disaster-related mortality data. The structural consequences of this heterogeneity include poor interoperability and coordination among systems and stakeholders, variability in SLTT practices for attributing and collecting data on a death, and issues related to the completion of the death record in the state EDRSs. These major challenges contribute cumulatively to the under-reporting of disaster-related deaths and dramatic differences between states that would experience similar events.

Poor Interoperability and Coordination Among Systems and Stakeholders

Poor interoperability and limited coordination among systems and stakeholders present major challenges to the uniform attribution of disaster-related mortality across the nation. Medicolegal death investigation systems and vital statistics systems were not designed to capture information in a way that facilitates interoperability and data sharing within and across the SLTT and federal levels (Borfitz, 2019; Hanzlick, 2006; Noe, 2018). Furthermore, medical certifiers of death and those responsible for recording deaths have siloed professional roles and work within siloed systems despite multiple efforts to address these issues (ASPE, 2013).

Variability in SLTT Practices for Attributing and Recording Data on a Death

There exists no national uniform practice for attributing and recording disaster-related deaths, and substantial differences persist across SLTT practices for attributing and collecting data on a death. Variations in state and local practices on attributing and recording direct and indirect disaster-related deaths—particularly for natural deaths that are not sent to the ME/C for review—affect the collection of descriptive data on the death record. Table 3-1 illustrates the variation in disaster-related deaths attributed to four natural disasters across different state and federal entities and non-governmental organizations between 2008 and 2013. Table 3-2 illustrates the extent of definitional variation in assessment practices for COVID-19 deaths across states and jurisdictions, which demonstrates the potential for variation in reported mortalities from state to state.

For example, there are policy differences at the administrative level regarding what counts as a disaster-related death. In some jurisdictions the death investigations systems have applied CDC's uniform case definitions for direct and indirect disaster-related deaths, but many systems use different case definitions of varying stringency and specificity. Many jurisdictions do not count indirect deaths at all, and almost none purposefully count deaths that are partially attributable to a disaster, per the framework proposed by the committee in Chapter 2. ME/C systems typically have clearly defined legal requirements for which cases are reported as being disaster-related; however, inconsistencies among different states' requirements affect the accuracy of national-level reporting. A literature review of medicolegal death scene investigations after natural disaster- and weather-related events found no consistent approach for attributing deaths to a disaster and significant variation in how death scene data collection tools were being used (Rocha et al., 2017).

TABLE 3-1 Variations in Reported Number of Deaths After Large-Scale Disaster Events

Disaster Event	State Response Agencies	Red Cross	FEMA	NOAA–NWS	Vital Statistics
Hurricane Ike, TX (2008)	74	38	104	20	4
April 27 tornado, GA (2011)	15	15	9	15	6
Hurricane Sandy, NJ (2012)	75	34	61	12	24
May tornadoes, OK (2013)	48	42	19	30	36

NOTE: FEMA = Federal Emergency Management Agency; NOAA–NWS = National Oceanic and Atmospheric Administration–National Weather Service; State response agencies = medical examiners and coroners and emergency operations centers; Vital Statistics = post-disaster review of death certificates in state-based vital statistics systems.
SOURCE: Noe, 2019.

TABLE 3-2 Variations in Assessment Practices for COVID-19-Related Deaths by Jurisdiction, June 2020

State/Jurisdiction	Criteria for Including Death as Attributable to COVID-19
Centers for Disease Control and Prevention	• If COVID-19 played a role in the death, this condition should be specified on the death certificate. In many cases, it is likely that it will be the underlying cause of death, as it can lead to various life-threatening conditions, such as pneumonia and acute respiratory distress syndrome. In these cases, COVID-19 should be reported on the lowest line used in Part I with the other conditions to which it gave rise listed on the lines above it. • In some cases, survival from COVID-19 can be complicated by pre-existing chronic conditions, especially those that result in diminished lung capacity, such as chronic obstructive pulmonary disease or asthma. These medical conditions do not cause COVID-19 but can increase the risk of contracting a respiratory infection and death, so these conditions should be reported in Part II and not in Part I. • In cases where a definite diagnosis of COVID-19 cannot be made, but it is suspected or likely (e.g., the circumstances are compelling within a reasonable degree of certainty), it is acceptable to report COVID-19 on a death certificate as "probable" or "presumed." In these instances, certifiers should use their best clinical judgment in determining if a COVID-19 infection was likely.
Colorado	• A death may be attributed to COVID-19 in the absence of testing if the decedent showed symptoms and was in close contact with an infected person.
Iowa	• Coronavirus disease 2019 or COVID-19 should be reported on the death certificate for all decedents where the disease caused or is assumed to have caused or contributed to death. All deaths suspected or confirmed of COVID-19 must be reported to the medical examiner. Once details of the case are reviewed, the medical examiner will determine if an investigation will be started or jurisdiction declined. • All positive test results for COVID-19 must be documented on the cause of death. If COVID-19 is confirmed by a positive test, the underlying cause of death should be COVID-19. If COVID-19 is diagnosed clinically but testing was not performed or results were not obtained, Probable or Presumed COVID-19 should be the underlying cause of death. • Laboratory test results are not typically reported on death certificates; however, it is imperative that all information be documented for deaths when the COVID-19 is suspected. o The following terminology should be used to describe the status of the COVID-19 testing. ▪ COVID-19 testing is PENDING ▪ COVID-19 is Suspected—testing was REJECTED ▪ COVID-19 is Suspected—testing was NOT POSSIBLE ▪ COVID-19 NOT SUSPECTED

continued

TABLE 3-2 Continued

State/Jurisdiction	Criteria for Including Death as Attributable to COVID-19
Montana	• Coronavirus disease 2019 or COVID-19 should be reported on the death certificate for all decedents where the disease caused or is assumed to have caused or contributed to death. When a death is due to COVID-19, it is likely the underlying cause of death and thus it should be reported on the lowest line used in Part I of the death certificate. Ideally, testing for COVID-19 should be conducted, but it is acceptable to report COVID-19 on a death certificate without this confirmation if the circumstances are compelling within a reasonable degree of certainty. • Montana's Department of Public Health and Human Services website provides sample death cases as examples of whether and how to certify a death as attributable to COVID-19.
Connecticut, Delaware, Ohio	• Deaths of people who were presumed infected but were not tested are reported as attributed to COVID-19.
Pennsylvania	• Deaths attributed to COVID-19 that have been confirmed through laboratory testing should be reported as "COVID-19" in the lowest line reported under Cause of Death—Part I. • If COVID-19 laboratory samples are pending at the time of reporting the death, enter the underlying cause as "pending COVID-19 testing." • COVID-19 should be reported for all decedents where COVID-19 caused or is assumed to have caused or contributed to death.

SOURCES: Brown et al., 2020; CDC, 2020c; Iowa Board of Medicine, 2020; Montana DPHHS, 2020; Pennsylvania Department of Health, 2020.

Differences between New York City and Texas illustrate how variation in city- and state-level vital statistics systems affects mortality reporting. Both New York City and Texas have mandated electronic death registration systems. In New York City—one of only two U.S. cities to have an independent vital records jurisdiction—medical certifiers must start a death record within 24 hours of death, and the funeral home must complete the record (note that funeral directors do not play a role in determining cause of death and contributing factors) and register the death within 72 hours. The city's centralized medical examiner office and rapid timeline for death registration are conducive to using death records for real-time mortality surveillance. In Texas, the death record must be registered within 10 days of death; the record is initiated by the funeral home, and then the designated medical certifier—depending on the county in question, this individual could be a coroner with little or no medical training—has 5 days to complete the medical portion of the death record.

Challenges Specific to the Completion of the Death Record

A host of challenges in capturing accurate individual-level mortality data relate specifically to issues concerning the completion of death records by ME/Cs and other medical certifiers and contribute to the under-reporting of disaster-related deaths in state and national databases. The consistency and quality of data captured on a death record are contingent on the consistency and quality of the data source. A lack of quality data limits the ability to assess individual mortality counts and, by extension, population estimates of mortality because state- and national-level mortality statistics are based solely on the information reported on the death record (NVSS, 2017).

Death Record Format

If the data entered into a death record by the certifier do not include the appropriate disaster-related terms (see Box 3-3), then NCHS cannot assign an ICD-10 code that attributes a death to a disaster.[2] Prior research has noted that the quality of basic data recorded on death certificates is poor overall (Noe, 2018; NVSS, 2017) and that many death records in state EDRSs do not include clear, precisely defined terms for attributing a death directly or indirectly to a disaster.[3] This can make it difficult for a medical certifier to record whether a disaster contributed to the death and to what degree. Evaluation studies have found that disaster-related deaths were under-reported on death certificates because they did not include key disaster terms to attribute a death as being related to a specific event (Issa et al., 2019; Kulkarni et al., 2015). Properly completing a death certificate is challenging for multiple reasons (Madsen and Begier, 2013), which are intensified in a disaster context (Madsen and Begier, 2013), and most death registration systems currently used across the country do not offer or require simple, precisely defined options for coding a death as directly, indirectly, or partially attributable to a specific disaster. See Figure 3-3 for a current example of the cause and manner of death entry fields in the District of Columbia EDRS.

---

[2] "Brief History of Centers for Disease Control and Prevention Disaster-Related Mortality Activities." Paper provided to the committee at the August 29, 2019, workshop in Washington, DC. Available by request from the Public Access Records Office by emailing PARO@nas.edu.

[3] *Ibid.*

CAUSE OF DEATH

Actions

Part I. Enter the diseases, injuries, or complications that caused the death. Do not enter the mode of dying, such as cardiac or respiratory arrest, shock, or heart failure. List only one cause on each line.

Immediate Cause
(Final disease or condition resulting in death)

Approximate Interval Between Onset and Death

A.

Due to (or as a consequence of)

Sequentially list conditions, if any, leading to immediate cause. Enter Underlying Cause (Disease or injury that initiated events resulting in death) last.

B.

Due to (or as a consequence of)

C.

Due to (or as a consequence of)

D.

Due to (or as a consequence of)

Part II. Other significant conditions contributing to death but not resulting in the underlying cause given in Part I.

(max 240 characters)

Manner of Death

Was an autopsy performed? ○ Yes ○ No ○ Unknown

Were the results of autopsy available to complete the cause of death?

○ Yes ○ No ○ Unknown

Manner of death

Did tobacco use contribue to death?

FIGURE 3-3 Example of content from the EDRS data entry screen for cause and manner of death from the District of Columbia Vital Records Division.
SOURCE: Personal communication, R. Anderson, NCHS, June 11, 2020.

Inadequate Training for Certifiers

In many cases, medical certifiers, such as medical personnel who typically treat living patients, are inadequately trained in determining the cause of death in ordinary circumstances (Madsen and Begier, 2013); the burden on inadequately trained certifiers is further intensified during a disaster context. Studies have found errors in attributing the cause or manner of death on about one-third of death records, largely due to physician inexperience and a lack of training in death registration (Brooks and Reed, 2015). As mentioned previously, no minimum professional qualification exists for medical certifiers, and many are unfamiliar with CDC's uniform disaster mortality case definitions. Due to the lack of training and vastly different levels of professional qualification (Brooks and Reed, 2015), death certifiers may underappreciate the importance of including the disaster details or terms on death. Even if a death record entered into an EDRS does offer an option for disaster attribution, certifiers are generally not provided with clear case definitions or decision-making tools for distinguishing between directly and indirectly related deaths. Furthermore, ME/Cs may not have sufficient information from the death scene to attribute a death to the disaster (Bryant, 2003), and medical certifiers outside the medicolegal system frequently do not have access to descriptive health and personal data about the decedent that could be used to inform their completion of the death record. In many cases of "natural" death, the physician in the hospital is often asked to complete the death certificate without any knowledge or training in reporting disaster-related fatalities.

Philosophical Differences Among Certifiers

The diversity in medicolegal death investigation systems and the variability in what "counts" as a disaster-related death at a state and local level create an environment conducive to significant philosophical differences across the ME/C profession as to how to attribute the cause and manner of death. While most professionals agree that direct exposure to disaster-related environmental forces can contribute directly to morbidity and mortality, there is less consensus about how to codify the impact of indirect exposures on adverse health outcomes (Combs et al., 1999). For instance, some ME/Cs do not believe that certain types of deaths—such as natural deaths due to exacerbation of a chronic condition—should be attributed to a disaster.[4] A study carried out at the annual meeting of the National Association of Medical Examiners (NAME) asked attendees to determine the relative contribution of a disaster to several deaths that had already been attributed by other medical examiners. Agreement with the previous

---

[4] *Ibid.*

attributions among the attendees ranged from 27 to 100 percent, with agreement less likely for cases of natural death or deaths due to indirect exposures linked to the disaster (Combs et al., 1999). The standardization of practices for attributing mortality and consensus of opinion among medical certifiers will address much of the variability in the completion of death records following disasters. The burden for adopting this improvement does not fall only on ME/Cs and other medical certifiers, but also on state registrars (Slavova et al., 2015), NCHS, and public health agencies that value access to robust disaster-related mortality data.

Conclusion 3-1: The heterogeneity of the nation's systems of death investigation and registration prevents the accurate recording and reporting of disaster-related mortality data and impedes the meaningful analysis and use of these data to improve disaster management. Adoption of uniform practices for collecting, recording, and reporting mortality data is needed, as is improved vertical coordination across stakeholders and improved interoperability of electronic systems among medical certifiers, state vital records offices, and the national vital statistics system.

Conclusion 3-2: The collection and recording of disaster-related mortality data require the medicolegal workforce to value the need for these data and to have the capacity and capability to adopt standardized definitions, practices, and systems.

Federal Efforts to Improve the Quality of Mortality Data

Attempts have been made at a federal level to improve the quality of data collection and reporting and to evaluate the impact of these changes and investments on data quality. In 1986, CDC established the Medical Examiner and Coroner Information Sharing Program (MECISP) in order to improve the quality of death investigations nationwide through the standardization of policies and practices to facilitate communication among stakeholders, and to promote the sharing and use of death investigation data collected by ME/C offices (see Box 3-4).[5] Since 1999, CDC has used the uniform disaster mortality case definitions that were developed by MECISP to categorize direct and indirect disaster-related deaths in a standardized manner (see Box 2-2 in Chapter 2) (Combs et al., 1999). The use of uniform case definitions and the inclusion of terms for the role of a disaster on death certificates would support certifiers in providing accurate information needed to improve state- and federal-level mortality statistics

[5] *Ibid.*

BOX 3-4
Medical Examiner and Coroner Information Sharing Program

The Medical Examiner and Coroner Information Sharing Program (MECISP) was a program administered by the Centers for Disease Control and Prevention with the primary goals of (1) improving the quality of death investigations in the United States and promoting more standardized practices concerning when and how to conduct these investigations; (2) facilitating communication among death investigators, the public health community, federal agencies, and other interested groups; (3) improving the quality, completeness, management, and dissemination of information regarding investigated deaths; and (4) promoting the sharing and use of medical examiner and coroner (ME/C) death investigation data.

Major MECISP projects included the periodic production of a directory of death investigators in the United States and Canada, creation of standard and generic death investigation report forms, development of death investigation datasets, and collection of death investigation data from ME/C offices. MECISP also conducted site visits to assist in office computerization, supported educational meetings and the development of training materials for death investigators, facilitated ongoing projects being carried out by relevant professional organizations, contributed publications to the death investigation literature, conducted surveillance of selected types of deaths, and responded to specific inquiries from medical examiners and coroners about administrative and practical death investigation issues.

SOURCE: Hanzlick, 1997.

(Noe, 2018). However, the adoption of CDC's uniform case definitions by SLTT death investigation systems remains limited.[6]

CDC engaged with the ME/C and vital statistics community and found that many are not aware of the case definitions and do not use them in their practice.[7] To address this gap, CDC's National Center for Environmental Health and NCHS released the *Reference Guide for Certification of Deaths in the Event of a Natural, Human-Induced, or Chemical/Radiological Disaster* (CDC, 2020b) in 2017. It provides guidance on the uniform case definitions and a step-by-step guide for attributing the cause of death and recording that information on the death certificate. CDC's Disaster-Related Death Scene Investigation Toolkit (CDC, 2017) was also released in 2017 to help improve the quality of data collection at a death scene. In death scene investigations, ME/Cs or other death scene investigators gather information on how and why a death occurred. Death certifiers—which

[6] *Ibid.*
[7] *Ibid.*

may be ME/Cs, justices of the peace, or other responsible parties—use that information to determine the cause and manner of death and judge whether the death was related to a disaster. Standardizing the practices for collecting information during death scene investigations could provide death certifiers with more accurate information for determining a death's disaster-relatedness and accurately reporting that information on the death certificate, which would improve the quality and utility of state and federal mortality statistics.[8] However, whether and when to collect data at the scene remains a contentious topic among death scene investigators as this involves resources that their offices do not have, particularly in a disaster. CDC has also provided support for transitioning to and strengthening electronic death registration data systems for mortality data and piloting system improvements.[9] In Oklahoma, CDC supported the implementation of an electronic flagging process within the state EDRS to capture data on tornado-attributed deaths (Issa et al., 2019), which is noted in this chapter as a best practice for individual-level disaster reporting.

The Public Health Emergency Preparedness (PHEP) cooperative agreement, which provides funding to strengthen SLTT public health departments, has provided stronger backing for CDC efforts to promote voluntary standardization efforts for mortality data collection and reporting. However, because of the heterogeneity of death investigation systems and the state-level control of death registration procedures, federal efforts to standardize these practices have not found much success.

Public Health Data Systems: COVID-19 Case Study

There are several differences between how morbidity and mortality are classified and reported during a pandemic versus other disasters, such as a fire, blizzard, or hurricane (see Appendix C for an analysis of different methods used during the COVID-19 pandemic). To begin with, the primary data source for morbidity and mortality during a pandemic comes not from vital statistics and the death registration system but rather from an entirely different data system, which is compiled by epidemiologists for public health purposes. Regardless of the presence of a pandemic or major infectious disease outbreak, each state maintains a list of notifiable diseases that require health care providers to report every individual case (i.e., morbidity) that meets the established definition of a notifiable condition to the local or state health department, which in turn maintains a database. Case definitions are established by public health authorities and typically include both the characteristic symptoms caused by the pathogen and a laboratory

[8] *Ibid.*
[9] *Ibid.*

test to confirm that an individual has either an active or previous infection with the pathogen of concern. The health department uses this list to identify individuals who may have been in contact with the known cases, test these contacts, and isolate those who are infected. These data are also used for surveillance—for example, to calculate the incidence of new cases and the prevalence of cases in the population. Because the purpose of this database is to manage the outbreak, the focus is on living cases; therefore, the number of deaths caused by the pandemic is based on tracking the survival of the known cases.

Novel pathogens that cause large-scale disasters, such as COVID-19 pose several challenges for counting cases and associated fatalities. Case definitions often include options for naming someone as a "probable" or "presumptive" case based on symptoms and a "confirmed" case only with a positive test, and these case definitions evolve as more is learned about the pathogen. At the peak of the COVID-19 outbreak in New York City, tests were not available in sufficient numbers, and as a result, many individuals with symptoms of COVID-19 were regarded as presumptive cases. While appropriate at the time, this decision resulted in the appearance of a sudden jump in COVID-19 cases and deaths in New York that did not reflect the epidemiological reality (Goodman and Rashbaum, 2020). Further fueling the inaccuracy of case counts is the fact that testing processes—and even case definitions (see Table 3-2)—have varied substantially from state to state. Additionally, when tests are conducted without a provider's orders, such as with home tests and at freestanding testing sites, it is not clear how positive results collected via these activities are reflected in official public health databases.

Beyond the barriers associated with the collection of reported individual cases and deaths and mirrored by similar operational challenges associated with capturing morbidity data in other natural disasters, the early months of the COVID-19 pandemic have demonstrated ongoing reporting challenges. In order to be included in a public health database, the patient first must seek health care, then the health care provider must decide to order a diagnostic test, then the test must be available, and, in many cases, the patient must then go somewhere else to obtain the test. For many infectious diseases, providers often make treatment decisions empirically, based on symptoms alone, and so test samples are not collected or sent to a laboratory for confirmation. As a result, these unconfirmed cases are not included in initial public health case counts. Because COVID-19 can also be treated empirically—and because tests have been scarce and some health systems have been overwhelmed—relatively healthy people with COVID-19 symptoms have until recently been encouraged to stay home without testing, and thus they remain uncounted. For example, Holtgrave et al. (2020) found that during the height of the COVID-19 outbreak in New York State, the proportion of those tested and diagnosed varied widely by race and ethnicity; only 6.5 percent of infected Hispanic adults were diagnosed compared to 11.7 percent and 10.1 percent of non-Hispanic Whites and Blacks respectively. As a result, the number of officially recorded COVID-19 cases in the United States almost certainly underestimates the true number of infections, perhaps dramatically. As testing capacity grew, so did the number of positive results, possibly catching up with actual cases and thus not reflecting a true rising incidence of new infections.

Because COVID-19 cases and deaths are likely to be undercounted by public health databases, vital statistics provide an important alternative source of mortality data for COVID-19. However, as discussed in Appendix C, vital statistics systems use different definitions and processes than public health surveillance systems. In early April 2020, NCHS issued guidance indicating that if COVID-19 played a role in a death, this condition should be specified on the death certificate either as the underlying cause of death, where warranted, or as probable or presumed if the circumstances were compelling within a reasonable degree of certainty, even if testing was not done (as it often was not, due to a lack of testing capacity) (CDC, 2020c). Consequently, vital statistics data, which are compiled from death record data, will include some deaths not included in public health case counts. However, as with other reporting for other disasters, some COVID-19 deaths will be missed in both public health case counts and on death records, and other deaths might be inaccurately attributed to COVID-19 on death records.

For instance, in April 2020 vital statistics reports indicated a large increase in individuals dying at home rather than in the hospital (Gillum et al., 2020), especially in New York City (CDC, 2020a; Hogan, 2020). One might infer that many of these in-home deaths were caused, directly or indirectly, by COVID-19, but most were never tested or reported and hence are not included in health department case counts. Some of these deaths might eventually appear in vital statistics reports, but most of these cases will never appear in public health case counts for COVID-19. In the other direction, there have been claims offered, without evidence, that doctors were coached to mark COVID-19 as the cause of death when certifying the death even when it was not in order to inflate the pandemic's death toll per the vested interests of involved stakeholders (Rosenberg and Rutenberg, 2020). In response, some states do not include deaths in the official count without a mention of COVID-19 in the death record, even if the person had tested positive and was included in the public health surveillance database. In Colorado, this corresponds to a 24 percent reduction, because only 878 of 1,150 deaths (as of May 15, 2020) will be counted (Ingold and Paul, 2020).

Differences in Assessment of Mortality and Morbidity: Pandemics Versus Natural Disasters

Fundamentally, the collection and recording of individual-level mortality and morbidity for pandemics and other natural disasters are similar in terms of approaches that can be used. The major difference is the matter of temporality: hurricanes or wildfires occur over a period of days or weeks (although recovery can take much longer), while a pandemic can stretch into months or years. In all disasters, attributed mortality and morbidity counts and estimates change over time for two reasons: some long-term consequences take time to occur, and all data systems have lags, which vary over time. In pandemics, both of these factors apply, but there is an additional dynamic of ongoing infections. For instance, for the reasons discussed above COVID-19 deaths are sometimes seen as more reliable than case counts. However, deaths lag hospitalizations, the onset of symptoms, and the time of infection by 3 to 4 weeks. The daily number of COVID-19 deaths, therefore, is a lagging indicator of the efficacy of control efforts, and thus a poor guide for deciding whether certain infection control measures, such as social distancing measures, can be relaxed. Deaths may present as a lagging indicator in other types of disasters, such as from radiation exposure following a nuclear disaster, whereas direct deaths may take several weeks to present following the initial impact (CDC, 2018).

Conclusion 3-3: In pandemics and other disasters that evolve over time, trend data on the incidence of new cases are needed to assess the impact of control measures. In these settings care must be taken so that lags and reporting delays and changes in reporting systems do not obscure actual temporal changes.

OPPORTUNITIES TO FACILITATE THE CAPTURE AND REGISTRATION OF INDIVIDUAL DISASTER DEATHS

The ultimate aim of recording and reporting disaster-related deaths is to provide timely, accurate information to support communities affected by the disaster through the disaster lifecycle as well as to help communities be better prepared and resilient when faced with future events. Many entities across this enterprise are working diligently toward the aim of using individual mortality counts to protect the health and well-being of communities, but these efforts would benefit from greater collaboration and coordination across all systems and stakeholders to enable the network of state and federal death investigation and registration systems to function more effectively. At the outset, accurate and descriptive information to indicate, if present, the relationship of a death to a disasters—direct, indirect, or partially attributable to a disaster—needs to be entered into the death record by the ME/C or medical certifier; these data must then be identified and then correctly coded by NCHS as a disaster-related death in the national databases. Ensuring that these systems function together is essential to improving mortality assessment and will require collaboration among all stakeholders involved with data collection and initial recording (e.g., death scene investigators, ME/Cs, medical certifiers) as well as those parties involved with the secondary recording and reporting of data, such as state and federal vital statistics offices. To work toward achieving this vision, the committee has identified several barriers and best practices in the areas of leadership, standardized attribution of disaster-related mortality, training of certifiers, stakeholder engagement, research, and systems interoperability.

Building Leadership

Above all, strong leadership will be needed to coordinate these efforts and shift the paradigm away from traditional, siloed thinking about death investigation and vital statistics systems. Support from leadership within the SLTT entities involved in death investigation and registration will be needed to develop and operationalize uniform approaches for assessing individual-level mortality. Furthermore, the purposeful inclusion of leaders and other stakeholders from these SLTT systems in the disaster management enterprise would be a step toward elevating the quality of disaster-related mortality data.

Conclusion 3-4: The implementation of an enterprise approach for improving the assessment of mortality and morbidity following large-scale disasters is essential to the implementation of systemic improvements involving multiple, siloed stakeholders. Leadership at all levels—federal, state, local, tribal, and territorial—will be responsible for championing change.

Standardizing Disaster-Related Mortality Attribution

Inconsistent processes for attributing disaster-related mortality is a key barrier that can be addressed by the adoption, in policy and in practice, of uniform case definitions for attributing disaster-related deaths and standardized methods for reporting those deaths across all professions and jurisdictions. Novel data systems developed specifically for this purpose are unlikely to be adopted and will add to the administrative burden of ME/Cs in particular. Therefore, using existing electronic reporting systems would offer greater benefit and be more likely to be supported by stakeholders. For instance, the ability of ME/C case management systems and state-based EDRSs to identify and collect information on individual disaster deaths could be enhanced through the use of electronic alerts, automatic prompts, or dropdown boxes that would provide real-time support to the medical certifier in determining whether a death is related to the disaster and to what degree, per the framework developed by the committee (see Recommendation 2-1 in Chapter 2). These tools, which could be triggered to automatically appear following a Stafford Act disaster declaration or at the request of state or local leadership, would provide in-the-moment decision-making support to medical certifiers, including inserting descriptive terminology into the death record and allowing vital records staff to code and track flagged deaths (see Figure 3-4). For example, within the death record, the medical certifier could be asked whether the death is disaster related (Y/N), with definitions provided along with further Y/N prompts to indicate whether the death is direct, indirect, or partially attributable.

Beyond working to reduce inter-professional variation in the capture of direct deaths, which are most likely to be captured by ME/Cs as part of the death investigation system, such tools could provide value to other medical certifiers who are more likely to encounter indirect or partially attributable deaths within the clinical care environment. Furthermore, efforts to improve access to background health data by medical certifiers, such as electronic medical records, would assist medical certifiers in making more nuanced determinations concerning indirect and partially attributable disaster deaths.

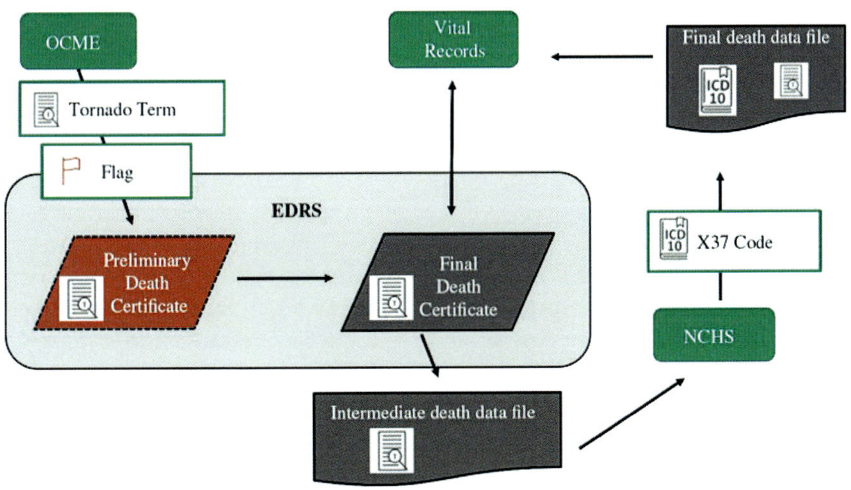

FIGURE 3-4 Flow of data in piloted system for improving the capture of tornado-related mortalities in Oklahoma.
NOTE: EDRS = electronic death registration system; NCHS = National Center for Health Statistics; OCME = Office of the Chief Medical Examiner.
SOURCE: Issa et al., 2019. Reproduced with permission.

Training Medical Certifiers

As described in the previous section, certain medical certifiers, such as medical doctors and nurse practitioners, typically receive little or no formal and recurring training in how to appropriately enter data into the death record, are unfamiliar with the data field, and are unaware of how to indicate the degree of attribution within the data fields of the death record (Brooks and Reed, 2015). Medical examiners and coroners are more likely to be familiar with how to enter data into EDRSs, but due to their professional philosophy, administrative policy, or training on disaster-death attribution they often fail to complete the death record accurately. Errors and missing information in the death record are an immediate barrier to the accurate recording and reporting of disaster-related deaths. Consequently, vital statistics offices encounter difficulty in coding the causes of death accurately and completely. Addressing this issue will require medical certifiers to receive better training that is tailored to their profession and to have access to resources within death investigation and registration systems to support them in carrying out this work—for example, and as described in the section above, user-friendly interfaces for e-filing death records and access to electronic health records (EHRs). In some cases, mandatory training may be felt to be less effective due to the lack of immediate salience for trainees, particularly those medical certifiers who are unlikely to regularly complete death records. In addition to requiring mandatory training, data systems should be designed to be intuitive and integrated into routine, day-to-day systems so that just-in-time training is sufficient. In terms of death registration training, lessons may be learned from the widespread implementation of mandatory training for opioid prescribers.

The use of existing disaster-related mortality tools developed by CDC and other agencies should also be promoted among medical certifiers, vital statistics staff, and emergency management staff alike. Importantly, most direct disaster-related deaths will be certified by a medical examiner or coroner because they are unnatural deaths. However, indirect or partially disaster-related deaths may not fall under the auspices of the ME/C, highlighting the critical importance of training and building capacity among all medical certifiers, not just those of the medicolegal death investigation system (e.g., ME/Cs), about how to appropriately handle disaster-related deaths. A standard system that can query for associated causation would assist providers who are not routinely involved in death investigations. Furthermore, the auditing of death records during declared disasters could offer an opportunity to clarify or add information. Enhancing training and support for medical certifiers involved in the medicolegal death investigation and death registration systems will require consistent funding and support. Additional resources will also be needed by state and local agencies to support quality assurance and investigations.

Engaging Stakeholders

The coordination, communication, and integration of efforts among ME/C, vital statistics, public health and epidemiology, emergency medical services, and emergency management stakeholders are fundamental to aligning efforts and enhancing collaboration to realize better mortality statistics. Leaders, decision makers, and practitioners at all levels need to understand the value of accurately collecting and reporting vital statistics data. Bringing together stakeholders from across the death registration system—particularly from the local and state levels—into the disaster planning, mitigation, response, and after-action sessions of EMS and law enforcement would also help to improve stakeholder buy-in.

The inclusion of ME/Cs in public health and disaster planning provides an opportunity for all entities to determine what data are most essential for local and regional use, what resources are needed, and how they can work together in both routine and emergency situations to carry out common goals. Several states have already made efforts to enhance partnerships across these siloed entities. In Florida, for example, partnerships among the state vital records system, county medical examiners, funeral directors, and professional associations are supported by state-level coordination by the State Commission. In Oklahoma, vital records officials are actively engaged in the emergency response and the immediate recovery period in order to provide death certificates on the spot to people who need them to access support services and settle legal affairs such as insurance claims and wills. Additionally, some medicolegal death investigation systems are sufficiently robust, such as Virginia and New Mexico, to have an epidemiologist on staff to initiate and organize disaster-related data collection and databases. In other systems, ME/Cs would benefit from developing a relationship with SLTT epidemiologists in order to mobilize epidemiology resources in anticipation of disasters typical for the regions as well as for pandemics and smaller infectious disease outbreaks. These functioning professional relationships provide a foundation for further collaboration to benefit data collection, recording, and use following disasters.

The multitude of stakeholders involved and the varied contexts in which they perform their work makes the adoption of new uniform methods for collecting and recording individual mortality data challenging. However, gaining stakeholder buy-in is especially critical for capturing indirect and partially attributable deaths, which are the most variable in mortality counts from disasters and which require a common approach for attribution and categorization by certifiers. Best practices for engaging stakeholders from across the enterprise include improving the function of these systems to reduce redundancy in data entry and facilitate easier attribution of disaster-related mortality by medical certifiers as well as providing clear evidence of the value of collecting and recording these data accurately and consistently. Access to training and the provision of active support by professional associations such as NAME and appropriate licensing boards and training by state registrars would also be beneficial, as these organizations play an important role in implementing change within these professions. There may be useful lessons that can be learned from the implementation of opioid death reporting systems (CDC, 2019).

Building an Evidence Base

Strengthening death investigation and registration systems has value beyond the collection of improved data for disaster-related deaths, but there is a lack of real-world evidence available to demonstrate the value of investing in these improvements. This lack can be addressed by conducting pilot projects and other real-world research to test modified practices and protocols for mortality reporting to improve the function of these systems and to increase stakeholders' capacity to consistently capture disaster-related mortality. These pilot projects can be followed with evaluation components to highlight the value of merging mortality and morbidity data over the lifecycle of various disasters and to provide critical information to planners and responders. Academic centers, specifically schools of public health, could potentially be used to determine assessment strategies and expand disaster epidemiology research capacity (see Chapter 4) without overburdening state and local public health and emergency response agencies.

Improving System Standards and Interoperability

Mortality data in the United States largely sit in silos because systems were not designed to be interoperable and share information with each other (Borfitz, 2019). Improving interoperability among ME/C case management systems, other mortality records systems, and state- and federal-level electronic death registration systems would enable data to be collected and reported more rapidly, reliably, and accurately. For instance, ME/C case management systems often include rich data that are not entered into death records created in the EDRS due to the administrative burden on ME/Cs to enter these data twice. Furthermore, individuals affected by disasters do not always remain in the declared disaster area and often cross jurisdictional and state lines, further underscoring the necessity of interoperability systems and easy data sharing across stakeholders.

Immediate opportunities to address this barrier include facilitating the transition to fully electronic ME/C case management and death registration systems that are interoperable and also developing and piloting new methods for flagging, including dropdown boxes, additional prompting for descriptive information about disaster-relatedness within those systems, and supporting in-the-moment decision making by medical certifiers as well as geocoding the place of death and place of residence. As mentioned previously, it is preferable to use and improve existing data systems rather than to develop novel systems. See Box 3-5 for examples of some of these efforts at the state level. Ultimately, mortality data need to be recorded and reported in a manner that can be fed back in meaningful ways to SLTT agencies and communities affected by disasters. As NVSS continues to strengthen and improve, there will be more opportunities to share data across and among states through better, more interoperable electronic data systems. Investing in the data infrastructure used for NVSS to collect, record, report, and use data on a daily basis will also strengthen disaster response capabilities. NCHS has worked with states to strengthen and improve the interoperability of their electronic death registration systems, and improving the quality of data captured on death records is a major priority for NCHS and NVSS. Vital statistics model law could be updated to incorporate data sharing and collection during disasters (e.g., standardized operation of electronic death records).

Technologies are also being developed to improve interoperability and support data sharing practices among ME/C systems, such as the Fast Healthcare Interoperability Resources standard for mortality reporting (Borfitz, 2019). An ideal integrated, interoperable system could provide immediate clinical decision support for death attribution, connectivity to

BOX 3-5
Brief Examples of Best Practices in State Death Investigation and Registration Systems

- Florida: This state has implemented a fully electronic vital record system and had developed a robust plan for continuity during periods without electricity. During these periods, PDF forms are distributed to certifiers to allow hard copies to be submitted and registered in the system. Vital records are geocoded within about 1 week and stakeholders use a system to facilitate regular communication between the vital statistics office and users to support hospitals, physicians, medical examiners, and funeral directors (Jones, 2019).
- California: California's electronic death reporting system includes more than 90 reportable diseases and conditions and efforts have been made to improve the function of the electronic death registration system to facilitate data access in real time and during inter-disaster periods (Bagwell, 2019).
- Louisiana: In Louisiana, birth and death records are now fully electronic by mandate after the experience of Katrina demonstrated the importance of electronic systems and vital records in emergency response and preparedness (DeSalvo and Petrin, 2017; Louisiana Department of Health, 2020).

funeral homes, and a real-time feedback loop to vital statistics and electronic death registration systems, with reports flowing to state authorities and NCHS. Better data sharing between EHRs and the electronic death registration systems could streamline processes and provide additional information on deaths. Challenges and opportunities with respect to data sharing for population-level mortality and morbidity data will be explored in more detail in Chapter 4.

Continuity of Data Collection and Recording During Disasters

The difficulty of maintaining electronic data systems' continuity during disasters is another barrier to the collection and reporting of individual-level mortality data. Flexible systems that are well tooled for day-to-day use are more effective than ad hoc systems or systems designed only for large-scale events. Research efforts should focus on evaluating continuity mechanisms for electronic systems so that these are robust enough for everyday use but also able to adapt and flex during a disaster. It is important to try to minimize the implementation of new procedures and practices during a crisis. For instance, Oklahoma has designed its electronic death registration system to be flexible for capturing information at large scale as well as for day-to-day use, for exercising the system, and for responding to smaller scale events (Baker, 2019). In Florida, surveillance systems are used continuously—not only deployed for disasters—and the system is flexible enough to expand beyond syndromic surveillance.

CONSIDERATIONS SPECIFIC TO THE COLLECTION OF MORBIDITY DATA

As described in Chapter 2, morbidity is a complex concept that covers a range of health outcomes from the physical to psychological, including cardiovascular, gastrointestinal, and respiratory diseases; physical injuries; and mental health outcomes. While a cause of death is sometimes difficult to determine, mortality itself is easier than morbidity to define. The collection and reporting of morbidity data, therefore, remains a persistent gap and the limited systems, tools, and practices associated with the collection of individual morbidity data cannot be evaluated to the same degree as mortality data. There are no standards or dedicated systems in place for the collection and recording of reported morbidities following disasters or for the use of data on morbidities. The collection of data about disaster-related morbidities in a uniform manner is challenging, given how broadly they are defined, the influence of pre-existing and co-morbid conditions on post-disaster health outcomes, the variation across disaster types, and the difficulties associated with mining morbidity data from across a broad network of unique federal, SLTT, and health care systems.

Although they are certainly in need of improvement, the basic systems, mechanisms, and processes for the collection and recording of disaster-related mortality data already exist to some degree; this is not, however, the case for disaster-related morbidity data at the individual level. As with mortality, the variability in the capacities of SLTT health departments—and the fact that many are under-resourced—makes the creation of a standard system for collecting individual-level morbidity data especially difficult.

There are many possible data sources for tracking morbidities, particularly within the health care systems, which already generates individual-level morbidity data. These include hospital admissions data, EHRs, syndromic surveillance systems, records from disaster medical assistance teams, and data from sheltering operations (CDC, 2016) (see Box 3-6). However, these data are not necessarily captured in a manner that would allow for disaster attribution. There is also no consensus as to what information about morbidities that end users such as public health or emergency planners, health care systems, and SLTT and federal agencies need in order to respond better to disasters. As a result, there is also no consensus on which morbidities, indicators of morbidities, or data sources should be consistently tracked in common types of disasters (e.g., hurricanes, blizzards, tornadoes, pandemics/epidemics) (CDC, 2016).

BOX 3-6
Possible Data Sources for Individual Counts of Disaster-Related Morbidity

Sources of data for morbidity include but are not limited to:

- public health case reports;
- insurance and disability claims;
- prescription monitoring;
- hospital admission and discharge data;
- emergency department and outpatient visit data (see Appendix C);
- incidence statistics for a given condition (e.g., suicide, cardiovascular disease);
- psychiatric inpatient admissions; and
- law enforcement reports (e.g., overdose, interpersonal violence).

Useful data to collect during morbidity surveillance include incidence rate, prevalence rate, and rates stratified by age, sex, and geographic location (CDC, 2016).

Conclusion 3-5: Collecting morbidity data presents an additional challenge due to the large quantity of possible outcomes and data available across multiple unique systems. Understanding which data are of greatest value and how these data can be used to inform disaster management requires more research.

Conclusion 3-6: Standards for morbidity data are needed across different types of disasters. A standard dataset by disaster type would dramatically improve the uniform collection of morbidity data. This will improve the usability and actionability of these data.

The lack of data sharing and the inadequate interoperability of systems at all levels remain substantial barriers. EHRs, the most obvious source of electronic data on morbidities, and the systems that contain them are varied. Many of these systems lack the capacity to push important data to relevant parties in real time. For many, it is not yet possible using available EHR technology to aggregate and analyze large volumes of morbidity data to support real-time decision making. While traditional data sources such as hospital discharge data, EHRs, reportable disease systems, and others could be tapped to develop estimates of morbidity, these systems can be easily disrupted by the disaster, may fail to capture those individuals who do not present for care in a clinical setting, and are currently not suited to rapidly collecting and pushing out morbidity data to public health and disaster management stakeholders (Schnall et al., 2011). The experiences of first responders during the 2018 Camp Fire in Paradise, California, illustrate the need of localities to have access to shared morbidity data through interoperable systems. As described by officials in Paradise, the lack of rapid access to actionable data from the county level required Paradise responders to rely on local hospital data to guide their initial response and recovery efforts. Other county health departments have invested heavily in data systems that allow for greater collection and use of real-time mortality and morbidity data and have benefited from embracing greater collaboration between the public health and emergency management departments at a county level (see Box 3-7). However, investment in these data systems is dependent on available resources and is, therefore, not a realistic opportunity for all health departments. Additional investment is required from the federal level to implement systems that allow for greater interoperability and coordination and to use existing data systems for the collection of morbidity data following disasters.

Addressing these operational challenges to the collection of disaster-related morbidity data will be necessary in order to systematically and accurately capture the effects of disasters on health and to guide the implementation of changes in response and recovery to future disasters.

BOX 3-7
Best Practice: Real-Time Health Surveillance Tracking in Ventura County, California

Following the passage of the Health Information Technology for Economic and Clinical Health Act (HITECH Act) in 2009, Ventura County, California, adopted the EpiCenter platform to manage public health data tracking. EpiCenter is a browser-based application that provides real-time and continuous health information access by automatically collecting, managing, detecting, and visualizing changes in public health as they occur (Health Monitoring, 2020). Because the application is web-based, it can be used and accessed in a variety of settings and locations without the need for access to physical health records and data.

The system was purchased with public health preparedness funds, supplemented by Hospital Preparedness Program and Public Health Emergency Preparedness cooperative funds. Now in its 10th year of use, Ventura County Public Health is able to receive syndromic surveillance data electronically from local acute-care centers using EpiCenter (Ventura County Health Care Agency, 2017). The data received via EpiCenter are integrated into an algorithm that alerts users via text or email if any statistical deviations in public health conditions occur. Most recently, the system was used during the COVID-19 pandemic to monitor suspected and confirmed cases in real time, allowing public health officials to run numerous reports and analyze the population. Other states, such as Connecticut (Connecticut State Department of Public Health, 2020) and New Jersey (New Jersey Department of Health, 2017) have also adopted EpiCenter to conduct statewide syndromic surveillance.

Standardizing data collection processes specific to morbidity after disasters can be built into the nation's operational disaster response function, in a way that is similar to (but with different collection procedures) that proposed for mortality data collection. Various strategies could be considered to more effectively and systematically capture existing data on significant disaster-related morbidities. For example, applied machine learning techniques from EHRs could reveal trends in emergency department and acute care facility use that may provide a better profile of morbidity. The implementation of these strategies will require substantial investment in the development of procedures and best practices related to the types of morbidity data to be collected (see Chapter 2) and the processes for recording such data.

Additionally, the absence of established standards and guidance regarding what types of morbidity data should be collected provides an opportunity for research to be conducted to determine what types of morbidities and morbidity indicators are most essential for collection following large-scale disasters (see Chapter 4 for further discussion on the use of morbidity data to develop population estimates). As described in Chapters 1 and 2, exclusively focusing on the collection of significant morbidities would likely fail to capture the data for less immediately critical but far more prevalent and costly morbidities related to the social determinants of health, such as respiratory diseases, mental health outcomes, and exacerbations of existing co-morbidities. See Appendix D for case studies describing the relationship between the social determinants of health and disaster-related morbidity and mortality. Defining which morbidity data to collect is a critical first step to building the capability within the system and stakeholders to collect and use these data. This foundation can then be developed further to facilitate the integration of data on social and environmental factors to better contextualize community vulnerabilities and programmatic targets for prevention and mitigation. Therefore, it will be necessary to invest in an ongoing process to develop, validate, and disseminate national standards for data collection concerning the key morbidities caused or exacerbated by specific types of disasters (see Recommendation 3-3).

Use of Electronic Health and Claims Data to Assess Morbidity: COVID-19 Case Study

The recent COVID-19 pandemic presents a potential model system for the recording and reporting of health data related to the virus, which could be replicated for morbidity data in future disasters. As noted in the section above on Public Health Data Systems, public health surveillance systems focus on cases (i.e., morbidity) rather than deaths. Nevertheless, much more needs to be known about the symptoms that these individuals exhibit, how many are hospitalized, and many other factors in order to comprehensively assess disaster-related morbidity. To address these issues, epidemiologists and health service researchers are using a variety of existing electronic data, such as claims data and EHRs. Accurately collecting, cleaning, and analyzing these data present enormous operational and analytical challenges for any type of large disaster. In the midst of a pandemic, these challenges need to be rapidly addressed due to an urgent need for these data to inform response.

Already, guidance has been developed concerning the use of COVID-19 health care claims data (Bohl and Roozeboom-Baker, 2020) and EHRs, which could be applied more broadly to other disaster-related mortalities and morbidities. It is important to consider a basic fact concerning these types of data: neither claims data nor EHR data were designed for the purposes of research. Claims data are designed for reimbursement purposes, and EHR data are designed for the recording of patient presentation, diagnosis, and treatment. Furthermore, as described earlier in this chapter, COVID-19 cases are likely widely under-reported, a deficit that will carry over to such data sources. However, the identification of many (but not all) patients admitted with COVID-19 can still be captured through a careful examination of individual claims (either using the newly released ICD-10 code for COVID-19 or by examining respiratory conditions common to COVID-19 infection) for hospital inpatient and outpatient services, skilled nursing and long-term care, and professional services (Bohl and Roozeboom-Baker, 2020). The use of EHR data presents its own unique challenges. The process used to extract, clean, and check COVID-19-related EHR records is painstaking and requires careful fact checking beyond the use of commonly employed software that sorts this type of data (Robbins, 2020). Nevertheless, in the absence of a formal reporting process for morbidity data, analysis of the types of data described here—and the processes being developed around COVID-19 identification—can inform future disaster morbidity research.

USE OF INDIVIDUAL-LEVEL MORTALITY AND MORBIDITY DATA TO INFORM DISASTER MANAGEMENT

As discussed in Chapter 2, individual-level mortality and morbidity data have a wide range of uses, but the data's primary value lies in preventing further health impacts of a disaster during response and recovery as well as in planning and mitigation to reduce the human impact of future disasters. These data have value for a broad range of stakeholders, including community members, public health practitioners, emergency management personnel, policy makers and political leadership, federal agencies such as FEMA, CDC, and the Department of Health and Human Services, and many others.

Barriers to and Best Practices for Use of Individual-Level Mortality and Morbidity Data

Data sharing and system interoperability within and across jurisdictions are major barriers to the operationalization of individual-level mortality data. Establishing data sharing agreements during interim periods between disasters as a best practice could address these barriers. In current practice, localities are often expected to share data with state and federal authorities without reciprocity. Instead, data sharing would benefit from the data flowing in a top-down as well as a bottom-up direction. A primary value of these data is to support local communities, so communities and local-level authorities should receive timely and actionable mortality data shared from the state and federal government systems.

Conclusion 3-7: Access to federal and state mortality and morbidity data is essential, but data access does not equate to actionability of these data at the local level. If data are to be actionable, localities require the tools needed to read, analyze, and display data received from the federal or state level in a meaningful way as well as the expertise and capacity to use these data in decision making.

Research Priorities for Individual Mortality and Morbidity Counts

Several research gaps related to the use of individual mortality data need to be addressed in order to improve the quality of the data and to increase the understanding of which types of data are most valuable for various stakeholders at different points in the disaster lifecycle. A body of practical evidence demonstrates how these data could be used to inform practice and could be included in pilot projects with evaluative components. Cost-effectiveness research would also be useful in gaining buy-in from policy makers and other stakeholders for investment system improvements, practices for collecting and reporting individual-level mortality data, and training for medical certifiers.

RECOMMENDATIONS

Recommendation 3-1: Strengthen Existing Systems to Improve Individual-Level Mortality Data Quality

The Centers for Disease Control and Prevention (CDC), through the National Center for Health Statistics (NCHS), should lead an enterprise-wide initiative to strengthen existing death registration systems to improve the quality of disaster-related mortality data at state, local, tribal, and territorial levels. These efforts should prioritize the standardization of methods for data reporting and recording and to improve the capacity of death investigation and registration systems to capture more detail on contributing causes of death following disasters.

The following immediate actions should be undertaken:

- NCHS should fund and support the transition of the remaining states and territories with paper-based death registration systems to electronic death registration systems (EDRSs) and lead, in collaboration with state vital records offices, the integration of best practices for capturing and coding disaster-related death data into state-based EDRSs.
- NCHS should directly fund improvements in and the standardization of medical examiner and coroner (ME/C) death e-filing systems and require interoperability with these systems and state EDRSs. Similarly, NCHS and state registrars should require that EDRSs adopt the following standard improvements:

- o Automatic filing of death information with state EDRSs via ME/C e-filing systems to reduce the administrative burden on ME/Cs;
- o Automated and uniform alert flags, prompts, drop-down options, and decision-making support for use by medical certifiers when entering data into a death record in both a routine and just-in-time capacity;
- o Offline data entry and other continuity mechanisms; and
- o Geocoding of deaths based on both place of residence and location of death.

The following long-term actions should be prioritized:

- NCHS should fund and adopt, where appropriate, artificial intelligence technologies to improve the throughput of its automated medical coding systems so as to improve the throughput of ME/C deaths to a level equivalent to that of other natural causes of death.
- State vital records offices and ME/C offices, with the support of CDC, should develop continuity plans to sustain the functions of these offices during emergencies.

Recommendation 3-2: Standardize Data Collection and Reporting of Individual-Level Reported Disaster-Related Mortality

The National Center for Health Statistics (NCHS), working with the states, should update the Model State Vital Statistics Act to drive uniformity of data collection and recording with respect to disaster-related mortality. To promote uniformity in definitions and practices for collecting and recording disaster-related mortality data and enhance the quality and comparability of these data, NCHS should revise the Model State Vital Statistics Act to provide clear guidance and data standards to state vital records offices and medical certifiers. These changes should include the use of automated flags, prompts, and drop-down options to collect data on the relationship of a death to a recent disaster and provide decision-making support for medical certifiers.

Recommendation 3-3: Develop a Set of Standards for Morbidity Data Collection

The Centers for Disease Control and Prevention, in collaboration with the Centers for Medicare & Medicaid Services, the Council of State and Territorial Epidemiologists, and the National Association of County & City Health Officials should establish and promulgate national standards for the collection of disaster-related morbidities before, during, and after disasters. These activities should include investment in research to identify common morbidities that occur as a result of or are exacerbated by the conditions of specific types of disasters (e.g., floods, hurricanes, blizzards, radiation events, pandemics, etc.) and across multiple disaster types. This should include the identification of minimum timelines for data collection, the development and validation of morbidity data systems for use by the disaster management enterprise, and pilot testing and implementation of approaches to collect these data in a standardized manner.

Recommendation 3-4: Strengthen the Capacity of the Medicolegal Death Investigation System to Assess Disaster-Related Mortality

The Centers for Disease Control and Prevention (CDC), in collaboration with state agencies and professional associations, should strengthen the value, capacity, and capability of the medicolegal death investigation system to improve investigation, training, data development and collection, and case management.

The following immediate actions should be undertaken:

- CDC should fund and re-launch the Medical Examiner and Coroner Information Sharing Program to provide guidance and support to medical examiners, coroners, and other medical certifiers.
- The National Association of Medical Examiners, the International Association of Coroners & Medical Examiners, the American Board of Medicolegal Death Investigators, and state-based medical examiner and coroner professional organizations should support the proposed framework for collecting and recording uniform mortality and morbidity data, encourage the use of existing CDC tools and guidance by all professionals, and provide continuing education courses for their members that reflect this guidance.
- CDC, through the National Center for Health Statistics, along with appropriate licensing bodies should provide standardized training and materials designed for medical certifiers (physicians, nurse practitioners, physician assistants, and others as applicable by state) who encounter natural deaths and are responsible for entering death information into the death record.
- Death investigation systems should develop relationships with state or university-based demographers and epidemiologists to formalize proactive data collection and sharing agreements for natural disasters that are typical for the state as well as mass mortality and morbidity due to disease.
- To promote more accurate death certification, the above agencies should incentivize and support the conversion of coroner systems to regionalized medical examiner systems staffed

by forensic pathologists and medicolegal death investigators professionally trained to identify and classify disaster-related deaths per the framework described in Recommendation 2-1.

Recommendation 3-5: Strengthen the Role of the Medicolegal Death Investigation and State Death Registration Systems in the Disaster Management Enterprise

State, local, tribal, and territorial public health and emergency management departments should integrate the professionals and agencies from the medicolegal death investigation and death registration systems in all aspects of preparedness and planning. This should involve the consideration of moving mortality management out of Emergency Support Function #8 (ESF8) and creating a separate ESF dedicated to mortality management. This new function could complement ESF8 and ensure focused attention on assessing mortality during and after disasters, while those charged with ESF8 responsibilities are focused on providing services to survivors. This new function could include the involvement of medical examiners, coroners, and other relevant professionals in planning drills for mortality management; effective, efficient, and unbiased data collection during disasters; training for family assistance centers; and standards for after-action reports and other mortality data reporting activities.

REFERENCES

ASPE (Assistant Secretary for Planning and Evaluation). 2013. *Assessing the status and prospects of state and local health department information technology infrastructure.* https://aspe.hhs.gov/basic-report/assessing-status-and-prospects-state-and-local-health-department-information-technology-infrastructure (accessed June 11, 2020).

Bagwell, D. 2019. *Session 4: Current capabilites in assessing and using morbidity and mortality data during the inter-disaster period.* Presentation at the August 29, 2019, public meeting of the National Academies of Sciences, Engineering, and Medicine's Committee on Best Practices in Assessing Mortality and Significant Morbidity Following Large-Scale Disasters, Washington, DC.

Baker, K. 2019. *Session 5: Looking forward—best practices and tools for assessing and using morbidity and mortality data during a large-scale disaster in real time.* Presentation at the August 30, 2019, public meeting of the National Academies of Sciences, Engineering, and Medicine's Committee on Best Practices in Assessing Mortality and Significant Morbidity Following Large-Scale Disasters, Washington, DC.

Bohl, A., and M. Roozeboom-Baker. 2020. *A COVID-19 primer: Analyzing health care claims, administrative data, and public use files.* https://www.mathematica.org/our-publications-and-findings/publications/a-covid-19-primer-analyzing-health-care-claims-administrative-data-and-public-use-files (accessed June 5, 2020).

Borfitz, D. 2019. CDC creating a "ruckus" around mortality reporting. *AITrends*, July 5. https://www.aitrends.com/ai-world-government/cdc-creating-a-ruckus-around-mortality-reporting (accessed July 1, 2020).

Brooks, E. G., and K. D. Reed. 2015. Principles and pitfalls: A guide to death certification. *Clinical Medicine & Research* 13(2):74–82.

Brown, E., B. Reinhard, and R. Thebault. 2020. Which deaths count toward the COVID-19 death toll? It depends on the state. *Washington Post*, April 16.

Bryant, C. D. 2003. *Handbook of death and dying*. Thousand Oaks, CA: Sage Publications.

CDC (Centers for Disease Control and Prevention). 2015. *Death investigation systems*. https://www.cdc.gov/phlp/publications/coroner/death.html (accessed July 16, 2020).

CDC. 2016. *A primer for understanding the principles and practices of disaster surveillance in the United States*. Atlanta, GA: Centers for Disease Control and Prevention.

CDC. 2017. *Death scene investigation after natural disaster or other weather-related events: A toolkit*. https://www.cdc.gov/nceh/hsb/disaster/docs/DisasterDeathSceneToolkit-P.pdf (accessed July 1, 2020).

CDC. 2018. *Determining deaths from a radiation emergency*. https://www.cdc.gov/nceh/radiation/emergencies/determinedeaths.html (accessed July 31, 2020).

CDC. 2019. *Enhanced state opioid overdose surveillance*. https://www.cdc.gov/drugoverdose/foa/state-opioid-mm.html (accessed June 5, 2020).

CDC. 2020a. *Preliminary estimate of excess mortality during the COVID-19 outbreak—New York City, March 11–May 2, 2020*. https://www.cdc.gov/mmwr/volumes/69/wr/mm6919e5.htm (accessed June 5, 2020).

CDC. 2020b. *Vital statistics reporting guidance*. https://www.cdc.gov/nchs/nvss/reporting-guidance.htm (accessed June 5, 2020).

CDC. 2020c. *Guidance for certifying deaths due to Coronavirus Disease 2019 (COVID-19)*. https://www.cdc.gov/nchs/data/nvss/vsrg/vsrg03-508.pdf (accessed July 1, 2020).

Combs, D. L., L. E. Quenemoen, R. G. Parrish, and J. H. Davis. 1999. Assessing disaster-attributed mortality: Development and application of a definition and classification matrix. *International Journal of Epidemiology* 28(6):1124–1129.

Connecticut State Department of Public Health. 2020. *Syndromic surveillance*. https://portal.ct.gov/DPH/Epidemiology-and-Emerging-Infections/Syndromic-Surveillance (accessed July 17, 2020).

DeSalvo, K., and C. Petrin. 2017. *From Katrina to wildfires: Leveraging technology in disaster response*. https://www.healthaffairs.org/do/10.1377/hblog20171113.545312/full (accessed June 5, 2020).

FEMA (Federal Emergency Management Agency). 2019. *Best practices for assessing mortlity and significant morbidity following large-scale disasters: Charge to the Committee*. PowerPoint Presentation. Presented at the May 28, 2019, public meeting of the National Academies of Sciences, Engineering, and Medicine's Committee on Assessing Mortality and Significant Morbidity Following Large-Scale Disasters. Washington, DC. http://webapp.nationalacademies.org/napar/projectview.aspx?key=51640#MeetingId11176 (accessed September 1, 2020).

Gillum, J., L. Song, and J. Kao. 2020. *There's been a spike in people dying at home in several cities. That suggests coronavirus deaths are higher than reported*. https://www.propublica.org/article/theres-been-a-spike-in-people-dying-at-home-in-several-cities-that-suggests-coronavirus-deaths-are-higher-than-reported (accessed June 5, 2020).

Goodman, J. D., and W. K. Rashbaum. 2020. N.Y.C. death toll soars past 10,000 in revised virus count. *The New York Times*, April 14.

Hanzlick, R. 1997. The Centers for Disease Control and Prevention's Medical Examiner/Coroner Information Sharing Program (MECISP). *Journal of Forensic Science* 42(3):531–532.

Hanzlick, R. 2006. Medical examiners, coroners, and public health: A review and update. *Archives of Pathology and Laboratory Medicine* 130(9):1274–1282.

Health Monitoring. 2020. *What is EpiCenter?* https://www.health-monitoring.com/syndromic-surveillance-epicenter (accessed July 17, 2020).

Hogan, G. 2020. *Staggering surge of NYers dying in their homes suggests city is undercounting coronavirus fatalities.* https://gothamist.com/news/surge-number-new-yorkers-dying-home-officials-suspect-undercount-covid-19-related-deaths (accessed June 5, 2020).

Holtgrave, D. R., M. A. Barranco, J. M. Tesoriero, D. S. Blog, and E. S. Rosenberg. 2020. Assessing racial and ethnic disparities using a COVID-19 outcomes continuum for New York State. *Annals of Epidemiology* 48:9–14. https://doi.org/10.1016/j.annepidem.2020.06.010.

Horney, J. 2017. *Disaster epidemiology: Methods and applications.* New York: Academic Press.

Ingold, J., and J. Paul. 2020. Nearly a quarter of the people Colorado said died from coronavirus don't have COVID-19 on their death certificate. *Colorado Sun*, May 15.

IOM (Institute of Medicine). 2003. *Medicolegal death investigation system: Workshop summary.* Washington, DC: The National Academies Press. https://doi.org/10.17226/10792.

Iowa Board of Medicine. 2020. *Guidelines for reporting and certifying COVID-19 deaths.* https://medicalboard.iowa.gov/document/guidelines-reporting-and-certifying-covid-19-deaths (accessed June 4, 2020).

Issa, A. N., K. Baker, D. Pate, R. Law, T. Bayleyegn, and R. S. Noe. 2019. Evaluation of Oklahoma's electronic death registration system and event fatality markers for disaster-related mortality surveillance—Oklahoma USA, May 2013. *Prehospital and Disaster Medicine* 34(2):125–131.

Jones, K. 2019. *Session 2: Florida system for assessing post-disaster mortality and significant morbidity—case study.* Presentation at the August 29, 2019, public meeting of the National Academies of Sciences, Engineering, and Medicine's Committee on Best Practices for Assessing Mortality and Significant Morbidity Following Large-Scale Disasters, Washington, DC.

Kulkarni, P. A., R. S. Noe, and M. Warner. 2015. *Sensitivity of disaster-related mortality surveillance after Hurricane Sandy—New Jersey, 2012–2013.* Paper presented at the 2015 Annual Meeting of the Council of State and Territorial Epidemiologists, Boston, MA.

Louisiana Department of Health. 2020. *LEERS electronic death registration—Information for physicians.* http://ldh.la.gov/index.cfm/page/913 (accessed July 1, 2020).

Madsen, A., and E. Begier. 2013. Improving quality of cause-of-death reporting in New York City. *Preventing Chronic Disease* 10:E118.

McKibben, B. 2020. Racism, police violence, and the climate are not separate issues. *The New Yorker.* https://www.newyorker.com/news/annals-of-a-warming-planet/racism-police-violence-and-the-climate-are-not-separate-issues (accessed September 1, 2020).

Montana DPHHS (Department of Public Health and Human Services). 2020. *Guidance for certifying COVID-19 deaths.* https://dphhs.mt.gov/vitalrecords/certificationofcovid-19 (accessed June 4, 2020).

NAPHSIS (National Association for Public Health Statistics and Information Systems). 2020a. *Jurisdictions.* https://www.naphsis.org/systems (accessed June 8, 2020).

NAPHSIS. 2020b. *State and Territorial Exchange of Vital Events (STEVE).* https://www.naphsis.org/steve (accessed July 1, 2020).

New Jersey Department of Health. 2017. *Meaningful use—syndromic surveillance.* https://www.nj.gov/health/meaningfuluse/syndromic.shtml (accessed July 17, 2020).

Noe, R. 2018. Chapter 5—Applications: Disaster-related mortality surveillance: Challenges and considerations for local and state health departments. In J. A. Horney (ed.), *Disaster epidemiology: Methods and applications.* London: Academic Press. Pp. 55–63.

Noe, R. 2019. *Session 3: Current capabilities in assessing and using morbidity and mortality data in real time during a large-scale disaster.* Presentation at the August 29, 2019, public meeting of the National Academies of Sciences, Engineering, and Medicine's Committee on Best Practices for Assessing Mortality and Significant Morbidity Following Large-Scale Disasters, Washington, DC.

NSTC (National Science and Technology Council). 2016. *Strengthening the medicolegal-death-investigation system: Improving data systems.* https://obamawhitehouse.archives.gov/sites/default/files/microsites/ostp/NSTC/strengthening_the_medicolegal_death_investigation_system_final.pdf (accessed July 3, 2020).

NVSS (National Vital Statistics System). 2017. *Vital statistics reporting guidance: A reference guide for certification of deaths in the event of a natural, human-induced, or chemical/radiological disaster.* https://www.cdc.gov/nchs/data/nvss/vsrg/vsrg01.pdf (accessed July 1, 2020).

Pennsylvania Department of Health. 2020. *Additional guidance for coroners & medical examiners: Reporting of deaths attributed to COVID-19.* https://www.health.pa.gov/topics/Documents/Reporting-Registries/SRN%202020-14%20Additional%20Guidance%20for%20Coroners%20and%20Medical%20Examiners%20-%20Reporting%20of%20Deaths%20Attributed%20to%20COVID-19.pdf (accessed July 1, 2020).

Robbins, R. 2020. *Hospital records hold valuable COVID-19 data. Making it usable is time-consuming work.* https://www.statnews.com/2020/05/27/mass-general-brigham-covid19-genetics-biobank (accessed June 5, 2020).

Rocha, L. A., C. Q. Fromknecht, S. D. Redman, J. E. Brady, S. E. Hodge, and R. S. Noe. 2017. Medicolegal death scene investigations after natural disaster- and weather-related events: A review of the literature. *Academic Forensic Pathology* 7(2):221–239.

Rosenberg, M., and J. Rutenberg. 2020. Fight over virus's death toll opens grim new front in election battle. *The New York Times*, May 9.

Ruiz, L., B. M. Posey, M. A. Neuilly, M. K. Stohr, and C. Hemmens. 2018. Certifying death in the United States. *Journal of Forensic Science* 63(4):1138–1145.

Schnall, A. H., A. F. Wolkin, R. Noe, L. B. Hausman, P. Wiersma, K. Soetebier, and S. T. Cookson. 2011. Evaluation of a standardized morbidity surveillance form for use during disasters caused by natural hazards. *Prehospital & Disaster Medicine* 26(2):90–98.

Slavova, S., D. B. O'Brien, K. Creppage, D. Dao, A. Fondario, E. Haile, B. Hume, T. W. Largo, C. Nguyen, J. C. Sabel, D. Wright, and members of the Council of State and Territorial Epidemiologists Overdose Subcommittee. 2015. Drug overdose deaths: Let's get specific. *Public Health Reports* 130(4):339–342.

Snohomish County. 2020. *Cause and manner of death.* https://snohomishcountywa.gov/806/Cause-Manner-of-Death (accessed July 31, 2020).

Ventura County Health Care Agency. 2017. *Acceptance of meaningful use data.* http://www.vchca.org/acceptance-of-meaningful-use-data#:~:text=Syndromic%20Surveillance%20Data%20Submission%3A,%3A%20805%2D981%2D5331 (accessed July 17, 2020).

4

Analytical Considerations for Population Estimates of Mortality and Morbidity

As indicated in the guiding precepts articulated in Chapter 1, the committee recognizes the importance of both individual counts and population-level estimates in assessing the impact of disasters. This chapter provides a review of major classes of techniques used to construct population-level estimates of disaster-related mortality and morbidity. This review is intended to be illustrative rather than a comprehensive evaluation of the whole of demographic and epidemiological research on disasters.

The committee's review of the methods encompassed by the population estimate approach is focused on three general classes of estimation techniques and methods that span a wide variety of analytical options that are particularly salient to measuring disaster effects. This chapter begins by discussing the issues associated with using conventional household or individual person *survey interviewing* for collecting data in disaster studies, whether to provide data on rates that can be scaled up to the level of the population or data to facilitate linkage of exposures to morbidity and mortality outcomes. Next, the chapter turns to the common practice of modeling *excess mortality* and significant morbidity effects—differences relative to baseline-level data and trends that may be attributed to a disaster. Finally, the chapter discusses some advanced survey and sampling methods for *estimating the size of hard-to-count or hidden populations* such as death, illness, or injury that is caused by a disaster but is not reported as such in the usual data sources. These methods require different kinds of information inputs and underlying assumptions, and each has strengths and weaknesses, but can be made more precise depending on attention to study design, comparison groups, available sample sizes, quality of supporting data sources, and statistical techniques for analysis. These methods and techniques can also be made more accurate with continuing research on the methods themselves.

Put in context, these classes of estimation methods related to disaster effects parallel those that have been applied to study mortality and morbidity in other settings, notably war. Jewell et al. (2018) provide an instructive framework for methods for measuring civilian war casualties, using the term *accounting* to refer to the general problem and differentiating between two major branches of inquiry. The first, *counting*, is exactly as the name implies—tallying fatalities one-by-one—while the second, *estimation*, "will usually mean using a statistical procedure, such as a sample survey, to extrapolate a total number from a subset of deaths that have been observed" (Jewell et al., 2018, p. 380). The Jewell et al. (2018, p. 390) framework lists six broad categories of measurement technique categories:

- *Documentation*, listing deaths person-by-person along with other information about the circumstances;
- Derivation of *excess mortality*, which is "the use of census and other population demographic information to estimate mortality potentially attributable to both direct and indirect losses;"
- The use of personal *survey interviewing* methods (through "epidemiologic or demographic household surveys") to estimate a count of deaths during and after an incident or incidents;
- Indirect estimation of death counts based on "assumed relationships" between incident-related deaths and information in *found data* ("data that happen to be available");
- *Crowdsourced* death reports, or a more free-form kind of self-report or observer-report data than a usual household survey; and
- The use of *multiple systems estimation*, using "distinct and separate listings" to arrive at an overall, statistically adjusted estimate.

The analogues of these measurement techniques to the study of disaster-related morbidity and mortality are clear. In particular, documentation corresponds directly to the counting-type measurement challenge described in Chapter 3, attempting to ensure that electronic death and health records include the information necessary to generate a complete, one-to-one itemization of deaths and harms arising from a disaster. The remaining classes of measurement techniques lie in the province of estimation and inference. Although this includes a broad range of methods, each with different strengths, weaknesses, and appropriate uses, the discussion of common issues and the attending conclusions and recommendations at the end of this chapter demonstrates that they do have much in common.

In countries where vital event recording systems are limited or nonexistent, techniques for estimating disaster-associated mortality and morbidity are essential because there is no viable alternative. In these settings, survey interviewing approaches are used to generate basic information on mortality levels. Even in countries like the United States, with a good system of collecting and recording vital statistics in place (though needing improvement, as detailed in Chapter 3), estimation methods based on statistical inference provide an important check on the completeness and accuracy of data produced solely by counting. Estimation methods are also important for quantifying the morbidity and mortality impacts of disasters over time and are therefore complements to (and not redundant of) counting techniques. Complex phenomena such as population health, crime, and the economy all require a variety of measurements to understand. Estimation techniques are well suited for capturing indirect mortality due to disasters. They may be the best reflection of deaths and morbidities that go unreported or misreported in records systems and may have greater utility in coordinating response to and recovery from subsequent disasters because when carefully implemented, they characterize well-defined populations known to be exposed to risk of the event. As with other approaches, these methods can be misleading when done improperly or too hastily. The advantages and disadvantages of all of these methods will be discussed later in this chapter.

SURVEY DATA COLLECTION IN THE WAKE OF DISASTERS

Collecting information from a sample of households or individuals and making inferences about the population for which that sample is designed to be representative is well established in public health and disaster research. Survey information can be relatively quick and inexpensive to generate, and survey data can play important roles in all stages of a disaster, from estimating potential impacts beforehand to forecasting long-term impacts well afterward. Surveys can be highly variable in their mode of administration (face-to-face interviewing, phone, Internet, mail) and their scope and structure, ranging from carefully tailored one-shot interviews to multiyear longitudinal interviews to banks of questions on the national household surveys that are a cornerstone of economic and social statistical indicators. It is also true and well known that survey data collection is facing some existential crises with an increasingly reluctant-to-participate public, and that much recent attention has been trained on harnessing data from administrative records or other sources. That said, in understanding disaster impacts as in other areas of study, surveys can be an indispensable resource.

As its form of a "rapid needs assessment" in the immediate wake of a disaster, the Centers for Disease Control and Prevention (CDC, 2014) advise completion of at least one Community Assessment for Public Health

Emergency Response (CASPER), a household survey meant to provide quick situational awareness of the disaster-affected population. The CDC guidance suggests two-stage cluster sampling as the best balance of feasibility and accuracy; in this approach the geographic assessment area of interest is partitioned into non-overlapping clusters, with a sample of clusters drawn in a structured, representative way and then a sample of households drawn within each cluster. The CDC CASPER toolkit echoes the World Health Organization's (WHO's) longstanding Expanded Programme on Immunization (EPI) approach of sampling 30 clusters in the first stage and conducting interviews with 7 households in each of those clusters, numbers chosen to provide reasonable precision—where reasonable means 10 percent in absolute difference from a true underlying population percentage (of immunization coverage, in its original application) with 95 percent confidence (CDC, 2014; Henderson and Sundaresan, 1982). However, most recent CASPER guidance usefully follows Malilay et al. (1996) and reacts to other criticism of the EPI approach (Marker, 2008; Turner et al., 1996) in emphasizing the importance of proper probability sampling in the second stage. The standard EPI approach is to interview consecutively within a cluster until a quota of seven households is reached. Instead, the CASPER preferred approach is to draw 30 clusters (typically census blocks in the U.S. context, selected with probability proportional to the number of housing units in the cluster) and 7 housing units drawn within each cluster (either by quickly generating an address list through field observation and sampling from it or by systematic sampling).

Malilay (2000) reviewed eight such initial survey-based assessments in the wake of disasters that were published in the *Morbidity and Mortality Weekly Report* from 1980 to 1999 (one each following an earthquake and an ice storm, and the others describing the impact of hurricanes). This review and the capsule description of the suggested CASPER process motivate a discussion of the key advantages and disadvantages of survey methods for studying disaster effects. On the advantages side of the ledger, the number and frequency of the survey studies reinforce the fact that surveys can be a relatively quick, inexpensive, and feasible mode of data collection—and, indeed, that rapid needs assessment has become a standard and accepted part of the disaster response playbook. Malilay (2000) found that the initial assessments were typically completed within 3–10 days of the disaster (reflecting the priority on obtaining information quickly). A second major advantage of survey methods is their flexibility in content relative to available death or health records. To wit, surveys provide the capacity to elicit information on personal and family exposures to the disaster in process, on their preparation for and personal response to the disaster, on experiences with utilities and medical services in the wake of the disaster, and on differential impacts within key subpopulations such as the ill or elderly. A particular strength of survey methods in the disaster context is the ability to study significant morbidity (relatively uncovered in records-based data sources) and mental health impacts, both in the short term and (with later administrations of the survey) in the longer term. A final advantage of surveys is that the data they generate may be vitally important as a grounding or starting point for more sophisticated estimation techniques such as those discussed later in the chapter.

Survey interviewing is best suited to the collection of information on personal experience and on things that are well known to the specific respondent, such as whether a family member, friend, or acquaintance was killed, sickened, or maimed by a disaster event. The mechanics and mathematics of familiar forms of sampling such as simple random sampling, as well as more complex designs such as stratified sampling (which permit, for instance, better accounting for heterogeneity in disaster exposure by varying sampling rates by demographic groups or geographic proximity from incident center), require an accurate, detailed, and up-to-date sampling frame or a listing of eligible sample units. The precision of sample survey estimates depends in large part on the sample size that is able to be gathered as well as on the adherence to the sampling protocols.

Taken together, these basic facts are essential to understanding some key disadvantages of survey methods in disaster impact analysis:

- If survey content focuses on topics about which respondents' knowledge is limited or error-prone, the resulting statistics will not be accurate—and, logically, survey measures of mortality or causes of death are necessarily proxy information provided by surviving respondents. Members of a household may know quite precisely whether other members perished in a disaster, particularly if they saw them die or identified the bodies afterward, but their knowledge of the circumstances may be incomplete. "Verbal autopsy" survey methods (see, e.g., Thomas et al., 2018) are used in some international settings where death registration systems are limited, and survey methods may reveal individuals who are missing or unaccounted for (and so may be disaster-related deaths). Of the disaster impact surveys reviewed by Malilay (2000), only one asked about mortality within the household while nearly all asked about morbidity.
- The sampling sizes and strategies that make disaster-affected survey work feasible in disaster-affected areas are typically meant to provide reasonable precision in percentages but not necessarily in point estimates of counts. Moreover, the tragic reality is that whole households (including single-person households) may perish in major disasters, and it may be difficult or impossible to collect

information on them (or, indeed, on whole geographic areas) in the wake of a disaster. What this means is that surveys after disasters are less well suited to generating counts (and death counts in particular) than in collecting information about the characteristics of those affected. Again, as borne out in disaster-specific assessments, Malilay (2000) observed that all of the survey-based studies estimated the proportion of needs or impacts in the affected areas but none of them made the extrapolation to the magnitude/number of impacts.

- The basic cluster sampling approach suggested for CASPER (CDC, 2014) works around the need for a detailed address list by hewing to statistical units (census blocks) and values (housing unit counts within those blocks) in the first stage of sampling—but even these may have accuracy and completeness issues.
- We return to this theme at the end of the chapter but, for now, it should be noted that targeted, survey-based assessments such as CASPER can only be useful if they are actually conducted. Absent resources and support (and a clearer statement of the informational benefits) and amidst the immediate logistical turmoil of the early disaster response stage, it can be a daunting task for state and local officials to field a rigorous and well-executed survey. If these officials are the only ones enlisted in such efforts then surveys may not be done.

In short, survey methods have advantages and disadvantages and the trade-offs can be weighed when other data are available, although in some instances they may be the only viable option. In other instances, they can serve as an independent reading or as a basic check on counting, records-based approaches; indeed, this is why Kishore et al. (2018), one of the major studies of excess mortality in Puerto Rico after Hurricane Maria, based their analysis on a sample survey. This is merely to sound a note of caution in interpreting the results of sample surveys. The direct estimation of mortality through surveys is returned to later in this section, as a lead-in to discussion of other statistical methods.

Other disadvantages of survey methods focused on disaster-related mortality and morbidity are both subtle and unavoidable but can be addressed by taking care in the construction of instruments and interpretation of results. Careful attention to the rules of scientific sampling yields results that can be extrapolated, with known error bounds, to a larger population. However, it may be impossible to follow those rules to the letter in conducting surveys in the immediate wake of a disaster, and this will provide grounds to challenge the true representativeness of the sample. Among these challenges is survivor bias: the people found in a CASPER or other post-disaster survey survived the disaster and are being contacted in close proximity (spatially and temporally) to the disaster, so there is inevitably concern as to how well they represent the sub-populations that were killed by the disaster or were displaced (voluntarily or not) by the disaster. It is also well known in survey research that the specific wording of questions or instructions, their exact ordering and appearance or the way in which they are asked verbally, and the interviewer's skill (or capacity) for building rapport with a respondent can have major effects on the results. Throughout this report, several terms are encountered that can mean different things to different people, such as "disaster-related" ("direct" or otherwise) or "significant injury" (morbidity). Translating abstract concepts into short, clear questions requires significant effort. Compounding this difficulty is that in a quick response to a major disaster, survey interviewing may need to be put into relatively unpracticed hands. Survey respondents may be unwilling to engage under the best circumstances, but this can be even more so at a time when their life and property is under direct threat. Survey interviewers and the agencies fielding the surveys must also take care to ensure that the selection probabilities underlying the survey are maintained. This is not always possible, however, which means making difficult decisions on how to handle sample households or even whole clusters that are physically inaccessible after a disaster (e.g., whether to track selected survey participants to new locations or to select alternative participants). Along those lines, a survey has great flexibility in terms of its possible content, and there may be great value in longitudinal, repeated interviews after the initial humanitarian concerns have been addressed following a disaster, but the trade-offs in time and respondent burden must be made carefully.

It is instructive to return to the analogous setting of measuring casualties and injuries in war because injury and death tolls after disasters are, like those in war, sensitive subjects that are subject to political misinterpretation—underscoring the importance of transparency in constructing surveys. Hence, it should be noted that survey-based estimates of civilian casualties in war are often disputed and highly controversial. In May–July 2006, 3 years after the March 2003 invasion of Iraq, Burnham et al. (2006) conducted a cluster sample survey to estimate the number of civilian casualties. They selected 50 clusters within Iraq's governates through two stages of probability-proportional-to-population sampling, sampling a residential street within the cluster through another staged process, and interviewing adjacent households from a randomly selected starting unit until 40 households were surveyed. The survey asked questions about deaths (and births and migration) between January 2002 and June 2006 (thus permitting before/during/after invasion estimates) and about the cause of death. Between February 2007 and March 2008, the British polling firm Opinion Research Business (ORB) conducted three surveys of adults in Iraq, asking about deaths since the 2003 invasion; Heald et al. (2010) observe that ORB provided little methodological description, other than specifying that the second survey (the focus of most attention) used multistage random sampling to arrive at a sample of 1,720 adults in Iraq. In contrast to the more nuanced studies of excess mortality described in the next section, the two war death surveys used relatively simple pre- and post-comparisons and yielded estimates much larger than other sources: Burnham et al. (2006) claiming 654,965 "excess Iraqi deaths as a consequence of the war" and ORB suggesting "1.2 million murders" of civilians resulting from the invasion, later revised downward to 1 million (Heald et al., 2010). Both surveys received heavy criticism and, in the case of Burnham et al. (2006), eventual censure from the American Association for Public Opinion Research of the study's principal investigator. Marker (2008) and Laaksonen (2008) both summarize many of the critiques of Burnham et al. (2006) over lack of transparency in describing the study's methodology while the journal *Survey Research Methods* featured a detailed methodological critique of ORB's study by Heald et al. (2010) and a colloquy between those authors and ORB (Heald et al., 2010). On one hand, the two Iraq War casualty surveys are commendable for what they were able to accomplish, conducting field interviews in extremely volatile and difficult conditions. But, with an eye toward studying disaster effects, the critiques suggest that potential coverage and measurement errors should give serious pause to those considering self-report measures of household mortality and make clear the need for a more nuanced analysis than simple before-and-after comparison of estimated fatality rates.

Similar themes are invoked by the Working Group for Mortality Estimation in Emergencies (2007), which argued for further research on survey-based mortality measures; the authors argued that survey interviewers should be better equipped and trained to elicit accurate temporal recall of deaths and household-member moves. Importantly, the Working Group also argued that the EPI-type two-stage cluster survey method is too frequently used as the cheapest, simplest method without considering alternatives, such as more careful stratified sampling. Doocy et al. (2013) provide a very useful example to consider in their study of the January 12, 2010, earthquake in Haiti. One year after the earthquake, they fielded a survey in metropolitan Port-au-Prince intended to study the effects of such risk factors as basic demography, age and composition of housing, and degree of crowding on mortality in the earthquake. The study was designed to permit comparison between the neighborhood population (still in their homes) and the population residing in displacement camps. Remote sensing had been used to estimate the extent of building damage in communes/districts of Port-au-Prince, and the resulting estimates of the population in heavily damaged areas were used to proportionally allocate sampling clusters across communes. Ultimately, Doocy et al. (2013) suggested that the camp and neighborhood populations did not experience significantly different odds of death in the earthquake, but extreme crowding and residence in multilevel structures did significantly increase the risk of death.

The studies that have arguably made the best use of survey methods to estimate disaster-related effects share some important common features: they play to the strengths of survey techniques and focus less on short-term mortality impacts and more on the longer-term impacts of disasters. Importantly, they have been able to build from or extend existing data collection efforts and thus have not needed to be built fully from scratch. For example, Phifer et al. (1988) report that in the early 1980s researchers in Kentucky already had a statewide panel survey in the field, interviewing a set of older adults (55 years of age and older) at 6-month intervals between early 1981 and early 1983 regarding their health and levels of stress. Southeastern Kentucky experienced major flooding in a 10-county area in June 1981 (halfway between waves 1 and 2 of the panel survey) and again, more severely, in May 1984. The researchers were able to conduct a sixth wave, re-contacting those survey subjects who had lived in one of the 10 counties affected by the 1981 floods (plus 5 adjacent counties) and adding questions about exposure to the floods and on subjects' assessment of their personal loss. They resolved a tricky conceptual problem—how best to elicit accurate recall of the longer-ago 1981 flood relative to the fresher-in-memory 1984 flood—by developing a narrative from 1981 newspaper accounts that was read to respondents. The unusual circumstances of the Kentucky study were such that they permitted examination of possible seasonal or time-decaying effects on health measures possibly attributable to the floods, but the effect of the flood/disaster intensity could also be studied (the 1984 flooding having been more damaging than the one in 1981). Similarly, Aida et al. (2017) report that the March 11, 2011, Great East Japan Earthquake and Tsunami occurred 7 months into data collection of the major Japan Gerontological Evaluation Study (JAGES), a nationwide cohort study focused on the health and social connectedness of adults aged 65 and older. The city of Iwanuma, one of the JAGES field sites, was particularly hard hit by the earthquake and because its Tamaura district was completely inundated by the tsunami, Tamaura residents became the focus of the disaster impact study. The Aida et al. (2017) example is different from the others examined here in that the survey information provided the necessary baseline and risk factor/predictor information, but the outcome variable being studied—all-cause mortality—was derived from Japan's national long-term care insurance database, to which local physicians are required to report via their municipal governments. Among the findings from the research is that elevated mortality was associated with depressive symptoms, which might be useful to consider in conducting disaster evacuations. Another example of disaster-related survey research building from extant data collections is the set of studies that have been done on data from the World Trade Center Health Registry, itself a voluntary enrollment registry open to people who were directly exposed to the World Trade Center disaster on September 11, 2001. Enrollment in the registry required the completion of a wave 1 general health survey in 2003–2004; thereafter, registry participants were administered follow-up surveys targeted to different age groups in wave 2 (2007–2008), wave 3 (2011), and wave 4 (2015, including a separate survey related to asthma). Registry members were also able to indicate their willingness to participate in other studies and surveys, and the registry has developed into a sampling frame for researchers examining the health after-effects of September 11. Studies born from the registry as sampling frame include the Jacobson et al. (2018) analysis of posttraumatic stress disorder and depression 14–15 years after the disaster; the registry has also facilitated studies such as Jordan et al. (2018) on the risks of mortality from various causes by degrees of September 11–related exposure (e.g., firefighters relative to commuters and passers-by).

An excellent example of a survey-based disaster impact study that vitally benefited from building from a solid baseline in the form of another survey data collection is the Study of the Tsunami Aftermath and Recovery (STAR) (Frankenberg et al., 2011). On December 26, 2004, a 9.3 magnitude earthquake struck off the coast of Sumatra, Indonesia, displacing 1 trillion tons of water and spawning massive tsunami waves affecting Indian Ocean coastline areas. The combined earthquake and tsunami disaster killed on the order of 170,000 Indonesians and displaced about 750,000, most within the province of Aceh, whose western coast parallels the 1,200-kilometer undersea rupture that generated the waves.

This longitudinal survey came to fruition because the national statistics office, Statistics Indonesia, allowed a sub-sample of its 2004 National Socioeconomic Survey (known by the acronym SUSENAS) to serve as a pre-tsunami baseline. The 2004 SUSENAS, an extensive, district-representative national survey, was fielded in February/March 2004, which was 9–10 months prior to the disaster. To facilitate the collection of unique longitudinal data from respondents from both affected and unaffected communities, Statistics Indonesia provided access to its sample to a project team from U.S. universities and SurveyMETER, an Indonesian survey research institution. The STAR team drew on household rosters for all households included in SUSENAS 2004 in 11 districts of Aceh with coastlines susceptible to tsunami inundation. The STAR project conducted five follow-up interviews on a roughly annual basis beginning in 2005, a 10-year follow-up in 2015, and interviews with a sub-sample in 2017–2018. STAR researchers made extensive efforts to track all (or obtain mortality information on all) of the eligible 2004 SUSENAS respondents, wherever they had relocated to after the disaster. STAR ascertained survival status for 98 percent of the original household members and has interviewed approximately 95 percent of survivors at least once. Detailed questionnaires were administered to each individual in the household. The STAR data collection included both community-level measures of disaster exposure (based on geographic proximity to coastline, elevation, observed tsunami wave height nearest that community's shore, and satellite imagery) and individual-level measures (e.g., whether individuals had lost family members in the disaster, had helped search for survivors, or saw people struggle in the tsunami waves). Because STAR covers communities devastated by the tsunami and communities where effects were limited, the data support analyses of the evolution of morbidity and mortality outcomes over time, differentiated by exposure to the disaster.

Papers written based on the STAR data have revealed a number of key findings regarding mortality at the time of the disaster and the evolution of health in its aftermath. In the most heavily damaged communities in the sample, more than 70 percent of the population perished in the tsunami (in comparison, in unaffected communities mortality between the 2004 and 2005 survey was 1.85 percent). Young children, older adults, and prime-age women were much more likely to die than prime-age men, but mortality risks were closely related to the demographic composition of the household, whereas higher levels of socioeconomic status were not protective (Frankenberg et al., 2011). The STAR data also shed light on how mortality risks evolved in the decade after the disaster among those who survived the tsunami. The evidence points to lower risks of subsequent mortality among those from communities in which tsunami mortality was high, but also to evidence of scarring for older men who experienced high levels of posttraumatic stress and for older women who lost a spouse in the disaster (Frankenberg et al., 2020). The evidence of elevated mortality due to psychological scarring did not emerge in analyses at the 5-year mark (Ho et al., 2017). With respect to psychosocial health, exposures to traumas at the time of the tsunami were clearly linked to the emergence of posttraumatic stress reactivity (Frankenberg et al., 2008). In addition, results for C-reactive protein and waist circumference, both aspects of health known to be associated with stroke and cardiovascular disease, indicate that stressful exposures at the time of the tsunami were associated with poorer health outcomes many years later (Thomas et al., 2018).

For coronavirus disease 2019 (COVID-19), efforts are under way to use survey methods to estimate the total impact of the virus. Understanding whether surveys or counting only test-positive cases from those presenting for care more accurately describes if the outbreak in a city or state is getting better or worse can inform a number of important policy questions. As described in Appendix C, sero-prevalence surveys identify and test randomly chosen individuals to determine the percentage of people in a community recently infected with COVID-19. In early April, CDC announced that such studies were under way in some of the nation's COVID-19 hot spots and would be extended to the rest of the country in the summer (Branswell, 2020). For example, Rosenberg et al. (2020) analyzed a statewide convenience sample of New York grocery store customers and estimated that the cumulative incidence of COVID-19 through March 29, 2020, was 14 percent. This rate varied substantially by geographic area (reaching 24 percent in New York City) as well as race and ethnicity. They also estimated that only 8.9 percent of individuals infected during this period were diagnosed, and that this fraction varied from 6.1 percent of individuals age 18–34 years to 11.3 percent of those 55 years or older. A number of sero-prevalence studies are now under way (Branswell, 2020; CDC, 2020a,b) and WHO is coordinating sero-prevalence studies in at least six countries (Vogel, 2020).

ESTIMATION OF EXCESS MORTALITY OR MORBIDITY

The basic idea behind an excess mortality study is to treat some focal, precipitating event—in this circumstance, the major disaster itself—as a statistical change-point. Mortality data series are obtained that cover a time window before and at least some period after the change-point/disaster. The pre-disaster, or baseline, data are modeled in some way in order to extrapolate or project an estimate of the expected number of deaths that would have occurred absent the change-point/disaster over some forecast time period. Excess deaths are then simply the difference between the observed mortality data after the disaster and the expected values, and the argument is that these excess deaths are attributable to the disaster.

These "excess" studies are a broad class that can be approached from many possible methodological directions, as crude as testing for differences in mean levels before and after the disaster yet sophisticated enough to include intricate time-series or regression structures in the pre- and post-disaster models. Case-control or propensity-matching studies, such as those discussed by Quast (2020), are another way of addressing the same basic issue, comparing different outcomes among disaster-affected cases with those among demographically similar but not disaster-affected baseline controls. So too are difference-in-difference analyses from the econometrics literature and general statistical models that permit change-points in parameter values. In short, there is no set, standard, universally appropriate method for completing the various steps in these analyses, and different approaches and sets of assumptions can yield different conclusions. Indeed, it is the resulting variety of estimates arising from excess mortality studies conducted in Puerto Rico in the wake of Hurricane Maria in September 2017 that was a major impetus for establishing this committee.

Excess mortality studies are tailored to estimate the volume of all deaths that are potentially attributable to the disaster, including those (in the committee's schema) that are indirectly or partially attributable and that may not be explicitly linked with the disaster in death records; that is, these studies are expressly intended to measure that which is not directly measurable. Moreover, the methodology depends critically on a loosely implied but unproven causal relationship that the detected excess deaths resulted from the disaster. In light of these major intangible factors, what keeps excess mortality studies from lapsing into post hoc ergo propter hoc fallacy is care in specification and documentation of assumptions. The credibility of excess mortality studies hinges on, among other factors:

- The quality, completeness, and sourcing of the pre- and post-disaster mortality data series;
- The care with which the baseline, pre-disaster mortality is measured and the resulting confidence that may be had in projecting expected death rates (absent the disaster) into the future;
- The degree to which the derivation of the baseline accounts for potential confounding factors and thus bolsters the claim that an excess is due to the disaster alone; confounding factors can include gross seasonal trends in the data, the differential presence of particularly vulnerable sub-populations in the study area (i.e., by age, sex, or proximity to the disaster), and the migration/displacement of the population;
- The length of the time window over which post-disaster events are studied, balancing the necessary tension between having too short a time window (some time is required for the events to manifest in the data) and too long a window (in which case the validity of projecting the expected, baseline levels would decay, straining the argument that all excess is truly disaster-related)—while recognizing that virtually any choice in window length will miss some events (such as injuries or disaster-exacerbated chronic conditions that ultimately result in death); and
- The extent to which the work is rigorously validated by assessing alternative counterfactuals/baselines or considering whether effects apply differently to different demographic groups.

In the balance of this section, some major exemplars of these excess mortality studies in the disaster arena are described, focusing on their handling of these design features. It should also be noted that the review in this section speaks exclusively about "excess mortality" because mortality has featured more prominently in the related literature to date than morbidity effects. Some studies have examined relevant cause-specific mortality (e.g., myocardial infarction or pneumonia) to permit some glimpse of possible disaster-related morbidity-leading-to-mortality effects and some studies have examined exposure-related morbidity effects in longer-term disasters (e.g., exposure to smoke and particulates in the wake of wildfires). That said, the classic pre- and post-disaster modeling, and derivation of estimates of excess death, should not be extended to examine the incidence of disaster-related significant morbidity in its own right.

This report has already described the high variation in estimated mortality counts in Puerto Rico following Hurricane Maria, which made landfall on the island on September 20, 2017. The following brief review highlights the choices made by various researchers in modeling excess deaths attributable to the storm. First as a preprint and soon revised as a note in the *Journal of the American Medical Association*, Santos-Lozada and Howard (2017, 2018) compiled vital statistics data on all deaths by month in Puerto Rico for 2010–2017, calculating a mean and 95 percent confidence interval for the observations for each calendar month (i.e., for all of the January counts, all of the February counts and so forth). Santos-Lozada and Howard (2018) recognized that major migration from Puerto Rico before the storm would have reduced the underlying population denominators, but they did not expressly account for that mobility in their analysis. Instead, they compensated in part by being conservative in calculating the excess, subtracting the upper 95 percent confidence bound from the observed all-cause death counts for September–November 2017 rather than the historical mean for the months. Santos-Lozada and Howard (2018) estimated 1,139 excess deaths for September–December 2017 that they argued were hurricane-related, substantially higher than the then-official death toll of 64 stipulated by the Puerto Rico government.

A report by Kishore et al. (2018), published in the *New England Journal of Medicine* and colloquially called the Harvard study, opted to construct a mortality estimate independent of Puerto Rico's death registration records, pending review of the quality of construction of those records following the hurricane. In January–February 2018, the researchers fielded a survey with a final sample size of 3,299 households—a survey involving some distinctive design and operational choices relative to conventional household surveys or those mortality/morbidity surveys described in the previous section. Puerto Rico's 900 barrios (administrative units used as clusters) were stratified into 8 categories based on values of a "remoteness index," measuring the road travel time to the nearest large city (50,000 population or more). Within each remoteness stratum, 13 barrios were chosen at random (adding 1 sampled barrio from each of the island municipalities of Vieques and Culebra); then, within each sampled barrio, 35 buildings or structures reported on available OpenStreetMap layers were selected. Whenever an interviewer visited a sampled structure location and could not complete a household interview—whether the structure was not a residence, the household declined to be interviewed, or no person was present at the time of the visit—interviewers were directed to pick at random "from all surrounding visible houses" and try to interview there. The survey questionnaire also differed from some conventional norms, including the rostering of household members. Many household surveys develop a household roster and then use that roster as reference or guide through the other survey questions; the Harvard survey asked about "each household member, including all persons who had moved in, moved out, been born, or died in 2017" but simultaneously did not record "any personal identifiers," leaving it unclear whether all pertinent questions were asked about each identified household member in turn or whether the interview looped through deaths and moves separately. (This is not to suggest any fault in the method but merely to mention one of the small contextual choices that are critical in survey practice.) The survey also asked about the number of deaths in the neighborhood (Kishore et al., 2018). Mortality rates for September 20–December 31, 2017, were estimated from the survey, with excess rates calculated relative to the official vital statistics death rate for the same date range in 2016; the researchers justified that choice by observing that the vital statistics mortality rates "showed seasonal but stable trends from 2010 through 2016" (Kishore et al., 2018). Ultimately, the Harvard research team would estimate 4,645 excess deaths attributable to Maria through the end of 2017—albeit with a 95 percent confidence interval of 793–8,498. Though the study would draw criticism for yielding too high an estimate of excess mortality and its large error bands, the authors conjectured that their estimate was likely an underestimate due to survivor bias and the conceptual difficulties noted in the previous section in estimating mortality in a survey. Logically, households in which there were no survivors (including single-person households) could not be included in the survey; hence, adjusting their rates using the 2016 vital statistics mortality rate in single-person households, Kishore et al. (2018) suggested that the true excess-death count could be 5,740 (95 percent confidence interval, 1,506–9,889).

The government of Puerto Rico commissioned the Milken Institute School of Public Health at The George Washington University (GWU) to conduct three studies related to deaths in Hurricane Maria, one component of which was an independent review of excess mortality attributed to the hurricane. The excess mortality portion of the broader GWU study is detailed in both the project's standalone report (GWU Milken Institute School of Public Health, 2018) and an article in *The Lancet Planetary Health* (Santos-Burgoa et al., 2018) and, importantly, has gone on to be accepted by Puerto Rico authorities as the official death toll for the commonwealth. The GWU study used all-cause mortality data by age, sex, and residential municipality in monthly time series from July 2010 through February 2018 as its source of mortality data. A subtle innovation made in the GWU study was setting the end point as the end of February 2018—a longer study period, over which estimated excess deaths are posited to be due to Hurricane Maria—than other studies. But the hallmark of the GWU study is the care and rigor with which the baseline, pre-disaster models were calculated. The data were grouped/stratified by age (three categories), sex, and a three-category breakout of a Municipal Socioeconomic Development Index used by the Puerto Rico Planning Board. The study team fit over-dispersed log-linear regression models to the July 2010–August 2017 data and ultimately assessed four different specifications of model interaction terms for each of two different methods for modeling seasonal and long-term trends before selecting a final form. Moreover, when projecting forward trends for September 2017–February 2018 against which to calculate excess deaths, Santos-Burgoa et al. (2018) compared a so-called "census counterfactual" (using U.S. Census Bureau population estimates for Puerto Rico) to a "displacement counterfactual." This approach decremented the population based on air travel data from the U.S. Bureau of Transportation Statistics and the Puerto Rico Planning Board to account for mass migration off the island. Ultimately, the researchers would conclude that the mobility effects were too substantial to ignore and accepted the displacement counterfactual. For comparison with the other researchers, Santos-Burgoa et al. (2018) estimated 2,098 excess deaths between September–December 2017, but the 2,975 excess deaths estimated through February 2018 is what has become accepted as the official toll in Puerto Rico. Shortly after the publication of Santos-Burgoa et al. (2018), Howard and Santos-Lozada (2019) would replicate their basic approach described above using the GWU team's compiled data, arguing that the displacement approach (subtracting out-mobility) overstates the mortality rate too much and makes the 2,975 estimate too high; in a rejoinder, Santos-Burgoa et al. (2019) reiterated their conclusion that failing to account for massive outmigration is itself a major bias.

In a more recent addition to the Hurricane Maria excess mortality literature, Cruz-Cano and Mead (2019) tightened the forecasting range, estimating excess mortality levels for only the months of September and October 2017. They fit a standard autoregressive integrated moving average (ARIMA) time-series model to monthly mortality rates from January 2008 to August 2017, themselves obtained from official vital statistics for Puerto Rico, thus exploiting the capacity of ARIMA models to capture broad time trends and seasonal effects. In addition to the time-series methodology, though, the Cruz-Cano and Mead (2019) analysis is distinctive for replicating the work for specific causes of death in an attempt to identify causes of death that may have been particularly exacerbated by the hurricane. Their overall estimate of 1,205 excess deaths for September–October 2017 is consistent with the GWU study's estimate of 1,271. The causes of death for which particularly strong excesses were detected included heart disease (253 deaths) and diabetes (195 deaths), along with a catch-all "other" causes (204 deaths), the chronic conditions suggesting that these might be death types where the hurricane indirectly contributed to the death by hindering access to regular treatment.

One particularly notable excess mortality study not focusing on Hurricane Maria and Puerto Rico was Morita et al. (2017), who investigated the after-effects of the triple disaster that struck Fukushima Prefecture, Japan, in 2011. On March 11, 2011, the Great East Japan Earthquake spawned a major tsunami in the Fukushima area; the earthquake had already caused internal electrical failure at the Fukushima Daiichi Nuclear Power Plant, and the tsunami waters inundated the plant and disabled the emergency generators, leading to multiple nuclear meltdowns and radioactive contamination between March 12–15, 2011, and forcing a wide evacuation zone around the plant. Mortality data for two cities in the prefecture for 2006–2015 (allowing for a very long 4-year post-disaster reaction period) were obtained from the nation's vital registration system, and Poisson regression models were fitted to the data (separately for each month from January through December in turn, as a check on seasonal effects). But the remarkable aspect of this triple-disaster response study was its embrace of the methodology's basic purpose to study the effects of indirect disaster-related deaths—to the extent that Morita et al. (2017) explicitly subtracted out direct disaster-related deaths before calculating the relative risks. Specifically, the researchers subtracted out numerous external-cause death types from the data for March 2011 that were likely due to the direct physical forces of the disaster, categories such as head injuries, burns and corrosions of multiple body regions, and any death that may have been coded as being "due to exposure to forces of nature;" deaths listed as being caused by drowning on March 11, presumably due to the tsunami, were also excluded (Morita et al., 2017). Though the lengthy time series permitted examination of both short- and long-term indirect health impacts, Morita et al. (2017) found that the estimated excess in indirect disaster-related deaths was concentrated in the first month following the disaster.

Not all studies that use the "excess deaths" nomenclature follow this pattern, but they adopt some unique approaches that are noteworthy nonetheless. An example of reconceptualizing the problem is the analysis by Kim et al. (2017) of excess mortality associated with Hurricane Sandy in New Jersey. The hurricane having made landfall in New Jersey on October 29, 2012, Kim et al. (2017) defined two post-disaster study periods of interest, the "Sandy month" (October 28, 2012–November 27, 2012) and the "Sandy quarter" (October 28, 2012–January 27, 2013). Obtaining mortality data from the state's electronic death registration system, the researchers aggregated deaths into monthly counts (months beginning on the 28th day of each calendar month). Negative binomial regression models were used to estimate death rates. The unique approach of this study was to study relative risks, the ratio of, for example, "Sandy month" to the corresponding month (October 28–November 27) across the years 2008–2011; the estimated relative risks were adjusted for seasonality and time trends based on the modeled rates for the pre-study period (the 11 months preceding "Sandy month") versus the pre-comparison period (the same 11 months across the years 2008–2011). Kim et al. (2017) performed separate analyses for all-cause mortality as well as analyses of some specific cause-of-death groups, and for the elderly separate from other ages, and they found consistent elevated risks in the Sandy-affected periods (though all-cause mortality excesses were statistically significant only for the "Sandy quarter," not the "Sandy month").

Another example of an atypical excess mortality–type study in the disaster context arose from work following Hurricane Katrina in August 2005. Noting the then-considerable delays in death reporting in greater New Orleans in Katrina's wake, Stephens et al. (2007) asked whether counts of death notices in the region's main newspaper (the *Times-Picayune*) might plausibly serve as a surveillance indicator for changing mortality trends. However, the study was mainly about whether death notice counts roughly correlated with historic death record totals and focused principally on death notice counts between January and June 2006, which themselves were considerably time-lagged relative to the disaster, rather than trying to estimate the extent of elevated mortality potentially attributable to Katrina. Still, the Stephens et al. (2007) study is distinctive for its attempt to use and corroborate a novel data resource—and for its lack of hubris in portraying its findings, emphasizing the preliminary and limited nature of the work.

A slightly different group of excess mortality–type studies is somewhat atypical in nature because the underlying natural disasters—heat waves and extreme temperature exposure—can develop and have intense effects over a more gradual time period than other disaster types. The exploratory data analysis of Henschel et al. (1969) on a July 1966 heat wave in St. Louis, Missouri, was an early entrant in the field, not positing any formal models but more bluntly examining spatial differences in deaths and recorded temperatures in parts of the region. Since 1969, studies of mortality in heat waves have grown more sophisticated in the ways that they try to control for demographic confounding effects (i.e., at-home deaths among the elderly) or for features of the built environment that may have major effects (e.g., housing conditions, locations of residences on upper floors of buildings). Further examples include Eisenman et al. (2016), Harduar Morano et al. (2016), Joe et al. (2016), Petitti et al. (2013), Vandentorren et al. (2006), and Zhang et al. (2017). The extreme heat waves that affected France in August 2003 (as well as in 2006 and 2009) have inspired a variety of studies on their own, including Pascal et al. (2012). Pascal et al. (2018) modeled the relationship between mortality and temperature in 18 French cities, with observations spanning 2000–2010, using a quasi-Poisson distribution and building other traditional confounding factors (e.g., population density and the percentage of the population age 75 and older) into their model. Accordingly, it stands as an intensive analysis of important baseline trends in mortality over time. Pascal et al. (2012) was a retrospective study to see whether daily changes in a set of candidate indicators (total mortality being one, but also including emergency room visits)—if available at the time of the less than severe 2006 and 2009 heat waves in France—might have shown enough excess activity (relative to values experienced in previous years, within some time window around the particular date) to trigger a "statistical alarm," and how the timing of those coincided with warnings of extreme warming from weather forecasts. Ultimately, Pascal et al. (2012) found that none of the chosen health indicators could have performed this early warning function well, even if they had existed in real time, though they still noted important trends in the potential indicators to analyze in broader scope following the heat waves.

As described in more detail in Appendix C, excess mortality analyses have played a prominent role in COVID-19. One method applied is an extension of CDC's standard method for determining the annual death toll for influenza. CDC regularly tracks the number of deaths from either pneumonia or influenza as a proportion of all deaths recorded each week, and these data are compared with typical seasonal patterns and departures above this pattern. CDC added COVID-19 deaths to this analysis and found that almost 25 percent of all deaths occurring during the week ending April 11, 2020, were due to pneumonia, influenza, or COVID-19. This is far above the traditional epidemic threshold of 7.0 percent, with sharp weekly increases from the end of February through mid-April (CDC, 2020b).

Efforts to use excess mortality methods to estimate the total number of deaths due to COVID-19 are under way. In an analysis originally published in *The Washington Post*,[1] Weinberger et al. (2020) conducted a similar analysis for the entire United States from March 1–May 30, 2020. They estimated that there were 122,300 more deaths than would typically be expected at that time of year, 28 percent higher than the official tally of COVID-19-reported deaths during that period. Woolf et al. (2020) analyzed mortality between March 1 and April 25, 2020, and estimated 87,001 excess deaths nationally, of which 65 percent were attributed to COVID-19.

[1] See https://www.washingtonpost.com/investigations/2020/04/27/covid-19-death-toll-undercounted/?arc404=true (accessed September 1, 2020).

The authors also identified substantial increases in mortality from heart disease, diabetes, and other causes, but few from pneumonia or influenza as underlying causes (Woolf et al., 2020).

One of the challenges in analyzing mortality data in real time is that deaths are reported weeks after the decedent was infected. In their COVID-19 excess mortality study, Weinberger et al. (2020) accounted for this by inflating reported deaths using weekly estimates of reporting delays. Reporting delays also are a problem for measures such as the case fatality rate that are derived from mortality data: at any given time, cases are more completely reported than deaths, so a simple ratio of deaths to cases will be biased downward. A not-yet-peer-reviewed analysis by members of a Centre for the Mathematical Modelling of Infectious Diseases working group on COVID-19[2] describes the adjustment of Russell et al. (2020) to account for this phenomenon and illustrates its impact.

SPECIALIZED METHODS FOR MEASURING HARD-TO-COUNT OR HIDDEN POPULATIONS

The full set of deaths or significant morbidities related to a disaster includes those incidences that are only indirectly related or partially attributable to the disaster as well as those that may be incorrectly noted as disaster-related in official records; these can be conceptualized as a "hidden finite set," or a hidden or hard-to-count population. That is, borrowing nomenclature from the review of the literature by Cheng et al. (2020, p. 1), it is a set whose "elements are not directly enumerable or [its] size cannot be ascertained via a deterministic query." Over the years, a wide array of techniques for estimating the size of such hidden sets have emerged and been widely used in a number of disciplines, including public health and epidemiology. Not all of these techniques, discussed briefly in this section, have been applied in the specific context of disaster impact and recovery, but to the extent that things like "people who died as an indirect result of a disaster" or "people who have various morbidities and co-morbidities" are hard-to-count populations, the techniques are methods that might be brought to bear in future disaster studies. Cheng et al. (2020) discuss these and other methodologies for estimating hidden populations, adopting common notation and focusing attention on the asymptotic properties of related estimators, in addition to citing their use in a wide array of substantive settings.

We particularly note three broad methods, following a hierarchy presented by McCormick (2020). Given interest in a hidden population (say,

---

[2] See https://cmmid.github.io/topics/covid19/global_cfr_estimates.html (accessed September 1, 2020).

disaster-affected individuals) for which there is no complete sampling frame (by definition), the next question is whether it is feasible or necessary to access the affected individuals directly. If not, and if indirect access would suffice, then the *network scale-up* method (NSUM) would be appropriate. On the other hand, if it is possible to access the affected individuals directly, then *capture–recapture* methods or *respondent-driven sampling* might be useful choices.

NSUM, which was introduced by Bernard et al. (1991) in early form, advanced in fuller form by Killworth et al. (1998), and summarized in the Bernard et al. (2010) overview paper, is a notable exception to other techniques listed here in that its first major application was actually in the context of assessing disaster impact—in that case, estimating the true number of deaths in the September 19, 1985, earthquake that struck Mexico City. NSUM is one of a class of methods that uses some implicit structuring within the hidden set to arrive at an adjusted estimate for the hidden population size. As the name implies, the particular structuring assumed by NSUM is based on a survey respondent's personal/social network size. For instance, survey respondents in the original Bernard et al. (1991) analysis were asked questions about how many members of five sub-populations (doctors, mailmen, bus drivers, television repairmen, and priests) they know—and how many victims of the earthquake they knew. The collected information can be used to estimate personal network size whether the true sub-population sizes are known (in the first Mexico City example, the numbers of workers in each of the five occupations was known) or unknown, in which case the queries turn to better-known but ideally mutually exclusive relationship categories (e.g., family, coworkers). The estimated network sizes for the designated sub-populations are reconciled with the network information on the phenomenon of interest (here, earthquake victims) to estimate a prevalence rate for and, in turn, the size of the hidden population. NSUM is applicable—and has been used—in many substantive settings, even though it does suffer some important shortcomings, as summarized by Bernard et al. (2010). Among these shortcomings are the assumptions that the survey respondents have accurate knowledge of the characteristics of people in their personal network circles (e.g., whether or not a contact has HIV/AIDS, if that is the hidden population trait of interest) and that they are willing to report that information accurately even if the target characteristic is particularly sensitive or stigmatizing. But, still, NSUM does have some distinct advantages, not least of which is that—being an indirect estimator—information is gathered from a basic probability sample of the general population and does not require resource-intensive searches for specific individuals or full sampling frames for (by definition) hard-to-enumerate groups. The survey questions necessary to perform NSUM analysis are simultaneously a benefit and a challenge: they can be rendered in such a way as to be relatively quick and easy to administer (and so may be easily slotted into a new or ongoing survey data collection), but they also assume that different respondents will interpret and assess what it means to "know" someone in the same way. Feehan and Salganik (2016) suggest a generalized scale-up estimator that is intended to curb some issues with normal NSUM (such as the imperfect knowledge of contacts' membership in the hidden population), but with a major departure: the generalized scale-up estimator requires samples from both the general/frame population and also the hidden population itself.

A longstanding methodology for estimating the size of hard-to-count sub-populations is *capture–recapture*, which takes its name from its original application area in wildlife studies. To estimate the number of fish in a pond, for instance, a sample of fish would be caught, tagged, and released back into the pond. On a return visit—sufficiently close in time that the composition within the pond would not be expected to change greatly—another sample of fish is collected and the number of tagged and untagged fish is recorded. Because the composition of the second sample should be proportional to the composition of the population as a whole, inference can be made about the total population size based on the two samples. The resulting *dual-systems estimation* methodology has become one of the principal ways in which the coverage of the U.S. decennial census is evaluated; an independently administered, carefully stratified follow-up survey is fielded and the results matched to a similarly carefully designed extract of census returns for the same sample areas, and the match rates between the two independent samples permit estimates of the undercount (or overcount) in the census. The capture–recapture or multiple systems estimation approach could be used in relatively pure form to estimate the true size of disaster-affected populations, though it stands to reason that (as discussed earlier in the chapter) if collecting one good sample survey in the context of a major disaster is difficult, collecting two or more (and properly accounting for mobility or shifts in population) would be even more so.

Finally, *respondent-driven sampling* (RDS) was inspired by the desire for methods to directly sample—exclusively—from some hidden population of interest. Particularly for hidden populations characterized by stigmatized or illegal behavior, studies have often had to resort to snowball or chain-referral sampling: on finding and completing a survey with a single member of the target, hidden population (the "seed"), the researchers then ask the person to name others in the population who might be interviewed. Then, each other person who completed the survey is asked to name others, and so on. Snowball sampling lacks grounding in effective probability sampling, and RDS, introduced by Heckathorn (1997, 2002) solves that problem.

Although the National Science Foundation (NSF) approves research that employs snowball sampling (NSF, 2020) some people recommended by the initial seed in a snowball sample may not want to be identified as a member of that particular hard-to-find or hard-to-count population. RDS solves that problem, too. RDS begins by finding a small number of subjects (members of the target hidden population) who are recruited to serve as "seeds." Upon completing the interview, the seeds are offered an incentive to recruit their peers (other members of the hidden population) into the survey. The new recruits, on arriving at the interview, are offered the chance to become new seeds and are thus doubly incentivized, both to complete the interview and to recruit new people from their personal networks. Sampling continues like this until the target sample size is reached or the recruit population is exhausted. The innovation made by Heckathorn (1997, p. 176) was in proving that the samples resulting from this process "are *independent of the initial subjects from which sampling begins*"—so that ultimately, it does not matter that the initial selection of seeds was a convenience sample. Implemented as instructed, the recruitment process can be treated as a Markov process, ultimately resulting in the surprising result of independence from the initial sample. In building the sample, it is critical to the calculations that key data items be recorded along with the survey—the coupon number returned by the recruit, which permits determination of who recruited whom, and the degree of each respondent (the stage at which the recruit entered the sample and, correspondingly, how many downstream recruits for whom they were ultimately responsible). Baraff et al. (2016), Green et al. (2020), and Raftery (2020) discuss a novel approach (a version of the bootstrap that preserves the tree structure of the seed/recruit process) for computing the variance of estimators from RDS data.

As another general approach along these lines, Bao et al. (2015)—and Raftery (2020) in his presentation to the committee—advocated a *Bayesian hierarchical model* as a potentially ideal form for estimating the size of hard-to-count populations, illustrating their proposal with a model intended to estimate the count of intravenous drug users in Bangladesh in 2004. The hierarchical model yielded both local and national estimates, and permitted the integration of "mapping data, surveys, interventions, capture-recapture data, estimates or guesstimates from organizations, and expert opinion" in an integrated framework (Bao et al., 2015, p. 125).

Johnston et al. (2015), for example, nested the same seed/recruit information and structure in a Bayesian framework, thus incorporating prior knowledge and approximations of the population size to yield a method called successive sampling–population size estimation. They applied the method to estimate sensitive and hard-to-count populations in six cities in Morocco, among them intravenous drug users and migrants from sub-Saharan Africa; Handcock et al. (2014) validated that approach by using it to estimate the size of known networked populations in the data files of the National Longitudinal Study of Adolescent to Adult Health, and Johnston et al. (2017) later applied the technique to estimate the number of women with sexual violence-related pregnancies in a province in the Democratic Republic of the Congo. Crawford et al. (2018) borrowed from the theoretical underpinnings of the network scale-up method and analyzed the tree/network structure generated by respondent-driven sampling using graph theory principles to generate a different take on estimating the number of intravenous drug users in St. Petersburg, Russia.

The field of estimation techniques for hidden and hard-to-count populations is developing quickly and will continue to improve—that is, make increasingly accurate estimates—as systematic research is applied on refining and improving the methodology. Feehan and Salganik's (2016) generalized NSUM offered conceptual advantages relative to the original. Other research has examined technical improvements to the base NSUM approach, including Habecker et al. (2015) and Maghsoudi et al. (2014). More recently, Verdery et al. (2019) combined elements of RDS (link tracing within respondent networks) and Feehan and Salganik's (2016) generalized NSUM to estimate the size of some sub-populations at risk of HIV/AIDS—all in the context of venue-based sampling (or time–space sampling), in which it is assumed that the target hard-to-count population tends to cluster in identifiable locations that can be sampled in meaningful ways. Much work remains to be done on venue-based sampling, but, just as with the other methods described in this section, systematic research on it promises improvements or efficiencies relative to currently used cluster sampling estimates.

COMMON ISSUES RELATED TO ESTIMATION TECHNIQUES

In its review of statistical estimation techniques for disaster-related mortality and significant morbidity, the committee reviewed the literature and, to supplement and close the review, hosted two public webinars on February 11 and 18, 2020, to gather input related to several of the studies and techniques (see Chapter 1). In particular, it invited several participants in the major research projects to summarize their work and offer their own thoughts on best practices (Ho, 2020; Irizarry, 2020; McCormick, 2020; Quast, 2020; Raftery, 2020; Zeger, 2020).

The main message derived from this review is that, in the measurement of disaster-related effects, as is true of virtually any area of scientific endeavor, there is not, nor can there be, a single universally correct or standard method for generating mortality or morbidity estimates. Instead, given the variation in ways for attributing the cause of any death and morbidity, there can be more than one appropriate approach to answering the question: "How many deaths and severe morbidities were caused by this disaster?" Just as with counting approaches, all of the estimation approaches described in this chapter make assumptions and are subject to bias. Accordingly, the best practices that can be specified for estimating disaster impacts are the same best practices that apply to research in general: (1) clarity in the specification of study objectives and definition of terms, (2) transparency in the statement of assumptions and the sourcing of data used in the study, (3) continued testing and improvement of the accuracy of measures, and (4) caution in advancing any particular measure or method as the single perfect solution. Any statistical indicator reflects a specific time period and geographic area, reflects a particular set of death or morbidity causes, and so forth, and the research should clearly specify these limits. Similar conclusions are drawn by Quarantelli (2001) in discussing high-level conceptual problems in disaster studies.

The preliminary needs assessment from CASPER-type surveys aside, the methods described in this chapter are generally retrospective and take time to implement well. Indeed, excess mortality studies only become possible and meaningful after some time has elapsed and post-disaster mortality data are available. Accordingly, these estimation techniques are not meant to be predictive indicators and are unlikely to be able to provide direct insight in the early disaster response phase, given how tightly focused natural disasters tend to be in space and time. But, with time to develop and care in specification, the estimation techniques are very useful in assessing the total impact of disasters and in planning for future disasters. In addition, the estimation methods described in this chapter can also provide more detail than case counts in terms of demographic and other disparities, types of illness and injuries experienced, and specific causes of death.

While the adoption of a standardized, universally applicable method for estimating the mortality and significant morbidity effects of major disasters is not recommended, there is value in some degree of standardization so that, as much as possible, observed differences reflect substantive differences rather than arbitrary methodological choices. Therefore, this suggests that there are very important avenues for information sharing and cultivation of best practices among researchers and state, local, tribal, and territorial (SLTT) disaster and public health officials for developing estimates and communicating them.

The field would benefit from a research program that begins with a discussion of advantages and disadvantages and a documentation of researchers' and policy makers' experience with choices that have worked particularly well (or not) in the past. Many of the estimates in the literature result from one-off efforts that do not build on or seek comparability with previous disasters. The first step in this research agenda requires that there be a careful comparison of different estimates from the same emergency to gain an understanding of how methodological choices and assumptions affect the estimates (see Recommendation 4-1).

This research program should consider such factors as:

- *Spatiotemporal boundaries of the study*—including the start and end of the study/disaster period, balancing the capacity to measure immediate/short-term/longer-term effects with respondents' or data providers' ability for accurate recall, as well as the precise geographic area being studied;
- Specification of a *comparison period or comparison population, or the handling of confounding or seasonal structure in the data*, for setting an appropriate counterfactual and bolstering the ability to argue that the estimated effects are attributable to the disaster;
- Determination of an accurate *sampling frame or an appropriate baseline* or careful elaboration of data collection protocols that ensure that the probabilities of selection and the assumptions underpinning accurate inference are adequately met;
- Development of *appropriate standard survey questionnaires* (and associated training materials) to promote consistency and comparability of results; and
- Crafting *appropriate statistical models* and documenting the results.

It has come up several times already but bears repeating: it is essential to develop *effective means of characterizing migration and population displacement* before, during, and in the immediate wake of the disaster, not only for estimation purposes but also to accurately calculate meaningful population rates.

In general, all of these estimation techniques rely on accurate and appropriate baseline, contextual data. Many of the techniques rely on vital records or vital statistics data—for example, the counting-based methods described in Chapter 3—so it is certainly true that improving the counting-type mortality and morbidity data is important to improving the quality of the estimates that use them. But an effective baseline for estimation techniques is broader than just these incident data. It includes data from the U.S. decennial census and the American Community Survey (ACS; the successor, since the 2010 census, to the census "long form" sample covering more detailed socioeconomic questions), other major federal surveys (such as the Current Population Survey and the National Health Interview Survey), and the growing array of administrative records-type data being compiled at the federal and state levels. Solid baseline data are essential in all of these estimation methods for a variety of purposes—to set denominators so that rates might be compared across time and geography, to reconstruct population as it was at the moment of disaster impact, to understand the sociodemographic characteristics of the disaster-affected population, to identify sampling frames for contact with survivors, and so forth. In this chapter, some of the more successful survey-based measures of disaster impacts documented had a strong *operational* baseline in that they were able to build from existing data resources, most notably the STAR tracking study that developed from (and inherited its representativeness from) a major Indonesian socioeconomic survey.

Accordingly, going forward, it will be useful to consider ways to nurture developments along several fronts related to the provision of both baseline and analytical data. First, the utility for disaster research of custom tabulation/estimation tools such as the Census Bureau's OnTheMap for Emergency Management,[3] which generates results from the ACS and other federal data sources for Federal Emergency Management Agency (FEMA)-designated disaster areas, and the CDC Wide-ranging ONline Data for Epidemiologic Research data portal should be examined. Second, it would be feasible (though very difficult at present) to replicate the STAR/Indonesia experience in the U.S. system, drawing on a federal household survey sample to implement a longitudinal survey of affected and comparison populations. Still, options for the better use of federal and state data resources should be examined; akin to the question modules and "pulse surveys" now being fielded by the Census Bureau in response to the COVID-19 epidemic, the capacity to add a module to an ongoing survey (to spark post-disaster data collection) or provisions for oversampling in disaster-affected areas (to be able to provide more area-specific survey estimates) on a short-term basis should be explored. The development of effective baseline data may also include exploring opportunities to use alternative and emerging data sources, such as cell phone location records and other administrative data, in ways that derive benefit from the new data resources while managing privacy and confidentiality concerns.

Developing an effective data and information structure for studying disaster impacts is not a basic research activity: it has immediate application value. It is and should be a cornerstone of the nation's operational disaster response function. It requires participation from actors in all levels of government as well as from outside government. To wit, some summary points:

- Research on analytical methods, based on the experience of past disasters, is essential to support good analytical choices in future disaster research. Research along these lines could be brokered by, among others, the National Institutes of Health (NIH) (as through

[3] See https://onthemap.ces.census.gov/em (accessed June 10, 2020).

the Biostatistical Methods and Research Design Study Section[4]) and NSF (as through the Methodology, Measurement, and Statistics Program).[5]

- The degree of analytical sophistication and the requirements for detailed data analysis and high-quality fieldwork are generally beyond the capabilities and time availability of most SLTT health departments—particularly in the immediate wake of a major disaster. Accordingly, it would be useful for CDC (perhaps through its Epidemic Intelligence Service), the Assistant Secretary for Preparedness and Response, and FEMA to pursue "jump teams" that might be brought in early in the disaster response cycle to supplement SLTT resources, helping to gather data and (importantly) begin the detailed analyses. Such practiced jump teams would help manage data collection in such a way as to not get in the way of first responders. Personnel in the National Disaster Medical System or Medical Reserve Corps could be part of these teams; the work could also be regionalized and partially accomplished with standing memoranda of understanding with epidemiology institutes and academic departments.
- Critical operational support is needed from federal agencies including the identification of appropriate mortality and morbidity datasets that might be brought to bear and pre-negotiation of data-sharing agreements to ensure access to these data when needed. As mentioned earlier, part of this operational support involves finding ways to use existing federal survey and data collection infrastructure, including identifying ongoing data collection programs to which disaster questionnaire modules could be piggy-backed (with appropriate adaption).
- Some of the survey procedures and data analyses suggested, particularly if building on data previously gathered for other purposes, may appear to conflict with consent procedures under the Common Rule, which guides human subject research, respondent burden issues under the Paperwork Reduction Act, which governs clearance of federal information collections, and the Health Insurance Portability and Accountability Act (HIPAA) Privacy Rule, which protects individual health information. While the committee believes that the public health benefits of accurate estimates of the mortality and morbidity effects of a disaster outweigh these concerns, it is useful to address these issues in advance and to ensure alternative arrangements (such as data disclosure rules in place at SLTT health departments) to protect privacy and confidentiality.

---

[4] See https://public.csr.nih.gov/StudySections/DABP/PSE/BMRD (accessed June 10, 2020).
[5] See https://www.nsf.gov/funding/pgm_summ.jsp?pims_id=5421 (accessed June 10, 2020).

Cultivating regional centers of excellence—possibly virtual in format, and possibly borrowing from CDC's previous experience in funding Preparedness and Emergency Response Learning Centers that paired academic institutions with SLTT officials—could be a useful step in facilitating many of these steps. A previous National Academies of Sciences, Engineering, and Medicine committee, tasked with the problem of deriving best practices for measuring community resilience to disasters, offered analogous guidance (NASEM, 2019). Concluding that there is no single, best measurement applicable to all communities and all elements of "resilience," that committee urged the development of a "resilience learning collaborative" in the Gulf of Mexico region, drawing together a variety of government, industry, academic, and nonprofit actors to coordinate measurement efforts and implement ongoing research (NASEM, 2019). This type of model may be useful to consider relative to the whole disaster cycle, not just resilience.

CONCLUSIONS AND RECOMMENDATIONS

Disasters are complex, so their health consequences are multifactorial, and no single number can sufficiently describe their impact. Because there can be more than one appropriate approach to answering the question "How many deaths and significant morbidities were caused by this disaster?" there cannot be a universally correct or standard method for generating mortality or morbidity estimates. While "estimation" might sound less precise than "counting," which is described in Chapters 2 and 3, methods used for counting provide imprecise results, which predictably undercount the total impact of disasters, especially with regard to specific sub-populations. While statistical estimation methods cannot determine whether any given dead or ill person died or became ill as a direct or indirect result of the disaster, those methods can generate a more complete picture of the total impact of the disaster on health outcomes.

In addition, excess mortality studies only become possible and meaningful after some time has elapsed and post-disaster mortality data are available. Accordingly, the estimation techniques discussed in this chapter are unlikely to be able to provide direct insight in the early disaster response phase. However, with time to gather data and develop proper specifications, the estimation techniques are useful in assessing the total impact of disasters and in planning for future disasters.

While there is no standardized, universally applicable method for estimating the mortality and morbidity effects of major disasters, there are best practices that can be specified. As for research in general, these include clarity in the specification of study objectives and definition of terms, transparency in the statement of assumptions and the sourcing of data used in the study, and caution in advancing any particular measure or method as a single solution. Thus, the field would benefit from a national research program that begins with a discussion of advantages and disadvantages and a documentation of researchers' and policy makers' experience with choices that have worked particularly well (or not) in the past (see Box 4-1 for selected research priorities for a national research program).

Conclusion 4-1: Given the variation in ways for attributing the cause of any death and morbidity, there can be more than one appropriate approach to answering the question: "How many deaths and severe morbidities were caused by this disaster?" Nevertheless, methodological best practices can be specified, and a national research program is urgently needed to identify, further develop, and validate these practices. As in all areas of research, these best practices are characterized by (1) clarity in the specification of study objectives and definition of terms, (2) transparency in the statement of assumptions and the sourcing of data used in the study, (3) continued testing and improvement of the accuracy of measures, and (4) caution in advancing any particular measure or method as the single perfect solution.

The counting-based methods described in Chapter 3 rely on accurate baseline and contextual data, including vital statistics data. Improving

BOX 4-1
Selected Research Priorities for a National Research Program

The research program could address factors such as:

- Specification of a comparison period or the handling of confounding or seasonal structure in the data;
- Determination of an accurate sampling frame;
- Comparison of different estimates from the same disaster to evaluate the effect of methodological choices and assumptions;
- Development of appropriate standard survey questionnaires;
- Creation of appropriate statistical models;
- Development of effective means of characterizing migration and population displacement before, during, and in the immediate wake of each common type of disaster;
- Furthering methodological research to lessen and characterize uncertainty in estimations;
- Exploration of modern causal inference techniques to determine appropriate causal estimands and methods for their estimation; and
- Development and evaluation of methods and tools for integrating social determinants of health data into estimations of disaster-related mortality and morbidity to produce more actionable and descriptive data.

these methods is thus essential for improving the quality of the estimates that use them—for setting denominators so that rates might be compared across time and geography, for reconstructing populations as they were at the moment of disaster impact, for understanding the sociodemographic characteristics of the disaster-affected populations, for identifying sampling frames for contact with survivors, and so forth. But an effective baseline for estimation techniques is broader than just these incident data and includes data from the U.S. decennial census, the ACS, other major federal surveys, and the growing array of administrative records–type data being compiled at the federal and state levels.

Developing an effective data and information structure for studying disaster impacts should be a cornerstone of the nation's operational disaster response function. It requires participation from actors in all levels of government as well as outside government. The research required for the development of the information structure could be brokered by, among others, NIH and NSF (as through the Methodology, Measurement, and Statistics Program).

The degree of analytical sophistication and the requirements for detailed data analysis and high-quality fieldwork are generally beyond the capabilities and time availability of most SLTT health departments—particularly in the immediate wake of a major disaster. Accordingly, it would be useful for CDC and FEMA to pursue jump teams that might be brought in early in the disaster response cycle to supplement SLTT resources, helping to gather data and (importantly) begin the detailed analyses.

> *Conclusion 4-2: Developing an effective data and information structure for studying disaster impacts on mortality and morbidity should be a cornerstone of the nation's operational disaster response function. Because the necessary analytical sophistication and high-quality fieldwork are generally beyond the capabilities and time availability of most SLTT health departments, it is essential that federal partners work to build and sustain the capacity of the nation's existing research and survey infrastructure to support the collection of survey data on the health effects of disasters.*

Critical operational support is needed from federal agencies, including the identification of appropriate mortality and morbidity datasets that might be brought to bear and the pre-negotiation of data-sharing agreements to ensure access to these data when needed. Some of the survey procedures and data analyses that are suggested, particularly if building on data previously gathered for other purposes, may appear to conflict with consent procedures under the Common Rule, which guides human subject research, respondent burden issues under the Paperwork Reduction Act, which governs clearance of federal information collections, and the HIPAA Privacy Rule, which protects individual health information. While the committee believes that the public health benefits of accurate estimates of the mortality and morbidity effects of a disaster outweigh these concerns, it is useful to address these issues in advance and to ensure alternative arrangements (such as data disclosure rules in place at SLTT health departments) to protect privacy and confidentiality.

Finally, academic departments and institutes can be more flexible in initiating and conducting studies, but care would be needed in specifying their work as part of the operational response (surveillance and evaluation function) of the National Incident Management System rather than pure or basic research. The involvement of academic, nongovernment units heightens the importance of being able to execute timely contractual agreements.

Recommendation 4-1: Fund and Conduct Research on Analytical Methods for Population Estimates

The Centers for Disease Control and Prevention, the National Institutes of Health, and the National Science Foundation should establish a national research program to advance analytical methods for conducting population-level estimates of mortality and morbidity related to disasters. This national research program should include the development and refinement of minimum standard methods and protocols for conducting population-level mortality and morbidity assessments as well as the creation and testing of tools for use by researchers, states, and localities to enhance their capabilities to carry out and use these analyses.

- Academic departments and institutes, which can be more flexible in initiating and conducting studies, should be included in these research efforts.
- Because many of the estimates in the literature result from "one-off" efforts that do not build on or seek comparability with previous disasters, an initial step in this research should be a careful comparison of different estimates from the same emergency to gain an understanding of how methodological choices and assumptions affect the estimates.

Recommendation 4-2: Enhance Capacity to Collect and Analyze Population Estimates for Mortality and Morbidity

The Department of Health and Human Services, together with state, local, tribal, and territorial (SLTT) agencies, should proactively develop partnerships to enhance the capacity to collect and analyze population-level disaster-related morbidity and mortality information. This includes the identification of appropriate mortality and morbidity datasets and sampling frames that might be brought to bear and the pre-negotiation of data-sharing agreements to ensure access to these data when needed.

The following immediate actions should be undertaken:

- The Secretary of Health and Human Services should push forward the collection of survey data on disaster-exposed and comparison populations to provide population-representative data on how disasters and their contributing stressors affect morbidity and to build the evidence base on differences in mortality and morbidity impacts across types of disasters.
- The federal statistical system, including the Centers for Disease Control and Prevention (CDC), the Substance Abuse and Mental Health Services Administration, and others should harness existing survey infrastructure and develop standard, Institutional Review Board (IRB)-approved sampling frames and methods for dealing with methodological challenges, such as population migration, for use by researchers conducting population estimates following large-scale disasters.
- The stakeholders listed above should address issues with informed consent procedures under the Common Rule, respondent burden issues under the Paperwork Reduction Act, and privacy under the Health Insurance Portability and Accountability Act Privacy Rule in advance and ensure that alternative arrangements are in place to protect privacy and confidentiality.
- SLTT agencies and academic research centers with the capability of conducting population estimates of disaster impact should formalize working relationships, data-sharing agreements, and IRB approvals in advance of a disaster to reduce delays in access to health data needed to conduct population estimates following a disaster and develop baseline assessments during the inter-disaster period.
- CDC and the Federal Emergency Management Agency should integrate frontline public health practitioners (e.g., epidemiologists and others) in the disaster response teams to help gather data and begin detailed analyses of mortality and morbidity data early in the disaster.

<u>Recommendation 4-3: Facilitate Access to and Use of Actionable Mortality and Morbidity Data by State, Local, Tribal, and Territorial (SLTT) Entities</u>

- **The Department of Health and Human Services (HHS) should work with the Centers for Disease Control and Prevention, the Federal Emergency Management Agency (FEMA), the Office of**

the Assistant Secretary for Preparedness and Response (ASPR), and other federal agencies to facilitate access to essential mortality and morbidity data to SLTT entities and academic research institutions throughout the disaster cycle. These data should be provided proactively and in a manner that is actionable for situational awareness and disaster response at state and local levels.

- **Additionally, state and federal agencies should fund the development and testing of analytical tools and work collaboratively with local entities to use mortality and morbidity data in meaningful ways.**
- The following immediate actions should be undertaken to ensure SLTT access to and use of mortality and morbidity data:
    - The National Center for Health Statistics (NCHS) should code and automatically provide, with the assistance of FEMA and ASPR, location-specific, baseline mortality data and up-to-date data on disaster deaths following a declared disaster and upon request, as well as offer ready-to-use tools within a set time frame following disasters to states and localities.
    - NCHS should make available to researchers and SLTT investigators the mortality data from the National Death Index.
    - NCHS and state vital records offices should retrospectively geocode death registry entries in select areas that were previously affected by large-scale disasters to provide sample data for modeling future impact and other research.
    - ASPR and CDC should provide state and local officials with guidance on standard practices for assessing mortality and morbidity and facilitate the analysis of these data by state and local health and emergency management officials.
    - CDC in collaboration with FEMA and ASPR should fund and conduct research to establish standard practices for analyzing disaster-related causes of death and its contributing causes, including guidance on standard timelines for data analysis (e.g., 30 days) and geographic parameters for defining a disaster's geographic scope.
    - CDC and the Centers for Medicare & Medicaid Services (CMS) should use existing systems to pilot the collection of relevant morbidity data following disasters to serve as an inter-disaster baseline.

- o CMS, in collaboration with electronic health record companies and health systems, should pilot and evaluate the inclusion of disaster-related *International Classification of Diseases, Tenth Revision* codes in electronic health records.
- o HHS should use both existing and novel data sources to improve mortality and morbidity data acquisition and reporting, including the use of surveys, artificial intelligence, machine learning, and other big data methods.

REFERENCES

Aida, J., H. Hikichi, Y. Matsuyama, Y. Sato, T. Tsuboya, T. Tabuchi, S. Koyama, S. V. Subramanian, K. Kondo, K. Osaka, and I. Kawachi. 2017. Risk of mortality during and after the 2011 Great East Japan earthquake and tsunami among older coastal residents. *Science Reports* 7(1):16591.

Bao, L., A. E. Raftery, and A. Reddy. 2015. Estimating the sizes of populations at risk of HIV infection from multiple data sources using a Bayesian hierarchical model. *Statistics and Its Interface* 8(2):125–136.

Baraff, A. J., T. H. McCormick, and A. E. Raftery. 2016. Estimating uncertainty in respondent-driven sampling using a tree bootstrap method. *Proceedings of the National Academy of Sciences* 113(51):14668–14673.

Bernard, H. R., E. C. Johnsen, P. D. Killworth, and S. Robinson. 1991. Estimating the size of an average personal network and of an event subpopulation: Some empirical results. *Social Science Research* 20(2):109–121.

Bernard, H. R., T. Hallett, A. Iovita, E. C. Johnsen, R. Lyerla, C. McCarty, M. Mahy, M. J. Salganik, T. Saliuk, O. Scutelniciuc, G. A. Shelley, P. Sirinirund, S. Weir, and D. F. Stroup. 2010. Counting hard-to-count populations: The network scale-up method for public health. *Sexually Transmitted Infections* 86(Suppl 2):ii11–ii15.

Branswell, H. 2020. CDC launches studies to get more precise count of undetected COVID-19 cases. *STAT*, April 4. https://www.statnews.com/2020/04/04/cdc-launches-studies-to-get-more-precise-count-of-undetected-covid-19-cases (accessed July 12, 2020).

Burnham, G., R. Lafta, S. Doocy, and L. Roberts. 2006. Mortality after the 2003 invasion of Iraq: A cross-sectional cluster sample survey. *The Lancet* 368(9545):1421–1428.

CDC (Centers for Disease Control and Prevention). 2014. *Disaster preparedness and response: Complete course. Facilitator guide, 1st ed.* Atlanta, GA: Centers for Disease Control and Prevention.

CDC. 2020a. *COVID-19 serology surveillance strategy*. https://www.cdc.gov/coronavirus/2019-ncov/covid-data/serology-surveillance/index.html (accessed June 2, 2020).

CDC. 2020b. *COVIDView—A weekly surveillance summary of U.S. COVID-19 activity*. https://www.cdc.gov/coronavirus/2019-ncov/covid-data/covidview/index.html (accessed July 13, 2020).

Cheng, S., D. Eck, and F. Crawford. 2020. Estimating the size of a hidden finite set: Large-sample behavior of estimators. *Statistics Surveys* 14:1–31.

Crawford, F. W., J. Wu, and R. Heimer. 2018. Hidden population size estimation from respondent driven sampling: A network approach. *Journal of the American Statistical Association* 113(522):755–766.

Cruz-Cano, R., and E. L. Mead. 2019. Causes of excess deaths in Puerto Rico after Hurricane Maria: A time-series estimation. *American Journal of Public Health* 109(7):1050–1052.

Doocy, S., M. Cherewick, and T. Kirsch. 2013. Mortality following the Haitian earthquake of 2010: A stratified cluster survey. *Population Health Metrics* 11(1):5.

Eisenman, D. P., H. Wilhalme, C. H. Tseng, M. Chester, P. English, S. Pincetl, A. Fraser, S. Vangala, and S. K. Dhaliwal. 2016. Heat death associations with the built environment, social vulnerability, and their interactions with rising temperature. *Health & Place* 41:89–99.

Feehan, D. M., and M. J. Salganik. 2016. Generalizing the network scale-up method: A new estimator for the size of hidden populations. *Sociological Methodology* 46(1):153–186.

Frankenberg, E., J. Friedman, T. Gillespie, N. Ingwersen, R. Pynoos, I. U. Rifai, B. Sikoki, A. Steinberg, C. Sumantri, W. Suriastini, and D. Thomas. 2008. Mental health in Sumatra after the tsunami. *American Journal of Public Health* 98(9):1671–1677.

Frankenberg, E., T. Gillespie, S. Preston, B. Sikoki, and D. Thomas. 2011. Mortality, the family, and the Indian Ocean tsunami. *Economic Journal* 121(554):F162–F182.

Frankenberg, E., C. Sumantri, and D. Thomas. 2020. Effects of a natural disaster on mortality risks over the longer term. *Nature Sustainability* 3(8):1–6. https://doi.org/10.1038/s41893-020-0536-3.

Green, A. K. B., T. H. McCormick, and A. E. Raftery. 2020. Consistency for the tree bootstrap in respondent-driven sampling. *Biometrika* 107(2):497–504.

GWU (George Washington University) Milken Institute School of Public Health. 2018. *Ascertainment of the estimated excess mortality from Hurricane Maria in Puerto Rico.* https://publichealth.gwu.edu/sites/default/files/downloads/projects/PRstudy/Acertainment%20of%20the%20Estimated%20Excess%20Mortality%20from%20Hurricane%20Maria%20in%20Puerto%20Rico.pdf (accessed July 12, 2020).

Habecker, P., K. Dombrowski, and B. Khan. 2015. Improving the network scale-up estimator: Incorporating means of sums, recursive back estimation, and sampling weights. *PLOS ONE* 10(12):e0143406.

Handcock, M. S., K. J. Gile, and C. M. Mar. 2014. Estimating hidden population size using respondent-driven sampling data. *Electronic Journal of Statistics* 8(1):1491–1521.

Harduar Morano, L. H., S. Watkins, and K. Kintziger. 2016. A comprehensive evaluation of the burden of heat-related illness and death within the Florida population. *International Journal of Environmental Research and Public Health* 13(6):551.

Heald, J., M. Spagat, and J. Dougherty. 2010. Discussion of "Conflict deaths in Iraq: A methodological critique of the ORB survey estimate." *Survey Research Methods* 4(1):17–19.

Heckathorn, D. D. 1997. Respondent-driven sampling: A new approach to the study of hidden populations. *Social Problems* 44(2):174–199.

Heckathorn, D. D. 2002. Respondent-driven sampling II: Deriving valid population estimates from chain-referral samples of hidden populations. *Social Problems* 49(1):11–34.

Henderson, R. H., and T. Sundaresan. 1982. Cluster sampling to assess immunization coverage: A review of experience with a simplified sampling method. *Bulletin of the World Health Organization* 60(2):253–260.

Henschel, A., L. L. Burton, L. Margolies, and J. E. Smith. 1969. An analysis of the heat deaths in St. Louis during July 1966. *American Journal of Public Health* 59(12):2232–2242.

Ho, J. 2020. *Methodological challenges and approaches for assessing the mortality impacts of disasters.* Presentation at the February 11, 2020, public meeting of the National Academies of Sciences, Engineering, and Medicine's Committee on Best Practices for Assessing Mortality and Significant Morbidity Following Large-Scale Disasters, conducted in webinar style. https://www.nationalacademies.org/event/02-11-2020/best-practices-in-assessing-mortality-and-significant-morbidity-following-large-scale-disasters-webinar-methodological-considerations-of-the-estimation-of-disaster-related-morbidity-and-mortality-at-a-population-level (accessed September 1, 2020).

Ho, J. Y., E. Frankenberg, C. Sumantri, and D. Thomas. 2017. Adult mortality five years after a natural disaster. *Population and Development Review* 43(3):467–490.

Howard, J. T., and A. R. Santos-Lozada. 2019. Mortality risk within counterfactual models: Puerto Rico and Hurricane Maria. *The Lancet Planetary Health* 3(5):e207–e208.

Irizarry, R. A. 2020. *Assessing mortality and significant morbidity following Hurricane Maria in Puerto Rico.* Presentation at the February 11, 2020, public meeting of the National Academies of Sciences, Engineering, and Medicine's Committee on Best Practices for Assessing Mortality and Significant Morbidity Following Large-Scale Disasters, conducted in webinar style. https://www.nationalacademies.org/event/02-11-2020/best-practices-in-assessing-mortality-and-significant-morbidity-following-large-scale-disasters-webinar-methodological-considerations-of-the-estimation-of-disaster-related-morbidity-and-mortality-at-a-population-level (accessed September 1, 2020).

Jacobson, M. H., C. Norman, A. Nguyen, and R. M. Brackbill. 2018. Longitudinal determinants of depression among World Trade Center health registry enrollees, 14–15 years after the 9/11 attacks. *Journal of Affective Disorders* 229:483–490.

Jewell, N. P., M. Spagat, and B. L. Jewell. 2018. Accounting for civilian casualties: From the past to the future. *Social Science History* 42(3):379–410.

Joe, L., S. Hoshiko, D. Dobraca, R. Jackson, S. Smorodinsky, D. Smith, and M. Harnly. 2016. Mortality during a large-scale heat wave by place, demographic group, internal and external causes of death, and building climate zone. *International Journal of Environmental Research and Public Health* 13(3):299.

Johnston, L. G., K. R. McLaughlin, H. El Rhilani, A. Latifi, A. Toufik, A. Bennani, K. Alami, B. Elomari, and M. S. Handcock. 2015. Estimating the size of hidden populations using respondent-driven sampling data: Case examples from Morocco. *Epidemiology* 26(6):846–852.

Johnston, L. G., K. R. McLaughlin, S. A. Rouhani, and S. A. Bartels. 2017. Measuring a hidden population: A novel technique to estimate the population size of women with sexual violence-related pregnancies in South Kivu Province, Democratic Republic of Congo. *Journal of Epidemiology and Global Health* 7(1):45–53.

Jordan, H. T., C. R. Stein, J. Li, J. E. Cone, L. Stayner, J. L. Hadler, R. M. Brackbill, and M. R. Farfel. 2018. Mortality among rescue and recovery workers and community members exposed to the September 11, 2001 World Trade Center terrorist attacks, 2003–2014. *Environmental Research* 163:270–279.

Killworth, P. D., C. McCarty, H. R. Bernard, G. A. Shelley, and E. C. Johnsen. 1998. Estimation of seroprevalence, rape, and homelessness in the United States using a social network approach. *Evaluation Review* 22(2):289–308.

Kim, S., P. A. Kulkarni, M. Rajan, P. Thomas, S. Tsai, C. Tan, and A. Davidow. 2017. Hurricane Sandy (New Jersey): Mortality rates in the following month and quarter. *American Journal of Public Health* 107(8):1304–1307.

Kishore, N., D. Marqués, A. Mahmud, M. V. Kiang, I. Rodriguez, A. Fuller, P. Ebner, C. Sorensen, F. Racy, J. Lemery, L. Maas, J. Leaning, R. A. Irizarry, S. Balsari, and C. O. Buckee. 2018. Mortality in Puerto Rico after Hurricane María. *New England Journal of Medicine* 379(2):162–170.

Laaksonen, S. 2008. Retrospective two-stage cluster sampling for mortality in Iraq. *International Journal of Market Research* 50(3):403–417.

Maghsoudi, A., M. R. Baneshi, M. Neydavoodi, and A. Haghdoost. 2014. Network scale-up correction factors for population size estimation of people who inject drugs and female sex workers in Iran. *PLOS ONE* 9(11):e110917.

Malilay, J. 2000. Public health assessments in disaster settings: Recommendations for a multidisciplinary approach. *Prehospital and Disaster Medicine* 15(4):167–172.

Malilay, J., W. D. Flanders, and D. Brogan. 1996. A modified cluster-sampling method for post-disaster rapid assessment of needs. *Bulletin of the World Health Organization* 74(4):399–405.

Marker, D. A. 2008. Review: Methodological review of "Mortality after the 2003 invasion of Iraq: A cross-sectional cluster sample survey." *Public Opinion Quarterly* 72(2):345–363.

McCormick, T. H. 2020. *Network scale-up and indirect methods for group size estimation.* Presentation at the February 11, 2020, public meeting of the National Academies of Sciences, Engineering, and Medicine's Committee on Best Practices for Assessing Mortality and Significant Morbidity Following Large-Scale Disasters, conducted in webinar style. https://www.nationalacademies.org/event/02-11-2020/best-practices-in-assessing-mortality-and-significant-morbidity-following-large-scale-disasters-webinar-methodological-considerations-of-the-estimation-of-disaster-related-morbidity-and-mortality-at-a-population-level (accessed September 1, 2020).

Morita, T., S. Nomura, M. Tsubokura, C. Leppold, S. Gilmour, S. Ochi, A. Ozaki, Y. Shimada, K. Yamamoto, M. Inoue, S. Kato, K. Shibuya, and M. Kami. 2017. Excess mortality due to indirect health effects of the 2011 triple disaster in Fukushima, Japan: A retrospective observational study. *Journal of Epidemiology and Community Health* 71(10):974–980.

NASEM (National Academies of Sciences, Engineering, and Medicine). 2019. *Building and measuring community resilience: Actions for communities and the Gulf Research Program.* Washington, DC: The National Academies Press.

NSF (National Science Foundation). 2020. *Frequently asked questions and vignettes.* https://www.nsf.gov/bfa/dias/policy/hsfaqs.jsp#snow (accessed June 10, 2020).

Pascal, M., K. Laaidi, V. Wagner, A. B. Ung, S. Smaili, A. Fouillet, C. Caserio-Schönemann, and P. Beaudeau. 2012. How to use near real-time health indicators to support decision-making during a heat wave: The example of the French heat wave warning system. *PLOS Currents* 4:e4f83ebf72317d.

Pascal, M., V. Wagner, M. Corso, K. Laaidi, A. Ung, and P. Beaudeau. 2018. Heat and cold related-mortality in 18 French cities. *Environment International* 121:189–198.

Petitti, D. B., S. L. Harlan, G. Chowell-Puente, and D. Ruddell. 2013. Occupation and environmental heat-associated deaths in Maricopa County, Arizona: A case–control study. *PLOS ONE* 8(5):e62596.

Phifer, J. F., K. Z. Kaniasty, and F. H. Norris. 1988. The impact of natural disaster on the health of older adults: A multiwave prospective study. *Journal of Health and Social Behavior* 29(1):65–78.

Quarantelli, E. L. 2001. Statistical and conceptual problems in the study of disasters. *Disaster Prevention and Management* 10(5):325–338.

Quast, T. 2020. *Excess mortality of older individuals with diabetes following Hurricanes Katrina and Rita.* Presentation at the February 18, 2020, public meeting of the National Academies of Sciences, Engineering, and Medicine's Committee on Best Practices for Assessing Mortality and Significant Morbidity Following Large-Scale Disasters, conducted in webinar style. https://www.nationalacademies.org/event/02-18-2020/best-practices-in-assessing-mortality-and-significant-morbidity-following-large-scale-disasters-webinar-methodological-considerations-for-estimating-excess-mortality-and-morbidity (accessed September 1, 2020).

Raftery, A. E. 2020. *Methods for estimating hard to count populations.* Presentation at the February 11, 2020, public meeting of the National Academies of Sciences, Engineering, and Medicine's Committee on Best Practices for Assessing Mortality and Significant Morbidity Following Large-Scale Disasters, conducted in webinar style. https://www.nationalacademies.org/event/02-11-2020/best-practices-in-assessing-mortality-and-significant-morbidity-following-large-scale-disasters-webinar-methodological-considerations-of-the-estimation-of-disaster-related-morbidity-and-mortality-at-a-population-level (accessed September 1, 2020).

Rosenberg, E. S., J. M. Tesoriero, E. M. Rosenthal, R. Chung, M. A. Barranco, L. M. Styer, M. M. Parker, S-YJ Leung, J. E. Morne, D. Greene, R. Holtgrave, D. Hoefer, J. Kumar, T. Udo, B. Hutton, and H. A. Zucker. 2020. Cumulative incidence and diagnosis of SARS-CoV-2 infection in New York. *Annals of Epidemiology* 48:23–29. doi: 10.1016/j.annepidem.2020.06.004.

Russell, T. W., N. Golding, J. Hellewell, S. Abbott, L. Wright, C. A. B. Pearson, K. van Zandvoort, C. I. Jarvis, H. Gibbs, Y. Liu, R. M. Eggo, J. W. Edmunds, and A. J. Kucharski. 2020. Reconstructing the early global dynamics of under-ascertained COVID-19 cases and infections. *medRxiv* 2020.07.07.20148460. doi: https://doi.org/10.1101/2020.07.07.20148460 [preprint].

Santos-Burgoa, C., J. Sandberg, E. Suárez, A. Goldman-Hawes, S. Zeger, A. Garcia-Meza, C. M. Pérez, N. Estrada-Merly, U. Colón-Ramos, C. M. Nazario, E. Andrade, A. Roess, and L. Goldman. 2018. Differential and persistent risk of excess mortality from Hurricane Maria in Puerto Rico: A time-series analysis. *The Lancet Planetary Health* 2(11):e478–e488.

Santos-Burgoa, C., J. Sandberg, E. Suárez, C. M. Pérez, and L. Goldmann. 2019. Mortality risk within counterfactual models: Puerto Rico and Hurricane Maria—Authors' reply. *The Lancet Planetary Health* 3(5):e209.

Santos-Lozada, A. R., and J. T. Howard. 2017. Estimates of excess deaths in Puerto Rico following Hurricane Maria. *SocArXiv*. doi: 10.31235/osf.io/s7dmu.

Santos-Lozada, A. R., and J. T. Howard. 2018. Use of death counts from vital statistics to calculate excess deaths in Puerto Rico following Hurricane Maria. *JAMA* 320(14):1491–1493.

Santos-Lozada, A. R., and J. T. Howard. 2019. Excess deaths after Hurricane Maria in Puerto Rico—Reply. *JAMA* 321(10):1005–1006.

Stephens, K. U., Sr., D. Grew, K. Chin, P. Kadetz, P. G. Greenough, F. M. Burkle, Jr., S. L. Robinson, and E. R. Franklin. 2007. Excess mortality in the aftermath of Hurricane Katrina: A preliminary report. *Disaster Medicine and Public Health Preparedness* 1(1):15–20.

Thomas, L. M., L. D'Ambruoso, and D. Balabanova. 2018. Verbal autopsy in health policy and systems: A literature review. *BMJ Global Health* 3(2):e000639.

Turner, A. G., R. J. Magnani, and M. Shuaib. 1996. A not quite as quick but much cleaner alternative to the Expanded Programme on Immunization (EPI) cluster survey design. *International Journal of Epidemiology* 25(1):198–203.

Vandentorren, S., P. Bretin, A. Zeghnoun, L. Mandereau-Bruno, A. Croisier, C. Cochet, J. Ribéron, I. Siberan, B. Declercq, and M. Ledrans. 2006. August 2003 heat wave in France: Risk factors for death of elderly people living at home. *European Journal of Public Health* 16(6):583–591.

Verdery, A. M., S. Weir, Z. Reynolds, G. Mulholland, and J. K. Edwards. 2019. Estimating hidden population sizes with venue-based sampling: Extensions of the generalized network scale up estimator. *Epidemiology* 30(6):901–910.

Vogel, G. 2020. "These are answers we need." WHO plans global study to discover true extent of coronavirus infections. *Science Magazine*, April 2. https://www.sciencemag.org/news/2020/04/these-are-answers-we-need-who-plans-global-study-discover-true-extent-coronavirus (accessed July 12, 2020).

Weinberger, D. M., J. Chen J., T. Cohen, F. W. Crawford, F. Mostashari, D. Olson, V. E. Pitzer, N. G. Reich, M. Russi, L. Simonsen, A. Watkins, and C. Viboud. 2020. Estimation of excess deaths associated with the COVID-19 pandemic in the United States, March to May 2020. *JAMA Internal Medicine* 180(10):1336–1344.

Woolf, S. H., D. A. Chapman, R. T. Sabo, D. M. Weinberger, and L. Hill. 2020. Excess deaths from COVID-19 and other causes, March–April 2020. *JAMA* 324(5):510–513.

Working Group for Mortality Estimation in Emergencies. 2007. Wanted: Studies on mortality estimation methods for humanitarian emergencies, suggestions for future research. *Emerging Themes in Epidemiology* 4(1):9.

Zeger, S. L. 2020. *Comments on prediction of causal effects of disasters on morbidity and mortality.* Presentation at the February 18, 2020, public meeting of the National Academies of Sciences, Engineering, and Medicine's Committee on Best Practices for Assessing Mortality and Significant Morbidity Following Large-Scale Disasters, conducted in webinar style. https://www.nationalacademies.org/event/02-18-2020/best-practices-in-assessing-mortality-and-significant-morbidity-following-large-scale-disasters-webinar-methodological-considerations-for-estimating-excess-mortality-and-morbidity (accessed September 1, 2020).

Zhang, Y., M. Nitschke, A. Krackowizer, K. Dear, D. Pisaniello, P. Weinstein, G. Tucker, S. Shakib, and P. Bi. 2017. Risk factors for deaths during the 2009 heat wave in Adelaide, Australia: A matched case–control study. *International Journal of Biometeorology* 61(1):35–47.

5

Meeting the Mission

In the wake of a large-scale disaster, from the initial devastation through the long tail of recovery, protecting the health and well-being of the affected individuals and communities is paramount. Obtaining accurate and timely information about mortality and significant morbidity related to the disaster is critical to supporting the efforts of the disaster management enterprise at all stages to save lives and prevent further health impacts and specifically to guide response and recovery priorities and to ensure a common operating picture, real-time situation awareness, public health messaging, and protection of vulnerable populations. Conversely, failure to capture mortality and significant morbidity data accurately and comprehensively undercuts the nation's capacity and moral obligation to proactively protect its population and acknowledge human suffering in a fair and consistent manner. Additionally, the increasing frequency and intensity of disasters underscores the financial imperative to reduce the direct and indirect costs of disaster by deploying data-guided mitigation and response practices informed by historical and prospective models of mortality and morbidity data. During the interim phase between disasters, mortality and morbidity data provide the foundation for evaluation, prevention, mitigation, and preparedness activities designed to reduce morbidity and mortality during future events. Beyond merely counting and attributing deaths and morbidities more accurately, better data on both the extent and causes of morbidity and mortality can be used to drive changes in policy, practice, and behavior.

Disasters are complex and their health consequences are multifactorial. The foundational challenge in the assessment of mortality and morbidity data is the reality that many different approaches exist for quantifying the impact of a disaster and the persistence of the expectation that each disaster is represented by a singular toll. There is no one approach for assessing a disaster's impact that can be applied across all disasters, and this inherently exposes mortality counts to manipulation and confusion concerning the true impact of a disaster. Individual counts, which estimate the total number of reported cases at an individual level and attribute the degree of relationship to the disaster for each, and population estimates, which apply statistical methods such as excess death to estimate the disaster impact at a population level, are the two main approaches for estimating mortality and morbidity. As discussed in Chapter 2 and in the subsequent chapters, each approach to assessment has unique benefits, weaknesses, and contexts for application. However, to avoid confusion and limit opportunities for manipulation, the processes for vital statistics, public health, and emergency response data systems must be improved.

Extracting the maximum value from these data is dependent on having standard practices and systems in place for collecting and reporting accurate information, analyzing it appropriately, and translating data into action. However, it is difficult to coordinate these efforts effectively and uniformly across the disaster management enterprise, which is composed of a vast and intricate network of federal and state, local, tribal, and territorial (SLTT) systems as well as a plethora of stakeholders ranging from emergency management, health care, government agencies, the general public, policy makers, and the public and private sectors. The practices and systems currently in place are not robust, coordinated, or reliable enough to use mortality and significant morbidity data to their fullest potential. Instead, these systems and stakeholders are often splintered, siloed, and unable to rapidly disseminate information to one another. Mortality and morbidity data that are not captured uniformly across jurisdictions and agencies mean that identical incidents can generate differing mortality and morbidity figures depending on jurisdiction. Data collected under these circumstances are less conducive to comparative analysis and may exclude valuable data about deaths and morbidities that are indirectly or partially attributable to a disaster. In some cases, available data about mortality and significant morbidity are squandered because they are not or cannot be used to add value to disaster management or because existing systems are not deriving the optimal value from the data. Additionally, the accurate, consistent collection of disaster-related mortality and morbidity data is often not prioritized because critical stakeholders involved may not be aware of its importance.

Despite this diverse set of challenges, there exist real opportunities to build stakeholder partnerships and cultivate adaptive systems for assessing morbidity and mortality, including using improvements within existing data (e.g., electronic medical records and claims data) and state and federal reporting systems. There is also great opportunity in investing in and conducting research to test and refine analytical approaches for developing population estimates as well as an opportunity to encourage a broader view of disaster morbidity and mortality and, by extension, a more nuanced understanding of the impact of disasters on human lives.

MOVING FORWARD

In its review of the current landscape of practices, systems, and tools for assessing mortality and significant morbidity following large-scale disasters, the committee identified several persistent, systemic challenges (see Box 5-1) as well as potential best practices that could be brought to scale. This final chapter of the report responds to these findings with a series of crosscutting recommendations that are intended to serve as a blueprint for moving forward. These recommendations couple short-term actions, which can be undertaken immediately for rapid impact, with long-term priorities, which are geared toward investments in the capacity and capability of the nation to capture, track, and use mortality and morbidity data to inform disaster management and save lives.

Recommended immediate actions needed to address current gaps in policy, practice, and infrastructure for mortality and morbidity assessment include

BOX 5-1
Foundational Challenges to the Assessment of Mortality and Morbidity Following Large-Scale Disasters

- Pervasive variation across the nation in data collection and recording and reporting practices for mortality and significant morbidity at the state, local, tribal, and territorial (SLTT) levels (see Chapters 2 and 3).
- A lack of prioritization of the accurate and consistent collection, recording, reporting, analysis, and use of data on mortality and significant morbidity by stakeholders across the enterprise (see Chapters 3 and 4).
- Poor functionality of data systems to effectively capture, record, and report mortality and morbidity data across multiple stakeholders in a uniform manner (see Chapter 3).
- A need for enabling and training on data collection, recording, and reporting and other support for medicolegal death investigation system professionals and SLTT agencies (see Chapters 3 and 4).
- Individual counts and population estimation data that are available are not being used or lack usability for providing value to disaster management, and SLTT entities lack access to actionable data (see Chapters 3 and 4).
- A need for additional research to develop and evaluate analytical methods for assessing mortality and morbidity and to create and test new tools (see Chapter 4).

1. Adoption and use of a uniform framework for collecting, recording, and reporting mortality and morbidity data (Recommendations 2-1 and 2-2).
2. Investment in improvements to data systems and tools for collecting, recording, and reporting individual count data at an SLTT level (Recommendations 3-1 and 3-2).
3. Update of the Model State Vital Statistics Act and Regulations to facilitate more robust and uniform mortality data collection across the nation (Recommendation 3-2).
4. Creation of a process to develop, validate, and promulgate national standards for reporting on a core set of morbidity impacts specific to the common types of major disasters (Recommendation 3-3).
5. Investment in and development of the capacity to collect and analyze the data necessary for population estimates of mortality and morbidity (Recommendation 4-2)
6. Implementation of new tools and approaches to share and use mortality and morbidity data (Recommendation 4-3).
7. Consideration of a separate Emergency Support Function dedicated to mortality management (Recommendation 3-5).

Recommended future priorities to strengthen the nation's ability to prepare for and respond to disasters and emergencies of all types via the enhanced assessment of individual counts and population estimates of mortality and morbidity include

1. Integration of new technologies, as these become available, into existing electronic data systems and tools (Recommendation 3-1).
2. Investment in research to advance the science of mortality and morbidity assessment (Recommendations 3-1, 4-1, and 4-2).
3. Development and dissemination of resources for training professionals in the medicolegal death investigation system and for inclusion in SLTT disaster management (Recommendations 3-4 and 3-5).

Applicability of the Committee's Recommendations Beyond the Stafford Act

As described in Chapter 1, the Statement of Task narrowed the intended focus of this report to disasters declared under the Robert T. Stafford Disaster Relief and Emergency Assistance Act (Stafford Act), with infectious disease-related disasters determined to not be the primary focus of the committee's deliberations.[1] While the committee's report reflects this guidance, the recommendations laid out in this chapter are broadly applicable to all types of disasters, including those of infectious origin, such as the coronavirus disease 2019 (COVID-19) pandemic. The committee shaped its recommendations around the development of the capabilities needed at SLTT and federal levels to improve the function and value of the nation's systems and structures for mortality and morbidity assessment and to improve the use of the data from these assessments, regardless of disaster type or even the presence of a disaster. Therefore, investment in the implementation of the policies and practices laid out in these recommendations represents a broader investment in the overall function and flexibility of the nation's existing death investigation and registration system, in novel opportunities to collect and use data to protect human life and health and in supporting the kind of cross-agency coordination and partnership that can be tapped in a time of crisis.

Guiding System Precepts

In developing its recommendations, the committee members defined a series of guiding precepts that synthesize the ethos and key characteristics of their vision for a highly effective and responsive system (see Box 5-2) and the discrete steps that should be taken to move toward achieving this vision. These precepts prioritize access to detailed data to support mortality and morbidity attribution for all cases; real-time availability of data; interoperable data systems; functional tools to aid decision making using mortality and morbidity data; access to training and professional support; and universal stakeholder buy-in, among others.

CONCLUSIONS AND RECOMMENDATIONS[2]

Organizational Leadership and an Enterprise Approach

Critical to the success of the recommendations presented in this report is that the coordination of these disparate yet essential changes across multiple systems cannot be the responsibility of any one entity. All stakeholders

[1] The Stafford Act has very rarely been used to access federal support due to an infectious disease pandemic or epidemic. Unlike a natural disaster, which is likely to be localized or regionalized in its impact, a pandemic is likely to—and in the case of the ongoing COVID-19 pandemic shown to—rapidly and simultaneously overwhelm states, localities, tribal areas, and territories across the nation, necessitating coordinated federal assistance (see Chapter 1).

[2] Note that conclusions and recommendations are indicated in Chapter 5 by the chapter number and then by the order in which they first appear in that chapter. For example, Recommendation 3-1 is the first recommendation found in Chapter 3. The committee has developed 12 recommendations, which are presented collectively in this final chapter of the report.

BOX 5-2
Guiding System Precepts

A highly effective system for assessing morbidity and mortality of major disasters would:

Collect and use data for community health protection as an essential component across all phases of disaster management

The fundamental responsibilities of emergency management and public health—at every level and capacity—are to protect human health, support recovery, and prevent similar consequences from occurring in the future. High-quality mortality and morbidity data can improve preparedness, mitigation, response, and recovery capabilities if they are widely accessible, appropriately analyzed, and used effectively. Efforts to improve the timeliness and accuracy of mortality and morbidity data should be underpinned by the broader ethos of saving lives, protecting health, and preparing for future disasters.

Incorporate both individual counts and population estimates to better understand a disaster's true effect

The two primary approaches for assessing disaster-related mortality and morbidity, individual counts and population estimates, have important and complementary value. The committee sought to balance the two approaches in contributing to a comprehensive picture of a disaster's true effects. These estimation approaches have different uses, advantages, and drawbacks, but both are critical for accurately and comprehensively assessing and describing a disaster's impact on human health and for developing and improving approaches to limit the future consequences of disasters.

Leverage morbidity data as well as mortality data to support response, recovery, mitigation, and preparedness

Focusing exclusively on disaster-related mortality—the traditional outcome of interest—is shortsighted. Using morbidity data—both during the crisis and in the inter-disaster period—to evaluate and guide disaster management efforts provides greater opportunities for reducing future mortality outcomes and increasing the resilience of the community.

are needed to commit to a coordinated enterprise approach, which allows all entities to overcome fragmentation, particularly in a time of crisis, and work toward a mutual goal. At present there is no singular federal entity or standard system that exists to oversee the operation of disaster-related mortality and morbidity reporting practices; these duties are largely in the domain of states, territories, and counties, and there are inadequate incentives for collaboration. However, when a major disaster happens, federal agencies, which have existing systems and capabilities to carry out their non-disaster-related missions, could pivot and apply these resources to improved disaster reporting (e.g., Census Pulse survey; Epidemic Intelligence Service). This will require focused and clear leadership at the federal level.

Build on and use existing systems, capacities, and methodologies

Efforts to drive systems-level improvements benefit from using existing capabilities and capacities as well as identifying shared goals and existing resources to support stakeholders across fields and disciplines. Failure to strengthen the broader system for collecting, recording, and reporting mortality and morbidity data weakens the ability of the nation to respond effectively to changing health threats. Changes that occur only in siloes or at certain levels will be insufficient to optimize the use of mortality and morbidity data.

Commit to the continuous improvement of systems over time

Access to valuable individual counts and population estimates of morbidity and mortality is foundational to understanding a disaster's impact. The specific data needs, appropriate tools, effective practices, and key stakeholders evolve over time; thus, systems need to respond by evolving in parallel. Adopting a systems-level learning approach can provide a foundation for continuously improving the integrity and interpretation of mortality and morbidity data, thus enabling greater protection of human life.

Adopt an enterprise approach to activate stakeholders and systems in times of crisis as well as during the inter-disaster period

Effectively collecting and using mortality and morbidity data requires collaboration across the disparate institutions and organizations that are directly and indirectly involved in disaster response, recovery, mitigation, and preparedness. An enterprise approach across the disaster management enterprise would unite stakeholders under common goals and mitigate the complexity of operationalizing improved practices and methods.

Support the resilience and strength of historically disadvantaged populations by using data to understand, mitigate, and eliminate inequalities in disaster impacts

Mortality and morbidity data can offer valuable contextual information about population-specific vulnerabilities and provide evidence for targeted mitigation and preparedness efforts in order to protect and improve the resilience of these populations.

Such action will also encourage SLTT agencies to coordinate their efforts, develop and promulgate national standards for case definitions, adopt guidance on death record reporting, compile cross-state data, provide rapid training and develop education, and support materials for medical certifiers, among other outcomes.

The organizational and logistical complexity of this problem will require all stakeholders—government agencies, medicolegal systems, public health offices, emergency preparedness offices, etc.—and particularly the leadership of each of these groups, to look beyond the day-to-day function of their respective independent agencies and organizations and apply, with creativity and purpose, those tools that they have at their disposal to force change for the benefit of the nation. While it is essential that federal agencies' leadership consistently champion and invest in these improvements, the committee acknowledges that SLTT entities have a corresponding obligation to recognize the value of these changes and facilitate their operationalization. The committee stresses that no lasting change will be possible without this mutual commitment and coordination across systems and stakeholders. The individual recommendations presented in this chapter assign certain key actors to specific actions, but the successful implementation of these recommendations will require broad commitment from all entities and their leadership to rise up to meet the challenge of their collective mission.

> *Conclusion 3-4: The implementation of an enterprise approach for improving the assessment of mortality and morbidity following large-scale disasters is essential to the implementation of systemic improvements involving multiple, siloed stakeholders. Leadership at all levels—federal, state, local, tribal, and territorial—will be responsible for championing change.*

> *Conclusion 5-1: Times of crisis necessitate the adoption of cross-agency responsibilities designed to meet the mission for domestic action during disasters and emergencies.*

Uniform Framework and Terminology for Attribution

Prior chapters have explored the multitude of terms that have been used to denote total mortality and to attribute the degree of a relationship between a death, injury, or illness and disaster as well as the reasons for the variety of terms. There is widespread variation in *what* is being assessed and the *context* in which it is being assessed as well as in how to record the strength of association of a case to a known disaster (see Chapter 2). Fundamentally, the lack of a consistently used framework of approaches for attributing mortality and morbidity across the nation results in inconsistent collection and reporting of data on the scope and causes of mortality and morbidity over time and across disasters.

> *Conclusion 2-1: Current terminology and case definitions used to describe disaster-related mortality and morbidity fail to capture the differences in assessment methods used and the totality and temporality of disaster-related deaths and significant morbidity. The lack of a uniform framework for assessing disaster-related health impacts undermines the quality and usability of these data in informing disaster management.*

In response to this critical gap, the committee has provided a framework as a guide, which is based on the two main approaches for assessing disaster-related mortality and morbidity—individual counts and population estimates—and parses out individual case definitions to characterize the level of attribution for all deaths (see Recommendation 2-1).

The committee also emphasizes that each approach—individual counts and population estimates—represents an estimation of impact at a distinct point of time, within a specific context, and based on particular assumptions. Both approaches encompass distinct methods and techniques. Individual counting methods are valuable for understanding the immediate impact of disasters but are susceptible to weaknesses in the accuracy of recorded and reported data, and they fail to count certain individuals, such as those who die of natural causes during a disaster but who would not have died but for the disaster. By contrast, population estimates are critical for obtaining a full understanding of the health impact of a disaster, but they cannot say which individuals died of the disaster and which would have died even if the disaster had not arisen (see Chapter 2). The adoption of a framework that acknowledges the value of both individual counts and population estimates for quantifying and describing morbidity and mortality is foundational to the development of uniform practices for collection, reporting, and recording of robust data that can be used to save lives. As such, adoption of and compliance with this framework may necessitate dedicated federal funding.

Recommendation 2-1: Adopt and Support the Use of a Uniform Framework for Assessing Disaster-Related Mortality and Morbidity

The Department of Health and Human Services and the Department of Homeland Security, including the Office of the Assistant Secretary for Preparedness and Response, the Centers for Disease Control and Prevention, the Centers for Medicare & Medicaid Services, and the Federal Emergency Management Agency, should adopt and support the use of a uniform framework for assessing disaster-related mortality and morbidity before, during, and after a disaster by state, local, tribal, and territorial (SLTT) entities; public health agencies; and death investigation and registration systems. To implement this uniform framework nationally, the National Center for Health Statistics in conjunction with state and local vital records offices, medical examiners and coroners, medical certifiers, and all relevant professional associations should jointly adopt and apply this framework to practice, including the routine use of uniform case definitions and data collection, recording, and reporting practices. Additionally, all Stafford Act declarations should require affected states and regions to comply with the reporting requirements for individual count and population estimation approaches as described in the framework. Timely guidance should be disseminated to SLTT entities regarding the proper certification of individual deaths with provision for direct, indirect, and partially attributable deaths following a large-scale disaster.

The following terminology and approaches for defining mortality and morbidity following large-scale disasters should be adopted immediately:

- **Total reported mortality and morbidity estimation using individual counts:** Individual counts are point-in-time estimates of disaster-related mortality and morbidity derived from reported cases.
    - o *Direct death or morbidity*: A death or morbidity directly attributable to the forces of the disaster or a direct consequence of these forces.
    - o *Indirect death or morbidity*: A death or morbidity not from a direct impact but due to unsafe or unhealthy conditions around the time of the disaster, including while preparing for, while responding to, and during recovery from the disaster.
    - o *Partially attributable death or morbidity*: A death or morbidity that cannot be tied definitively to the disaster but where the disaster more likely than not has played a contributing role in the death.
    - o *Unrelated death or morbidity*: A death or morbidity that is unassociated with or cannot be attributed to the forces of a disaster.
- **Total mortality and morbidity derived from population estimates:** Population estimates are point-in-time estimates of the impact of a disaster at a population level derived using various statistical methods and tools, including sampling.

<u>Recommendation 2-2: Report Both Individual Counts and Population Estimates</u>

Both individual counts and population estimates should be used as accepted standards for reporting by state, local, tribal, and territorial entities and supported by the federal agencies as indicators of mortality and morbidity to determine the impact of disasters over time. State and federal reporting of total mortality and morbidity estimates following disasters should use both individual counts of direct and indirect deaths and population estimates of mortality and morbidity as these data become available following a disaster. Individual count data should be referred to as *reported cases* or *reported deaths* and should not be referred to as reflecting *total mortality* or a *death toll.*

Total mortality estimates should be derived from population estimation methods, which provide a more complete assessment of overall impacts of large-scale disasters.

Strengthening Systems and Practices for Conducting Individual Counts

The collection of consistent and accurate mortality and morbidity data is dependent on the function and ability of the systems used to do so. Therefore, the absence of standard practices for attributing and recording reported individual-level disaster-related mortality information across SLTT entities is a significant barrier to the accurate estimation of disaster impact and the use of these data to save lives. As outlined in the chapter, there are several structural, operational, and philosophical reasons for the persistence of inconsistent policies and practices for the attribution and reporting of disaster-related mortality. Most challenging of these is the decentralized structure of the nation's medicolegal death investigation and death registration systems, which provides an environment in which a diversity of data collection and recording practices is dependent on the structure of the local or state medicolegal system, the professional philosophies of the policy makers and practitioners within each system, and local professional education and training requirements (see Chapter 3). The committee stresses that the disjointed nature of the death investigation and registration systems is a detriment to the uniform and accurate collection and recording of mortality data and that uniform practices, systems, tools, and professional standards are needed to strengthen the collection and attribution of individual disaster deaths at the local level.

Conclusion 3-1: The heterogeneity of the nation's systems of death investigation and registration prevents the accurate recording and reporting of disaster-related mortality data and impedes the meaningful analysis and use of these data to improve disaster management. Adoption of uniform practices for collecting, recording, and reporting mortality data is needed, as is improved vertical coordination across stakeholders and improved interoperability of electronic systems among medical certifiers, state vital records offices, and the national vital statistics system.

The committee recognizes that the inherent variation in death investigation systems and death certification significantly impairs the collection of quality mortality data and that medicolegal death investigation systems that feature a centralized medical examiner system may be better equipped to address the needs of the medicolegal system and specifically the assessment of disaster-related mortality (see Recommendation 3-4). However, the committee also acknowledges that the restructuring of the nation's medicolegal death investigation systems is a long-term process that would require considerable federal intervention and legislative changes. Therefore, in the following recommendations the committee highlights other actions that could be undertaken immediately to address the need for uniformity in data collection and to move toward the development of coordinated or regionalized medical examiner systems as standard. These include the implementation of expanded responsibilities for federal agencies and SLTT entities to develop standards for and make improvements to data collection and reporting practices and systems. Recommendations 3-1 and 3-2 address a variety of operational, administrative, and data system challenges noted by committee members over the course of their deliberations. These challenges result from the breadth of different terminology and attribution practices in use across SLTTs and by different medical certifiers (also see Recommendation 2-1 for the committee's recommended framework and terminology), poor prioritization of robust disaster-related mortality and morbidity data collection and recording, data system inadequacies for both medical examiner and coroner electronic data systems and state electronic death record systems, a lack of access to data and tools for decision-making support, and the absence of a federal requirement for inclusion of disaster death information in the death registration process (see Chapter 3).

Significant opportunity exists to rapidly enhance the baseline quality of data collected on mortality and morbidity following all disasters by SLTT entities through the universal adoption of a uniform process for data collection and reporting. In the case of individual-level mortality assessment, the committee feels strongly that these changes are unlikely to be achieved through mere modifications to the death certificate, which is a legal document that is legislated by each individual state. Instead, the committee recommends that the National Vital Statistics System should directly initiate the introduction of minimum data requirements by updating the Model State Vital Statistics Act to require medical certifiers to supply certain types of descriptive data to improve the attribution of a death to a particular disaster (see Chapter 3). Electronic data system improvements represent another area of promise for mortality assessment, specifically in relation to the reduction of the administrative burden on medical examiners and coroners, to the enhancement of coordination across systems and stakeholders, and to the improvement of electronic decision-making support for all medical certifiers. Efforts should be made to improve and build onto exiting systems wherever possible, rather than developing new data systems.

Recommendation 3-1: Strengthen Existing Systems to Improve Individual-Level Mortality Data Quality

The Centers for Disease Control and Prevention (CDC), through the National Center for Health Statistics (NCHS), should lead an enterprise-wide initiative to strengthen existing death registration systems to improve the quality of disaster-related mortality data at state, local, tribal, and territorial levels. These efforts should prioritize the standardization of methods for data reporting and recording and to improve the capacity of death investigation and registration systems to capture more detail on contributing causes of death following disasters.

The following immediate actions should be undertaken:

- NCHS should fund and support the transition of the remaining states and territories with paper-based death registration systems to electronic death registration systems (EDRSs) and lead, in collaboration with state vital records offices, the integration of best practices for capturing and coding disaster-related death data into state-based EDRSs.
- NCHS should directly fund improvements in and the standardization of medical examiner and coroner (ME/C) death e-filing systems and require interoperability with these systems and state EDRSs. Similarly, NCHS and state registrars should require that EDRSs adopt the following standard improvements:
  - o Automatic filing of death information with state EDRSs via ME/C e-filing systems to reduce the administrative burden on medical examiners and coroners;
  - o Automated and uniform alert flags, prompts, drop-down options, and decision-making support for use by medical certifiers when entering data into a death record in both a routine and just-in-time capacity;
  - o Offline data entry and other continuity mechanisms; and
  - o Geocoding of deaths based on both place of residence and location of death.

The following long-term actions should be prioritized:

- NCHS should fund and adopt, where appropriate, artificial intelligence technologies to improve the throughput of its automated medical coding systems so as to improve the throughput of ME/C deaths to a level equivalent to that of other natural causes of death.
- State vital records offices and ME/C offices, with the support of CDC, should develop continuity plans to sustain the functions of these offices during emergencies.

Recommendation 3-2: Standardize Data Collection and Reporting of Individual-Level Reported Disaster-Related Mortality

The National Center for Health Statistics (NCHS), working with the states, should update the Model State Vital Statistics Act to drive uniformity of data collection and recording with respect to disaster-related mortality. To promote uniformity in definitions and practices for collecting and recording disaster-related mortality data and enhance the quality and comparability of these data, NCHS should revise the Model State Vital Statistics Act to provide clear guidance and data standards to state vital records offices and medical certifiers. These changes should include the use of automated flags, prompts, and drop-down options to collect data on the relationship of a death to a recent disaster and provide decision-making support for medical certifiers.

Standards for Morbidity Data Collection

Collecting data about disaster-related morbidities presents its own set of challenges, given the broad definition of disaster-related morbidities; the influence of pre-existing and co-morbid conditions on post-disaster health outcomes; variation across disaster types; and logistical challenges associated with mining morbidity data from across a broad network of unique federal, SLTT, and local health care systems. Assessing health outcomes is a critical component in improving rapid responses following a disaster though the allocation of resources and targeted public health messaging as well as for improving prevention and mitigation activities during the inter-disaster period. When acted on appropriately, morbidity data can help to reduce mortality (i.e., by preventing morbidities from becoming mortalities) and can be used to help shape public health messaging and medical preparedness. For end users in the field of disaster management, in particular, estimates of morbidity resulting from a disaster may actually be of more value than mortality data in informing life-saving mitigation and preparedness activities and in enhancing real-time response. An exclusive focus on mortality data, the traditional outcome of interest, at the expense of morbidity data is tantamount to focusing only on the worst cases.

Morbidity data collection and recording presents different challenges than the collection and recording of mortality data. First, although mortality data collection and recording systems require extensive improvement, the basic structure of these systems and their supporting administrative and methodological processes for collecting individual-level mortality data already exist. This is not the case for disaster-related morbidity data. Additionally, morbidity involves a wider range of data and data sources, such as hospital admissions data, electronic health records and syndromic surveillance systems, records from disaster medical assistance teams, and data from sheltering operations. The types and severity of the significant morbidities that occur following a disaster also vary widely and tend to be disaster-specific (e.g., burns are not likely to spike following a major flood and near-drowning incidents are unlikely to occur during a wildfire) making it difficult, but not impossible, to standardize policies and practices for data collection for reported cases of morbidities. Despite this variation, past research into disaster-related morbidity suggests that key morbidities may exist across common types of disasters and further suggests that these morbidities could be used to define a standard set of data that could be tracked to inform disaster management policy and practice. Defining what morbidity data to collect is a critical first step to building the capability to collect and use these data. Therefore, investment in an ongoing process is needed to develop, validate, and disseminate national standards for data collection of key morbidities caused or exacerbated by specific types of disasters.

Conclusion 3-5: Collecting morbidity data presents an additional challenge due to the large quantity of possible outcomes and data available across multiple unique systems. Understanding which data are of greatest value and how these data can be used to inform disaster management requires more research.

Conclusion 3-6: Standards for morbidity data are needed across different types of disasters. A standard data set by disaster type would dramatically improve the uniform collection of morbidity data. This will improve the usability and actionability of these data.

<u>Recommendation 3-3: Develop a Set of Standards for Morbidity Data Collection</u>

The Centers for Disease Control and Prevention, in collaboration with the Centers for Medicare & Medicaid Services, the Council of State and Territorial Epidemiologists, and the National Association of County & City Health Officials should establish and promulgate national standards for the collection of disaster-related morbidities before, during, and after disasters. These activities should include investment in research to identify common morbidities that occur as a result of or are exacerbated by the conditions of specific types of disasters (e.g., floods, hurricanes, blizzards, radiation events, pandemics, etc.) and across multiple disaster types. This should include the identification of minimum timelines for data collection, the development and validation of morbidity data systems for use by the disaster management enterprise, and pilot testing and implementation of approaches to collect these data in a standardized manner.

Improving the Use of Analytical Methods for Population Estimates

Statistical estimation methods, in contrast to individual counting approaches, generate a more complete picture of the total impact of a disaster on health outcomes, but they do not yield an allocation of individual cases into mutually exclusive categories of death or illness resulting from the disaster versus from other causes. Given the variation in ways of attributing the cause of any death and morbidity, there can be more than one appropriate approach for answering the question "How many deaths and severe morbidities were caused by this disaster?" Still, these estimates can be more complete than those derived from case-counting methods, which tend to systematically undercount morbidity and mortality in major disasters, and they are thus critical for understanding the total impacts of disasters. There is no standard method for generating mortality or morbidity estimates. Nevertheless, methodological best practices can be specified, and a national research program is vital to further develop and validate these and to indicate appropriate circumstances for their uses. As in all areas of research, these practices would benefit from clarity in the specification of study objectives and definition of terms, by transparency in the statement of assumptions and the sourcing of data used in the study, and by great caution in advancing any particular measure or method as a perfect solution.

> *Conclusion 4-1: Given the variation in ways for attributing the cause of any death and morbidity, there can be more than one appropriate approach to answering the question "How many deaths and severe morbidities were caused by this disaster?" Nevertheless, methodological best practices can be specified, and a national research program is urgently needed to identify, further develop, and validate these practices. As in all areas of research, these best practices are characterized by (1) clarity in the specification of study objectives and definition of terms, (2) transparency in the statement of assumptions and the sourcing of data used in the study, (3) continued testing and improvement of the accuracy of measures, and (4) caution in advancing any particular measure or method as the single perfect solution.*

Developing an effective data and information structure for studying disaster impacts on mortality and morbidity should be a cornerstone of the nation's operational disaster response function. Because the necessary analytical sophistication and high-quality fieldwork are generally beyond the capabilities and time availability of most SLTT health departments, the Department of Health and Human Services (HHS) should build and sustain the capacity of the nation's existing research and survey infrastructure to support the collection of survey data on the health effects of disasters.

Conclusion 4-2: Developing an effective data and information structure for studying disaster impacts on mortality and morbidity should be a cornerstone of the nation's operational disaster response function. Because the necessary analytical sophistication and high-quality fieldwork are generally beyond the capabilities and time availability of most SLTT health departments, it is essential that federal partners work to build and sustain the capacity of the nation's existing research and survey infrastructure to support the collection of survey data on the health effects of disasters.

<u>Recommendation 4-1: Fund and Conduct Research on Analytical Methods for Population Estimates</u>

The Centers for Disease Control and Prevention, the National Institutes of Health, and the National Science Foundation should establish a national research program to advance analytical methods for conducting population-level estimates of mortality and morbidity related to disasters. This national research program should include the development and refinement of minimum standard methods and protocols for conducting population-level mortality and morbidity assessments as well as the creation and testing of tools for use by researchers, states, and localities to enhance their capabilities to carry out and use these analyses.

- Academic departments and institutes, which can be more flexible in initiating and conducting studies, should be included in these research efforts.
- Because many of the estimates in the literature result from "one-off" efforts that do not build on or seek comparability with previous disasters, an initial step in this research should be a careful comparison of different estimates from the same emergency to gain an understanding of how methodological choices and assumptions affect the estimates.

<u>Recommendation 4-2: Enhance Capacity to Collect and Analyze Population Estimates for Mortality and Morbidity</u>

The Department of Health and Human Services, together with state, local, tribal, and territorial (SLTT) agencies, should proactively develop partnerships to enhance the capacity to collect and analyze population-level disaster-related morbidity and mortality information. This includes the identification of appropriate mortality and morbidity datasets and sampling frames that might be brought to bear and the pre-negotiation of data-sharing agreements to ensure access to these data when needed.

The following immediate actions should be undertaken:

- The Secretary of Health and Human Services should push forward the collection of survey data on disaster-exposed and comparison populations to provide population-representative data on how disasters and their contributing stressors affect morbidity and to build the evidence base on differences in mortality and morbidity impacts across types of disasters.
- The federal statistical system, including the Centers for Disease Control and Prevention (CDC), the Substance Abuse and Mental Health Services Administration, and others should harness existing survey infrastructure and develop standard, Institutional Review Board (IRB)-approved sampling frames and methods for dealing with methodological challenges, such as population migration, for use by researchers conducting population estimates following large-scale disasters.
- The stakeholders listed above should address issues with informed consent procedures under the Common Rule, respondent burden issues under the Paperwork Reduction Act, and privacy under the Health Insurance Portability and Accountability Act Privacy Rule in advance and ensure that alternative arrangements are in place to protect privacy and confidentiality.
- SLTT agencies and academic research centers with the capability of conducting population estimates of disaster impact should formalize working relationships, data-sharing agreements, and IRB approvals in advance of a disaster to reduce delays in access to health data needed to conduct population estimates following a disaster and develop baseline assessments during the inter-disaster period.
- CDC and the Federal Emergency Management Agency should integrate frontline public health practitioners (e.g., epidemiologists and others) in the disaster response teams to help gather data and begin detailed analyses of mortality and morbidity data early in the disaster.

Access to and Use of Mortality and Morbidity Data

The committee strongly believes that the collection of mortality and morbidity data should be founded on the intention to use those data for the protection of human life and, in particular, that the data should be used in a manner that supports the resilience of vulnerable populations. Because disaster-related mortality and morbidity data are not yet systematically used in disaster management by SLTT entities, significant opportunity exists to formalize the use of mortality and morbidity data as an essential component of the practice of disaster management. The successful operationalization of accessing and using mortality and morbidity data on a large scale highlights the need for the adoption of an enterprise approach by all relevant stakeholders and support for leadership to initiate change (see Conclusion 3-4).

In their review of current practices and barriers, the committee noted the need for improved access to actionable data by SLTT stakeholders to federal data and tools before, during, and after a disaster. Because the capability to analyze and act on these data and access to resources varies across SLTTs, certain entities may require greater support, beyond just data access, from federal agencies than others. Several current and proposed practices have been identified that could be brought to scale to facilitate access to actionable data that could be used at the SLTT level (e.g., the data systems used by Ventura Country).

For example, stakeholders, particularly those at the state and local levels, could establish data-sharing agreements during the inter-disaster period to facilitate data access across actors and systems during an emergency. There is often an expectation that localities are responsible for providing data to state and federal authorities without reciprocity. The committee instead encourages the bi-directional flow of data because the fundamental purpose of collecting data is its meaningful use. However, streamlining data access is insufficient without supporting under-resourced local entities in developing the tools and capacities needed to analyze and act on these data. Without prioritizing actionability alongside access, the delivery of large quantities of federal or state data is a distraction at best (see Conclusion 3-7). Additionally, investment in research is needed to develop an understanding of what data are most valuable to various stakeholders at different times and to demonstrate how these data could be used to inform policy and practice throughout the disaster management cycle.

For example, certain contextualizing data delivered alongside morbidity data could provide critical information about the characteristics of a specific zip code and lead to enhanced responses through more targeted public health interventions that raw individual counts of morbidity would be unable to provide alone. Research priorities include the initiation of pilot projects with evaluative components, cost-effectiveness research to secure the support of policy makers, and implementation research to evaluate the function of data systems and practices for using individual- and population-level mortality and morbidity data. The development and piloting of new tools, such as data dashboards and other electronic tools for analysis by lay users, for acting on mortality and morbidity data to inform decision making by local entities is also needed (see Chapter 3).

Conclusion 3-7: Access to federal and state mortality and morbidity data is essential but data access does not equate to actionability of these data at the local level. If data are to be actionable, localities require the tools needed to read, analyze, and display data received from the federal or state level in a meaningful way as well as the expertise and capacity to use these data in decision making.

Recommendation 4-3: Facilitate Access to and Use of Actionable Mortality and Morbidity Data by State, Local, Tribal, and Territorial (SLTT) Entities

- **The Department of Health and Human Services (HHS) should work with the Centers for Disease Control and Prevention, the Federal Emergency Management Agency (FEMA), the Office of the Assistant Secretary for Preparedness and Response (ASPR), and other federal agencies to facilitate access to essential mortality and morbidity data to SLTT entities and academic research institutions throughout the disaster cycle. These data should be provided proactively and in a manner that is actionable for situational awareness and disaster response at state and local levels.**
- **Additionally, state and federal agencies should fund the development and testing of analytical tools and work collaboratively with local entities to use mortality and morbidity data in meaningful ways.**
- The following immediate actions should be undertaken to ensure SLTT access to and use of mortality and morbidity data:
  - The National Center for Health Statistics (NCHS) should code and automatically provide, with the assistance of FEMA and ASPR, location-specific, baseline mortality data and up-to-date data on disaster deaths following a declared disaster and upon request, as well as offer ready-to-use tools within a set time frame following disasters to states and localities.
  - NCHS should make available to researchers and SLTT investigators the mortality data from the National Death Index.
  - NCHS and state vital records offices should retrospectively geocode death registry entries in select areas that were previously affected by large-scale disasters to provide sample data for modeling future impact and other research.
  - ASPR and CDC should provide state and local officials with guidance on standard practices for assessing mortality and morbidity and facilitate the analysis of these data by state and local health and emergency management officials.

- o CDC in collaboration with FEMA and ASPR should fund and conduct research to establish standard practices for analyzing disaster-related causes of death and its contributing causes, including guidance on standard timelines for data analysis (e.g., 30 days) and geographic parameters for defining a disaster's geographic scope.
- o CDC and the Centers for Medicare & Medicaid Services (CMS) should use existing systems to pilot the collection of relevant morbidity data following disasters to serve as an inter-disaster baseline.
- o CMS, in collaboration with electronic health record companies and health systems, should pilot and evaluate the inclusion of disaster-related *International Classification of Diseases, Tenth Revision* codes in electronic health records.
- o HHS should use both existing and novel data sources to improve mortality and morbidity data acquisition and reporting, including the use of surveys, artificial intelligence, machine learning, and other big data methods.

Use of Morbidity Data

Currently, electronic health records and systems are exceptionally varied, and many lack the capability to push priority data on morbidities to the relevant parties in real time. Therefore, the aggregation and analysis of large volumes of morbidity data to support real-time decision making across these disparate data systems is not yet a reality. As with mortality data, data-sharing challenges and the lack of interoperability of data systems at all levels remain substantial barriers to the use of morbidity data. Opportunities exist to use existing federal systems, such as CMS data systems, to collect valuable morbidity data following emergencies. Testing and then implementing processes for monitoring, evaluation, and assessment of the collection and use of morbidity data would help to identify gaps and best practices in order to guide the evolution of existing electronic systems to be able to capture and report morbidity data.

Professional Training and Support

Medicolegal professionals, charged with completing death certificates for unnatural or unexplained deaths, are not universally equipped to implement the preceding recommendations. As described above and in Chapter 3, the medicolegal death investigation system within the United States is composed of a patchwork of different systems and professionals at the SLTT level that are responsible for establishing their own policies and practices and setting standards for the minimum professional requirements for medical examiners, coroners, justices of the peace, and other medical certifiers. Many different stakeholders are involved in the collection and recording of mortality data, and each requires the appropriate training and professional support. Although there is no federal agency responsible for the oversight of these SLTT medicolegal systems, CDC, in collaboration with state vital records offices and professional organizations, is well positioned to serve in this training and support role.

The collection and recording of disaster-related mortality data require the medicolegal workforce to value the need for these data and to have the capacity and capability to adopt standardized definitions, practices, and systems. The committee recognizes that medical examiners are key to the function of the system and, because of their medically oriented education and professional backgrounds, are best suited to perform the essential functions of the medicolegal death investigation system and support the consistent and accurate assessment of individual deaths following disasters. However, the number of individuals in this profession is in decline. Therefore, while outside of the direct scope of the report, it is critical to the integrity of the medicolegal system that the challenges facing the medical examiner profession, in particular burnout and lack of access to basic resources to perform job functions, be addressed.

Conclusion 3-2: The collection and recording of disaster-related mortality data require the medicolegal workforce to value the need for these data and to have the capacity and capability to adopt standardized definitions, practices, and systems.

<u>Recommendation 3-4: Strengthen the Capacity of the Medicolegal Death Investigation System to Assess Disaster-Related Mortality</u>

The Centers for Disease Control and Prevention (CDC), in collaboration with state agencies and professional associations, should strengthen the value, capacity, and capability of the medicolegal death investigation system to improve investigation, training, data development and collection, and case management.

The following immediate actions should be undertaken:

- CDC should fund and re-launch the Medical Examiner and Coroner Information Sharing Program to provide guidance and support to medical examiners, coroners, and other medical certifiers.
- The National Association of Medical Examiners, the International Association of Coroners & Medical Examiners, the American Board of Medicolegal Death Investigators, and state-based medical examiner and coroner professional organizations

should support the proposed framework for collecting and recording uniform mortality and morbidity data, encourage the use of existing CDC tools and guidance by all professionals, and provide continuing education courses for their members that reflect this guidance.

- CDC, through the National Center for Health Statistics, along with appropriate licensing bodies should provide standardized training and materials designed for medical certifiers (physicians, nurse practitioners, physician assistants, and others as applicable by state) who encounter natural deaths and are responsible for entering death information into the death record.
- Death investigation systems should develop relationships with state or university-based demographers and epidemiologists to formalize proactive data collection and sharing agreements for natural disasters that are typical for the state as well as mass mortality and morbidity due to disease.
- To promote more accurate death certification, the above agencies should incentivize and support the conversion of coroner systems to regionalized medical examiner systems staffed by forensic pathologists and medicolegal death investigators professionally trained to identify and classify disaster-related deaths per the framework described in Recommendation 2-1.

Recommendation 3-5: Strengthen the Role of the Medicolegal Death Investigation and State Death Registration Systems in the Disaster Management Enterprise

State, local, tribal, and territorial public health and emergency management departments should integrate the professionals and agencies from the medicolegal death investigation and death registration systems in all aspects of preparedness and planning. This should involve the consideration of moving mortality management out of Emergency Support Function #8 (ESF8) and creating a separate ESF dedicated to mortality management. This new function could complement ESF8 and ensure focused attention on assessing mortality during and after disasters, while those charged with ESF8 responsibilities are focused on providing services to survivors. This new function could include the involvement of medical examiners, coroners, and other relevant professionals in planning drills for mortality management; effective, efficient, and unbiased data collection during disasters; training for family assistance centers; and standards for after-action reports and other mortality data-reporting activities.

Appendix A

Preliminary Literature Review Strategy

The committee conducted a primary literature review at the beginning of its deliberations and the articles obtained by this preliminary literature review were then assessed by the committee and staff for relevance to the committee's charge. The search parameters for this primary review of the literature are detailed below. This is not an exhaustive list of all research conducted as additional, targeted searches were conducted throughout the course of the committee's work as new areas of focus emerged and additional information was gathered through public sessions, workshops, and webinars.

Search Parameters

- Date range: 1980–present
- Type: Peer-review/grey literature
- Range: International, English only

Databases Reviewed

- Cochrane Database of Systematic Reviews
- Embase
- Medline
- News Abstracts
- PAIS
- Periodicals Abstracts
- ProQuest
- PsycInfo
- PubMed

- Scopus
- SocINDEX
- Worldcat

Primary Search Terms

- Morbidity
- Mortality

AND

Primary Search Terms

- Disaster impact
- Disaster preparedness
- Disaster-related
- Hazard
- Large-scale disasters
- Natural disasters
- Natural hazard

AND KEY WORDS

Causalities

- Chronic illness/injury/disease
    - Cancer
    - Diabetes
    - Dialysis
    - End-stage renal disease
    - Noncommunicable diseases
    - Nursing homes
- Death certification
- Death certification process
- Death certification timeliness
- Death counts
- Death data
- Death scene investigation
- Death statistics
- Death tolls
- Direct deaths/injury
- Disability
- Excess death
- Excess morbidity
- Excess mortality

- Indirect deaths/injury
- Infectious diseases
- Quality-adjusted life-year

Crisis Coordination
- Agency capacity
- Capacity
- Crisis coordination
- Crisis management
- Disaster mortuary operation teams
- Incident Command System
- Incident management
- Medical examination
- Military government coordination
- Red Cross
- Risk assessment
- Risk planning

Emergency Preparedness
- Displacement
- Emergency management
- Emergency preparedness
- Emergency responders
- Emergency response

Human-Induced Disaster
- Bioterrorism
- Biowarfare
- Mass shootings
- Terror attacks
- Terrorism
- Warfare

Infrastructure
- Collapses
- Infrastructure failure
- Structural failures

Insurance
- Funeral assistance
- Home insurance
- Life insurance

Medicolegal

- Medical law
- Medicolegal

Natural Disasters

- Avalanche
- Blizzard
- Cold wave
- Cyclone
- Drought
- Earthquake
- Floods
- Heat wave
- Hurricane
- Landslide
- Mudslide
- Sinkhole
- Tornado
- Typhoon
- Volcano
- Wildfire
- Winter storm

Psychosocial Health

- Interviews
- Medical examinations
- Psychosocial health

Public Health

- Community mental health
- Lasting effects of disasters
- Medical examination
- Neighborhood social processes
- Public health communications
- Public health policies

Social Determinants of Health

- Social capital
- Social networks

Survey Implementation/Data Collection

- Centers for Disease Control and Prevention
- Data collection capabilities
- Disaster data collection
- Electronic death registration system
- Electronic health records
- Federal Emergency Management Agency
- Formative assessment
- National Center for Health Statistics
- Network scale-up method
- Sampling
- Summation method
- Survey monitoring
- Years of potential life lost

Vulnerable Populations

- Affected populations
- At-risk
- Culturally appropriate
- Disability
- Hidden populations
- Marginalized
- Vulnerability assessment
- Vulnerable populations

PubMed Search Strategy Example

((((“disasters”[MeSH] OR “weather”[mesh] OR “geological phenomena”[mesh] OR disaster*[tiab] OR post-disaster[tiab] OR “relief planning”[tiab] OR “climatic processes”[MeSH] OR “climatic processes”[tiab] OR hurricane*[tiab] OR tornado*[tiab] OR typhoon*[tiab] OR cyclone*[tiab] OR earthquake*[tiab] OR flood*[tiab] OR storm*[tiab] OR drought*[tiab] OR tsunami*[tiab] OR snow[tiab] OR rain[tiab] OR “tidal wave”[tiab] OR “tidal waves”[tiab] OR landslide*[tiab] OR wildfire*[tiab] OR “forest fire”[tiab] OR “forest fires”[tiab] OR avalanche*[tiab] OR volcan*[tiab] OR blizzard*[tiab] OR lightning[tiab] OR windstorm*[tiab] OR snowstorm*[tiab] OR fire[tiab] OR windstorm*[tiab] OR “heat wave”[tiab] OR “heat waves”[tiab] OR heatwave*[tiab] OR blizzard*[tiab] OR sinkhole*[tiab]

Appendix B

Public Workshop Agendas

First Committee Meeting
May 28, 2019

500 Fifth Street, NW
Washington, DC 20001
Keck Center, Room 103

1:00 p.m. Welcome to the Open Session
Ellen MacKenzie, Committee Chair
Johns Hopkins Bloomberg School of Public Health

1:10 p.m. Presentations and Discussion on the Scope and Context of Study Charge
(20 minutes of opening remarks followed by a 45-minute question-and-answer period)

Alex Amparo
Assistant Administrator, National Preparedness Directorate
Federal Emergency Management Agency

Anthony Macintyre
Senior Medical Advisor, Department of Homeland Security
Office of Health Affairs
Medical Liaison Officer, Federal Emergency Management Agency

Justin Pelletier
Legislative Director, Congresswoman Nydia Velazquez (NY-07)

2:15 p.m. Assessing Mortality After Disaster—Hurricane Maria Case Study

- Provide the background and context for your study of mortality following Hurricane Maria in Puerto Rico.
- Discuss the main considerations for selecting the study design and the major challenges associated with its implementation.
- Identify lessons learned for the future in terms of quantifying mortality and serious morbidity following large-scale disasters.
  (20 minutes of opening remarks followed by a 55-minute question-and-answer period)

Lynn Goldman
Dean, Milken Institute School of Public Health, The George Washington University

Caroline Buckee
Associate Professor, Harvard T.H. Chan School of Public Health

3:30 p.m. ADJOURN

Second Committee Meeting
DAY 1: August 29, 2019
OPEN SESSION

9:00 a.m. Welcome and Opening Remarks
Ellen MacKenzie, Committee Chair, Johns Hopkins Bloomberg School of Public Health

SESSION 1: HURRICANE MARIA IN PUERTO RICO—CASE STUDY

90 minutes (5 minutes for opening remarks followed by moderated discussion and Q&A)

9:15–10:45 a.m. Moderator: **Maureen Lichtveld,** Committee Member, Tulane University School of Public Health and Tropical Medicine

Panelists:

- **Francisco Murphy Rivera,** Physician, Adjuntas, Puerto Rico
- **José Cordero,** Department Head, Epidemiology and Biostatistics, University of Georgia
- **Maria M. Juiz Gallego,** Supervisor of the Division of Quality Assurance, Demographic Registry of Puerto Rico
- **Judith Mitrani-Reiser,** Director of the Disaster and Failure Studies Program, National Institute of Standards and Technology

10:45–11:00 a.m. BREAK

SESSION 2: FLORIDA SYSTEM FOR ASSESSING POST-DISASTER MORTALITY AND SIGNIFICANT MORBIDITY—CASE STUDY

90 minutes (5 minutes for opening remarks followed by moderated discussion and Q&A)

11:00 a.m.–12:30 p.m. Moderator: **Charles Rothwell,** Committee Member, National Center for Health Statistics (retired)

Panelists:

- **Carina Blackmore,** State Epidemiologist and Director, Division of Disease Control and Health Protection, Florida Department of Health
- **Kenneth Jones,** State Registrar, Florida Department of Health
- **Stephen Nelson,** District 10 Medical Examiner and Chairman of the Florida Medical Examiners Commission

- **Sandon Speedling,** Health Officer, Florida Department of Health

12:30 p.m. LUNCH

SESSION 3: CURRENT CAPABILITIES IN ASSESSING AND USING MORBIDITY AND MORTALITY DATA IN REAL TIME DURING A LARGE-SCALE DISASTER

90 minutes (5 minutes for opening remarks followed by moderated discussion and Q&A)

1:15–2:45 p.m. Moderator: **Sue Anne Bell,** Committee Member, University of Michigan School of Nursing

Panelists:

- **Tara Das,** State Registrar, Texas Department of State Health Services
- **Edward Kilbane,** Physician–Forensic Pathologist, National Disaster Medical System
- **Mac McClendon,** Director of Public Health Preparedness and Response, Harris County Public Health
- **Rebecca Noe,** Epidemiologist, Capacity Building Branch, Center for Preparedness and Response, Centers for Disease Control and Prevention

2:45–3:00 p.m. BREAK

SESSION 4: CURRENT CAPABILITIES IN ASSESSING AND USING MORBIDITY AND MORTALITY DATA DURING THE INTER-DISASTER PERIOD

90 minutes (5 minutes for opening remarks followed by moderated discussion and Q&A)

3:00–4:30 p.m. Moderator: **W. Craig Vanderwagen,** Committee Member, East West Protection, LLC

Panelists:

- **Dee Ann Bagwell,** Policy and Planning Director, Los Angeles County Department of Public Health
- **Carla Britton,** Senior Epidemiologist, Alaska Native Tribal Health Consortium
- **Devin George,** State Registrar, Louisiana Department of Health
- **Amy Davidow,** Associate Professor, Rutgers School of Public Health
- **Chesley Richards,** Deputy Director for Public Health Science and Surveillance, Centers for Disease Control and Prevention

4:30 p.m. ADJOURN Open Session

DAY 2: August 30, 2019
OPEN SESSION

8:30 a.m. Welcome and Opening Remarks
Ellen MacKenzie, Committee Chair, Johns Hopkins Bloomberg School of Public Health

SESSION 5: LOOKING FORWARD—BEST PRACTICES AND TOOLS FOR ASSESSING AND USING MORBIDITY AND MORTALITY DATA DURING A LARGE-SCALE DISASTER IN REAL TIME

90 minutes (5 minutes for opening remarks followed by moderated discussion and Q&A)

8:45–10:15 a.m. Moderator: **Richard Serino,** Committee Member, Harvard T.H. Chan School of Public Health

Panelists:

- **Tegan Boehmer,** Chief, Health Studies Section, National Center for Environmental Health, Centers for Disease Control and Prevention
- **Kelly Baker,** Registrar, Vital Records, Oklahoma State Department of Health
- **Frank DePaolo,** Deputy Commissioner for Forensic Operations, City of New York

10:15–10:30 a.m. BREAK

SESSION 6: LOOKING FORWARD—BEST PRACTICES AND TOOLS FOR ASSESSING AND USING MORBIDITY AND MORTALITY DATA DURING THE INTER-DISASTER PERIOD

90 minutes (5 minutes for opening remarks followed by moderated discussion and Q&A)

10:30 a.m.–12:00 p.m. Moderator: **Elizabeth Frankenberg,** Committee Member, University of North Carolina

Panelists:

- **Steven Schwartz,** Director, Division of Vital Statistics, National Center for Health Statistics, Centers for Disease Control and Prevention
- **Umair Shah,** Director, Harris County Public Health
- **Skip Skivington,** Vice President of Health Care Continuity Management and Support Services, Kaiser Permanente
- **Kevin Yeskey,** Principal Deputy Assistant Secretary, Office of the Assistant Secretary for Preparedness and Response

PUBLIC COMMENT

30-minute session

12:00–12:30 p.m. Moderator: **Ellen MacKenzie,** Committee Chair, Johns Hopkins Bloomberg School of Public Health

- Members of the public are invited to sign up to provide comments on the workshop topic (3 minutes each)

12:30 p.m. ADJOURN Open Session

Third Committee Meeting
DAY 1: October 7, 2019
OPEN SESSION

SESSION 1: COMMITTEE BREAKFAST

9:00–10:00 a.m. Moderator: **Ellen Mackenzie,** Committee Chair, Johns Hopkins Bloomberg School of Public Health

Panelist: Sacramento County Coroner Kimberly Gin will join the committee breakfast to discuss her office's work during the Camp Fire in Paradise.

10:00 a.m. ADJOURN and DEPART for Paradise

SESSION 2: PARADISE TOWN HALL

1:00–2:30 p.m. Moderator: **Ellen Mackenzie,** Committee Chair, Johns Hopkins Bloomberg School of Public Health

Panelists: Various representatives from the fire department, law enforcement, health care providers and administrators, civil leaders, town hall staff, and key community members will come to discuss their experiences during the Camp Fire in Paradise.

2:45 p.m. ADJOURN and DEPART for Butte County

SESSION 3: BUTTE COUNTY HEALTH DEPARTMENT

3:15–4:45 p.m. Moderator: **Ellen Mackenzie,** Committee Chair, Johns Hopkins Bloomberg School of Public Health

Panelists: Various representatives from the fire department, law enforcement, health care providers and administrators, civil leaders, town hall staff, and key community members will come to discuss their experiences during the Camp Fire in Paradise.

5:00 p.m. ADJOURN and DEPART for Sacramento

Webinar: Methodological Considerations for the Estimation of Disaster-Related Morbidity and Mortality at a Population Level

Tuesday, February 11, 2020
2:30–4:30 p.m. ET

The National Academies of Sciences, Engineering, and Medicine Committee on Best Practices for Assessing Mortality and Significant Morbidity Following Large-Scale Disasters is hosting this webinar as part of the committee's broader effort to learn from the perspectives of researchers who are using a variety of analytical approaches to estimate population size and disaster impact on human health. The committee's Statement of Task can be found on the last page of this agenda. The committee is specifically interested in learning more about the following:

1. Generalizing from your experience with custom analyses of individual disasters, what best practices or standards may exist for estimating disaster-related mortality and morbidity across different disaster types, sizes, and locations?
2. Experiences with the challenge of measuring disaster exposure and selecting methodological approaches for addressing issues like in- and out-migration.
3. Perspectives on using existing federal surveys (barriers, necessary data items, etc.) in such studies, as well as the essential role of spot, custom survey data collection.
4. Potential roles that researchers can play to support state and local stakeholders in analyzing morbidity and mortality data.
5. Recommendations on what is needed (resources, tools, partnerships, etc.) to develop more accurate and timely estimates of disaster impact.

2:30 p.m.	Welcome and Panel 1 Introduction **Elizabeth Frankenberg,** Carolina Population Center, Committee Member
2:40 p.m.	Panel 1: Survey-Based Methods for Assessing Mortality and Morbidity **Rafael Irizarry,** Harvard University **Jessica Ho,** University of Southern California
3:00 p.m.	Discussion with Committee
3:30 p.m.	Panel 2 Introduction **H. Russell Bernard,** Arizona State University, Committee Member

3:40 p.m.	Panel 2: Methods for Estimating Hard-to-Count Populations **Adrian Raftery,** University of Washington **Tyler McCormick,** University of Washington
4:00 p.m.	Discussion with Committee
4:30 p.m.	Adjourn Webinar

Webinar: Methodological Considerations for Estimating Excess Mortality and Morbidity

Tuesday, February 18, 2020
2:30–4:00 p.m. ET

The National Academies of Sciences, Engineering, and Medicine Committee on Best Practices for Assessing Mortality and Significant Morbidity Following Large-Scale Disasters is hosting this webinar as part of the committee's broader effort to learn from the perspectives of researchers who are using excess mortality to assess disaster impact. The committee's Statement of Task can be found on the last page of this agenda. Rather than the findings from the research, the committee is specifically interested in learning more about the methodological challenges researchers face in conducting such research and how these challenges can be addressed, including:

1. Critical assumptions that must be made and what is needed to make better informed assumptions.
2. The identification of accurate baseline data and coping with a lack of baseline data.
3. The selection of exposed and comparison populations across different disaster contexts, determinations of which outcomes to measure (including causes of death and morbidity), when to measure them, and for how long.
4. Selection of statistical methods when using large databases that lead to more precise estimates.
5. Addressing privacy and confidentiality concerns and other barriers to data sharing and use.
6. Potential roles that researchers can play to support state and local stakeholders and federal policy makers in analyzing morbidity and mortality data.
7. Recommendations on what is needed (resources, tools, partnerships, etc.) to develop more accurate and timely estimates of disaster impact.

2:30 p.m.	Welcome and Panel Introduction **Michael Stoto,** Georgetown University, Committee Member **Sue Anne Bell,** University of Michigan, Committee Member
2:40 p.m.	Panel Presentations **Scott Zeger,** Johns Hopkins University **Troy Quast,** University of South Florida
3:00 p.m.	Discussion with Committee
4:30 p.m.	Adjourn Webinar

Appendix C

Assessing Morbidity and Mortality Associated with the COVID-19 Pandemic: A Case Study Illustrating the Need for the Recommendations in This Report

Authored by M. A. Stoto and M. K. Wynia, July 22, 2020

INTRODUCTION AND SUMMARY

In a crisis, the public wants to know what is happening and policy makers want good data for decisions. The coronavirus disease 2019 (COVID-19) pandemic has generated a sea of numbers: cumulative totals and daily numbers of new cases, individuals hospitalized and recovered, deaths and death rates, numbers tested, testing capacity, and undiagnosed and asymptomatic cases. Policy makers seek to use these and other data to know whether we have "flattened the curve," to assess which non-pharmaceutical interventions—social distancing, mask wearing, restrictions on gatherings, and so on—are most effective, and to serve as metrics for relaxing or tightening restrictions. The pandemic has dramatically illustrated the high level of public interest in the total numbers of reported cases and deaths, though it is widely acknowledged by experts (and for reasons described in this report) that these early estimates typically underestimate the full effects of the pandemic.

The pandemic has also illustrated how numbers of deaths and illnesses associated with a disaster can inform critical decisions with public health, economic, and political implications, which can make the accuracy of these estimates a source of vigorous debate. In this regard, the pandemic has shone a spotlight on the need for accurate information to both guide disaster response and improve preparedness for the future. Yet, the plethora of COVID-19 numbers also reminds us that the consequences of any major disaster are far more complex than can be represented by a single number, the "death toll." Moreover, it shows that even the "death toll" cannot be fully captured in a single number except at a single point in time.

As described in the body of the committee's report, there are two basic approaches to assessing morbidity and mortality from disasters. Both approaches produce valuable information about disaster-related mortality and morbidity, though each has different strengths, weaknesses, and appropriate uses. One is to try to count casualties individually (whether deaths, injuries, or cases of illness) and determine whether each is directly or indirectly caused by, or associated with, the disaster. The second approach is to estimate the number of casualties using statistical means, either through sampling methods or by comparing observed deaths with deaths observed in the previous year or a comparison population.

The first approach (case counting) typically generates an underestimate of total morbidity and mortality, and the COVID-19 pandemic has shown that these numbers may be skewed even further downward when testing for the presence or absence of the condition in question is unavailable or unreliable. Yet, the counting approach is essential for contact tracing and for getting relief to specific individuals affected by the disaster. Case counts are also often the first set of numbers available to decision makers.

Meanwhile, the population estimation approach typically takes more time, and suffers from the additional weakness of not being useful for determining which specific individuals might have been affected and which would have died or become ill even in the absence of the disaster. However, population estimation methods provide a much more complete picture of the entire population affected by the disaster and are preferred (when available) for making policy decisions where this more comprehensive view is important, such as about reopening strategies and targeting aid to areas and populations most affected.

To reiterate: both approaches are scientifically legitimate, though they differ in their assumptions and data requirements, and as suggested in Recommendation 2-2, both should be used and reported. More important, the availability of alternative approaches does not mean that "anything goes"—the COVID-19 pandemic has shown the value of carefully considering each method's unique strengths, weaknesses, and appropriate uses (see Table C-1). Although we note below where some methods might be more appropriate for specific uses than others, we do not regard any given method as always better than the others; they are different.

TABLE C-1 Strengths, Weaknesses, and Intended Use of Different Methods for Assessing COVID-19 Mortality and Morbidity

Assessment Method	Strengths	Weaknesses	Most Useful for
Individual Counts			
Case counts, by public health and emergency operations	• Draw on state and local public health data systems used to manage the pandemic	• Only include patients actually tested for COVID-19, which may not be available or necessary for their own care	• Directing contact tracing • Informing time-sensitive policy decisions such as relaxation of social distancing and distribution of resources
Vital statistics, by death certificates	• Include some cases that were not tested or only indirectly related to COVID-19 (e.g., myocardial infarctions in patients who did not come to emergency departments) • Include data not in public health records (e.g., race and ethnicity)	• Require certifying physicians' inference that COVID-19 was a cause when testing may not have been done • Substantial lag until death occurs and delays until recorded	• In-depth analysis after the pandemic
Population-Based Estimates			
Sero-prevalence surveys	• Estimate total number of infected individuals, including those without symptoms or not tested • Identify trends and differences across sociodemographic groups	• Require testing scientifically selected representative samples of the population, including many who are not symptomatic	• Identify trends in infection rates • Assess impact of social distancing and other public health efforts • Assess levels of immunity in the population
Excess morbidity and mortality estimates	• Rely on existing data systems (vital statistics, electronic medical records, etc.)	• Require complex statistical modeling and assumptions, which take time	• In-depth analysis after the pandemic

We present this analysis as a case study that illustrates the issues raised in the committee's report[1] and provides real-time context and support for the its recommendations. This analysis draws from a rapid expert consultation from the National Academies of Sciences, Engineering, and Medicine, which describes the strengths and weaknesses of different types of COVID-19 data.[2] The COVID-19 situation is changing rapidly, so we note that this analysis reflects the situation as of July 22, 2020.

Counting Individual COVID-19 Cases and Deaths

The report notes that during and shortly after a natural disaster the focus is typically on trying to count the individuals injured or killed. This counting requires (1) a process to determine whether a particular death is directly or indirectly caused by the disaster and (2) a mechanism to report these deaths to a central office so they can be tabulated and analyzed. Individual deaths are classified as directly or indirectly caused by the disaster by physicians, medical examiners, or coroners. Some of these decisions are obvious. For instance, people who drown in a flood or are hit by flying debris in a tornado should be reported as "direct" deaths, while a person killed while clearing trees after a tornado should be counted as an indirect death. Yet, current methods for individual counting generally would not count as an indirect death someone who suffered a fatal heart attack triggered by the stress of the disaster. And some cases are even more challenging, such as the person who survived a wildfire but then returned to his burned-out home and committed suicide.[3]

With regard to reporting, as in normal times, deaths during disasters are reported to state health departments through vital registration systems, which can take days or even weeks. For this reason, deaths and injuries in disasters are also often reported to and rapidly tabulated by public health emergency operations centers. This becomes especially important in infectious disease outbreaks.

---

[1] The Statement of Task directed the committee to focus on non-infectious disease–related disasters as defined in the Robert T. Stafford Disaster Relief and Emergency Assistance Act (Stafford Act). However, the triggering of a Stafford Act Declaration in March 2020 in response to the COVID-19 pandemic brought the consideration of this disaster within the committee's scope. The study sponsor, the Federal Emergency Management Agency, gave its approval for the committee's consideration of COVID-19 in this report.

[2] National Academies of Sciences, Engineering, and Medicine. 2020. *Evaluating data types: A guide for decision makers using data to understand the extent and spread of COVID-19.* Washington, DC: The National Academies Press. https://doi.org/10.17226/25826.

[3] See https://sanfrancisco.cbslocal.com/2017/11/14/man-kills-himself-in-ruins-of-his-burned-out-santa-rosa-home (accessed September 1, 2020).

Using Public Health Case Counts

There are several differences between how morbidity and mortality are classified and reported during a pandemic versus a natural disaster such as a fire, blizzard, or hurricane. In many natural disasters the focus is on immediate deaths, while in a pandemic, public health epidemiologists often focus on live cases, since they pose an infectious risk to others. Still, the COVID-19 pandemic has shown the intensity of public and policy-maker interest in the numbers of deaths based on counts, even as experts acknowledge that early case counts typically provide underestimates (see below). For pandemics, individuals are included in the epidemiological "case count" if they meet an established case definition, which typically includes characteristic symptoms caused by the pathogen and a laboratory test confirming infection, if one exists. These definitions can evolve as more is learned, and they often include options for naming someone as a "probable," "presumptive," or "confirmed" case, which can be critical for carrying out effective contact tracing. Importantly, contact tracing is a primary purpose of public health surveillance: clinicians are required to report cases to local or state health departments, which use this information to trace case contacts and help stem the outbreak. With regard to mortality estimates, however, the total number of deaths from the outbreak derived from case counts is based on tracking the survival of only those cases known to the health department, and one must acknowledge that errors in diagnosis and reporting can arise at every step of this process.

With regard to morbidity estimates, the COVID-19 pandemic illustrates several problems related to diagnosis. For instance, with no preexisting diagnostic test for the virus, early COVID-19 case definitions in Wuhan, China, were based on symptoms and a characteristic pattern in a computed tomography (CT) scan.[4] Setting aside any questions about intentional misreporting, respiratory symptoms are common in the winter, some patients do not present for care, and CT scans are expensive and not always available in outpatient settings, so it is entirely predictable that many cases in Wuhan were not included in early official case counts. Similarly, at the peak of the outbreak in New York City, tests were not available in sufficient numbers to test everyone with symptoms, and many individuals with symptoms of COVID-19 were regarded as "presumptive cases." Adding these presumptive cases into the official case count was appropriate, though it resulted in what seemed like a sudden jump in COVID-19 cases

[4] Wu, P., X. Hao, E. H. Y. Lau, J. Y. Wong, K. S. M. Leung, J. T. Wu, B. J. Cowling, and G. M. Leung. 2020. Real-time tentative assessment of the epidemiological characteristics of novel coronavirus infections in Wuhan, China, as at 22 January 2020. *Euro Surveillance* 25(3):2000044.

and deaths in New York.[5] Thus, the pandemic provides several examples of uncertainties that can arise in case counting due to diagnostic uncertainty.

The COVID-19 pandemic also illustrates some common challenges related to accurate and timely reporting of known cases. While physicians have a responsibility to report COVID cases, and health departments publish guidance about what should be reported and how, the changing nature of this guidance has made it difficult for busy practitioners to know what to do. To mitigate the risk of physician under-reporting, laboratories are also required to report positive test results, so that health departments can reach out to their physicians to gather additional data. Still, for COVID and for other reportable conditions, cases can be missed. Although some testing locations no longer require a referral, in many cases the patient to be tested must first seek health care, then the physician must decide to order a diagnostic test, the test must be available, and in many situations the patient must then go somewhere else to obtain the test. Further fueling the inaccuracy of national case counts for COVID-19 have been that testing processes, and even case definitions, have varied substantially from state to state.[6]

For many reportable infections, provider reporting is far from complete[7] and sudden increases in the proportion of cases reported, as can arise during a local outbreak, can distort surveillance statistics.[8] For many infectious diseases, such as influenza, physicians often make treatment decisions "empirically," based on symptoms alone, so test samples are not collected or sent to a lab. As a result, these cases are not included in initial public health case counts. Because COVID-19 can also be treated empirically, and tests have been scarce and some health systems overwhelmed, relatively healthy people with compatible symptoms have until recently been encouraged to stay home without testing.[9] As a result, the number of

[5] Goodman, J. D., and W. K. Rashbaum. 2020. N.Y.C. death toll soars past 10,000 in revised virus count. *The New York Times*, April 14, 2020. www.nytimes.com/2020/04/14/nyregion/new-york-coronavirus-deaths.html?smid=em-share (accessed September 1, 2020).

[6] Brown, E., and B. Reinhard. 2020. Which deaths count toward the COVID-19 death toll? It depends on the state. *The Washington Post*, April 16. www.washingtonpost.com/investigations/which-deaths-count-toward-the-covid-19-death-toll-it-depends-on-the-state/2020/04/16/bca84ae0-7991-11ea-a130-df573469f094_story.html (accessed September 1, 2020).

[7] Fill, M. A., R. Murphree, and A. C. Pettit. 2017. Health care provider knowledge and attitudes regarding reporting diseases and events to public health authorities in Tennessee. *Journal of Public Health Management and Practice* 23(6):581–588.

[8] Piltch-Loeb, R., J. Kraemer, K. W. Lin, and M. A. Stoto. 2018. Public health surveillance for Zika virus: Data interpretation and report validity. *American Journal of Public Health* 108(10):1358–1362.

[9] Begley, S. 2020. States have a long way to go on testing, review shows. *The Boston Globe*, April 28. www.bostonglobe.com/2020/04/27/nation/states-have-long-way-go-testing-review-show (accessed September 1, 2020).

officially recorded COVID-19 cases in the United States almost certainly underestimates the true number of infections, perhaps dramatically.

Epidemiologists refer to the fact that only a proportion of infected individuals seek care, are diagnosed, and are reported as the "iceberg effect." This has occurred with COVID-19 and it is a natural phenomenon; it should not be regarded or portrayed as an attempt to hide the full extent of the pandemic. For example, Holtgrave et al. demonstrated this effect during the height of the COVID-19 outbreak in New York State, and they also found that the proportion of those tested and diagnosed varied widely by race and ethnicity. They estimated that only 6.5 percent of infected Hispanic adults were diagnosed compared to 11.7 percent and 10.1 percent of non-Hispanic Whites and Blacks, respectively. Hispanics and Blacks who were infected, on the other hand, were more than twice as likely to be hospitalized compared to Whites.[10] This study from the COVID-19 pandemic illustrates another reason for cautious interpretation of case count data; certain population subgroups may be disproportionately represented (or unrepresented) in counting mechanisms.

The pandemic also illustrates how changes in case counting methods over time can affect reported numbers. As testing capacity grew in April, May, and June, so did the number of positive results, possibly "catching up" with actual cases and perhaps not reflecting a true rising incidence of new infections. Similarly, reducing the amount of testing would be expected to reduce the reported case count, which led public health officials to adjust recommendations for reopening according to testing numbers. For instance, one of the criteria for relaxing social distancing in the White House plan was a "downward trajectory of positive tests as a percent of total tests within a 14-day period," but the volume of tests must be flat or increasing[11] to avoid this bias. During the surge in cases in the South and West in June and July, however, shortages of testing resources[12] and delays in obtaining results[13] emerged, perhaps re-creating undercounts of cases. Notably, a state-by-state analysis by Stat News showed that in 26 of the 33 states that saw cases increase between mid-May and mid-July, the case

[10] Holtgrave, D. R., M. A. Barranco, J. M. Tesoriero, D. S. Blog, and E. S. Rosenberg. 2020. Assessing racial and ethnic disparities using a COVID-19 outcomes continuum for New York State. *Annals of Epidemiology* 48:9–14. https://doi.org/10.1016/j.annepidem.2020.06.010.

[11] White House. 2020. Opening up America again. www.whitehouse.gov/openingamerica (accessed October 1, 2020).

[12] Mervosh, S., and M. Fernandez. 2020. Months into virus crisis, U.S. cities still lack testing capacity. *The New York Times*, July 7. www.nytimes.com/2020/07/06/us/coronavirus-test-shortage.html?smid=em-share (accessed September 1, 2020).

[13] Wu, K. J. 2020. Testing backlogs may cloud the true spread of the coronavirus. *The New York Times*, July 19. www.nytimes.com/2020/07/19/health/coronavirus-testing-viral-spread.html?smid=em-share (accessed September 1, 2020).

count rose because there was actually more disease, not because there was more testing.[14]

Finally, there have been multiple reports of U.S. patients diagnosed retrospectively with COVID-19 who had not been previously included in official case counts. Some individuals were thought to have the infection but tests were not available;[15] in others COVID-19 was not initially suspected.[16] Such reports are sometimes characterized as surprising, or even to suggest that cases had been intentionally hidden, but they are an expected occurrence in disease outbreaks, especially with a novel pathogen.

The differences in the way COVID-19 cases are classified and reported—among jurisdictions and over time—described in this section create challenges for local, state, and national public health experts monitoring the pandemic. Developing a set of national standards as called for in Recommendation 3-3 would help policy makers at all levels choose appropriate control strategies.

Using Vital Statistics Data to Count COVID-19 Mortality

COVID-19 has also illustrated both opportunities and challenges associated with using vital statistics data to count mortality from the pandemic. Because COVID-19 cases are likely to be undercounted by public health, so are COVID-19 associated deaths based on case counts.[17] An alternative source of individual-level mortality data is vital statistics, which uses different definitions and processes than public health case counting and is essentially complete (i.e., nearly every person who dies in the United States is accounted for on a death certificate). In early April 2020, the National Center for Health Statistics (NCHS) issued guidance[18] indicating that if COVID-19 played a role in a death, this condition should be specified on the death certificate

---

[14] Begley, S. 2020. Trump said more COVID-19 testing "creates more cases." We did the math. *STAT News*, July 20. https://www.statnews.com/2020/07/20/trump-said-more-covid19-testing-creates-more-cases-we-did-the-math (accessed September 1, 2020).

[15] Duhigg, C. 2020. Seattle's leaders let scientists take the lead. New York's did not. *The New Yorker*, May 4. www.newyorker.com/magazine/2020/05/04/seattles-leaders-let-scientists-take-the-lead-new-yorks-did-not (accessed October 1, 2020).

[16] Fuller, T., M. Baker, S. Hubler, and S. Fink. 2020. A coronavirus death in early February was "probably the tip of an iceberg." *The New York Times*, April 22. www.nytimes.com/2020/04/22/us/santa-clara-county-coronavirus-death.html?smid=em-share (accessed September 1, 2020).

[17] On the other hand, serious cases are more likely to seek health care and be tested, so the degree of undercounting is probably less. Thus, the Case Fatality Rate (the proportion of cases with a condition who die) calculated from these data is likely to be an overestimate, and the same is true for the proportion of infected who suffer severe symptoms and need to be hospitalized.

[18] NVSS (National Vital Statistics System). 2020. Guidance for certifying deaths due to coronavirus disease 2019 (COVID-19). *Vital Statistics Reporting Guidance*. https://www.cdc.gov/nchs/data/nvss/vsrg/vsrg03-508.pdf (accessed September 1, 2020).

either as the underlying cause of death where warranted or as "probable" or "presumed" if the circumstances were compelling within a reasonable degree of certainty, even if testing had not been done (as it often was not, due to lack of testing capacity). Consequently, vital statistics data, which are compiled from death certificate data, will include some deaths not in the public health case counts. But some COVID-19 deaths will be missed in both public health case counts and on death certificates, and other deaths might be inaccurately attributed to COVID-19 on a death certificate.

For instance, in April 2020, vital statistics reports indicated a large increase in individuals dying at home, rather than in the hospital,[19] especially in New York City.[20] One might infer that many of these in-home deaths were caused, directly or indirectly, by COVID-19, but most were never tested or reported and hence are not included in health department case counts. Some of these deaths might eventually appear in vital statistics reports, if physicians follow the NCHS guidance, but because death certificate data are not used for contact tracing, most of these cases will never appear in public health case counts.

The COVID-19 pandemic provides multiple examples of the political tensions that can arise around these numbers. For instance, there have been claims offered without evidence that doctors are being "coached" to mark COVID-19 as the cause of death on death certificates even when it is not, to inflate the pandemic's death toll for political purposes.[21] In response, some states elected to not include deaths without a mention of COVID-19 on the death certificate in their official counts, even if the person had tested positive and was included in the public health surveillance database. In Colorado, this corresponded to a 24 percent reduction in deaths from COVID-19, as only 878 of 1,150 deaths (as of May 15, 2020) had COVID-19 specifically noted on the death certificate.[22] Moreover, NCHS added an extra step in which humans instead of computers must verify the information on the

[19] Gillum, J., L. Song, and J. Kao. 2020. There's been a spike in people dying at home in several cities. That suggests coronavirus deaths are higher than reported. ProPublica. www.propublica.org/article/theres-been-a-spike-in-people-dying-at-home-in-several-cities-that-suggests-coronavirus-deaths-are-higher-than-reported (accessed September 1, 2020).

[20] Hogan, G. 2020. Staggering surge of NYers dying in their homes suggests city is undercounting coronavirus fatalities. *Gothamist*, April 7. www.gothamist.com/news/surge-number-new-yorkers-dying-home-officials-suspect-undercount-covid-19-related-deaths (accessed September 1, 2020).

[21] Rosenberg, M., and J. Rutenberg. 2020. Fight over virus's death toll opens grim new front in election battle. *The New York Times*, May 9. www.nytimes.com/2020/05/09/us/politics/coronavirus-death-toll-presidential-campaign.html?referringSource=articleShare (accessed September 1, 2020).

[22] Ingold, J., and J. Paul. 2020. Nearly a quarter of the people Colorado said died from coronavirus don't have COVID-19 on their death certificate. *The Colorado Sun*, May 15. www.coloradosun.com/2020/05/15/colorado-coronavirus-death-certificate/?mc_cid=7ed16a0b8b (accessed September 1, 2020).

death certificate before it is added to the tally, adding around 1 week of delay in formally recording COVID-19 deaths.[23]

COVID-19 also shows how mortality data based on counting methods, while valuable for some purposes, can also create inaccurate impressions of overall pandemic control efforts.[24] For instance, as the number of new cases started to increase throughout the South and West of the United States in June and July 2020, some took comfort that mortality remained low in those states. But deaths typically occur 2–3 weeks or longer after an individual is infected, and there is further delay until they are reported, so the increase in mortality appeared in July.[25] Thus, COVID-19 shows how deaths can be a "lagging indicator." In addition, recent COVID-19 trends demonstrate two other ways in which deaths can provide an incomplete picture. First, because COVID-19 cases tended to be younger in June and July than they had been in April and May,[26] the early case fatality rate in this "second wave" in the United States was lower. At the time of this writing however, the virus was spreading to older and more vulnerable individuals, and the case fatality rate will likely go up. Second, recent case fatality rates have probably also been lower because the medical care provided to infected individuals has improved, though as hospitals in the South and West become as overwhelmed with cases as those in the New York City area were in April and May, that effect too may diminish.[27,28]

As with case counts, differences in the way COVID-19 deaths are recorded and tabulated described in this section create challenges for monitoring the pandemic. Standardizing mortality data and reporting (Recommendation 3-2) and strengthening systems to improve the quality of these

---

[23] Arnold, C. 2020. How scientists know COVID-19 is way deadlier than the flu. *National Geographic*, July 3. www.nationalgeographic.com/science/2020/07/coronavirus-deadlier-than-many-believed-infection-fatality-rate-cvd (accessed September 1, 2020).

[24] Thompson, D. 2020. COVID-19 cases are rising, so why are deaths flatlining? *The Atlantic*, July 10. www.theatlantic.com/ideas/archive/2020/07/why-covid-death-rate-down/613945 (accessed September 1, 2020).

[25] Stockman, F., M. Smith, and G. McDonnell Nieto del Rio. 2020. Daily virus death toll rises in some states. *The New York Times*, July 10. www.nytimes.com/2020/07/10/us/daily-virus-death-toll-rises-in-some-states.html?referringSource=articleShare (accessed September 1, 2020).

[26] Bosman, J., and S. Mervosh. 2020. As virus surges, younger people account for "disturbing" number of cases. *The New York Times*, June 26. www.nytimes.com/2020/06/25/us/coronavirus-cases-young-people.html?action=click (accessed September 1, 2020).

[27] Bump, P. 2020. The White House's favorite new coronavirus metric—mortality rate—probably won't be a favorite for long. *The Washington Post*, July 13. www.washingtonpost.com/politics/2020/07/13/white-houses-favorite-new-coronavirus-metric-mortality-rate-probably-wont-be-favorite-long/?arc404=true (accessed September 1, 2020).

[28] Ritchie, H., and M. Roser. 2020. What do we know about the risk of dying from COVID-19? Our World In Data, March 25. www.ourworldindata.org/covid-mortality-risk (accessed September 1, 2020).

data (Recommendation 3-1) would provide policy makers at all levels with the ability to monitor the pandemic and make better decisions about controlling it.

In sum, experiences with COVID-19 to date have provided a number of valuable examples of ways in which individual-level counting methods can underestimate total mortality and morbidity in disasters. Experiences with the pandemic also demonstrate that even though case counts and death counts can be (and typically are) presented as precise numbers down to the single case—and even though individual counting methods are critical when it comes to certain tasks such as contact tracing and assigning death benefits to individuals—these statistics are in fact *estimates* of the true total mortality or morbidity. To illustrate this, consider that even the two primary sources of data for individual counts of deaths—public health case counts and vital statistics—can be expected to generate different totals.[29] The COVID-19 pandemic further demonstrates that when case counts are the product of evolving case definitions, testing procedures, and reporting processes, the estimates generated through case counting can change (and hopefully improve) over time, but they remain estimates; typically, they will produce underestimates of the total disaster impact.

Population Estimation Approaches

The COVID-19 pandemic has also provided valuable illustrations of how a complementary set of methods can provide useful data and better assessments of the total impact of the pandemic on morbidity and mortality. These methods include (a) surveys using representative or complex sampling of affected populations (i.e., surveillance data) and (b) estimates derived by comparing observed deaths or illness to expected numbers based on prior years or comparison populations. Because these methods include a broader range of associated illness and death, they often produce numbers larger than those determined using individual case counts.

While statistical estimation might sound less precise than case counting, recall that case count methods provide imprecise results that are also estimates of the true effect of a disaster. Statistical estimation methods also have both strengths and weaknesses. While they can provide a more complete picture of the total impact of the disaster on health outcomes, they are not useful for determining whether any given dead or ill person became dead or ill as a direct or indirect result of the disaster. As an extreme example of these trade-offs, following Hurricane Maria a group of analysts based

[29] Reinhard, B., and E. Brown. 2020. Which deaths count toward the COVID-19 death toll? It depends on the state. *The Washington Post*, April 16. www.washingtonpost.com/investigations/which-deaths-count-toward-the-covid-19-death-toll-it-depends-on-the-state/2020/04/16/bca84ae0-7991-11ea-a130-df573469f094_story.html (accessed September 1, 2020).

at Harvard University used survey sampling methods to estimate 4,645 (95% confidence interval [CI] 793–8,498) excess deaths among Puerto Ricans.[30] Another group based at The George Washington University used excess mortality methods to estimate 2,975 (95% CI 2,658–3,290) excess deaths for the period of September 2017 through February 2018.[31] These numbers are now widely agreed to be much more accurate estimations of the total impact of the hurricane than the case count method, which suggested only 64 people died as a result of the hurricane. While Hurricane Maria represents a particularly egregious case of inadequacy of counting methods, it is illustrative of the dramatic undercounting that is possible following disasters. Experiences to date with using statistical estimation methods to assess COVID-19 morbidity and mortality have shown smaller, but still very significant estimation differences between case counting and statistical estimation methods, as summarized below.

Using Survey Sampling Methods to Assess Total COVID-19 Morbidity and Mortality

Efforts are under way to use survey methods to assess total morbidity and mortality of COVID-19. These methods use information collected from samples of individuals, extrapolating this information to a population to estimate the total impact of COVID-19. These methods are being used to inform a number of important policy questions. For instance, random sample survey methods can determine whether a COVID-19 outbreak in a city or a state is getting better or worse, and how fast, more accurately than counting only positive test results from those presenting for care. Specifically, sero-prevalence surveys from randomly chosen individuals in the population can determine the real percentage of people in a community recently infected with severe acute respiratory syndrome coronavirus 2 (SARS-CoV-2), assuming an accurate serologic assay is available.[32,33] For example, Rosenberg et al. analyzed a statewide convenience sample of New

---

[30] Kishore, N. D., D. Marqués, A. Mahmud, M. V. Kiang, I. Rodriguez, A. Fuller, P. Ebner, C. Sorensen, F. Racy, J. Lemery, L. Maas, J. Leaning, R. A. Irizarry, S. Balsari, and C. O. Buckee. 2018. Mortality in Puerto Rico after Hurricane María. *New England Journal of Medicine* 379(2):162–170.

[31] Milken Institute School of Public Health. 2018. *Ascertainment of the estimated excess mortality from Hurricane María in Puerto Rico*. Washington, DC: Milken Institute School of Public Health, The George Washington University.

[32] Mostashari, F., and E. J. Emanuel. 2020. We need smart coronavirus testing, not just more testing. *STAT*, March 24. www.statnews.com/2020/03/24/we-need-smart-coronavirus-testing-not-just-more-testing (accessed September 1, 2020).

[33] Lipsitch, M. 2020. Opinion. "Serology" is the new coronavirus buzzword. Here's why it matters. *The Washington Post*, May 4. www.washingtonpost.com/opinions/2020/05/04/serology-is-new-coronavirus-buzzword-heres-why-it-matters (accessed September 1, 2020).

York grocery store customers and estimated that the cumulative incidence of COVID-19 through March 29, 2020, was 14 percent. This rate varied substantially by geographic area (reaching 24 percent in New York City) as well as race and ethnicity. They also estimated that only 8.9 percent of individuals infected during this period were diagnosed, and that this fraction varied from 6.1 percent of individuals 18–34 years of age to 11.3 percent of those 55 years of age or older.[34] Sero-prevalence studies have been conducted in California[35,36] and other countries (e.g., Geneva, Switzerland[37]). The World Health Organization is coordinating sero-prevalence studies in at least six countries.[38]

Experience with COVID-19 also shows how data from survey methods can inform clinical decision making. For example, "sentinel testing" on samples of individuals at high risk of infection, such as health care workers or contacts of known cases,[39] have helped improve understanding of viral transmission risk and risk factors for more severe disease.[40]

COVID-19 has demonstrated the value of ongoing surveillance efforts, such as the Centers for Disease Control and Prevention's (CDC's) Outpatient Influenza-like Illness Surveillance Network (ILINet), which provides data on visits for influenza-like illness (ILI) (fever and cough and/or sore throat) from

---

[34] Rosenberg, E. S., J. M. Tesoriero, E. M. Rosenthal, R. Chung, M. A. Barranco, L. M. Styer, M. M. Parker, S.-Y.J. Leung, J. E. Morne, D. Greene, R. Holtgrave, D. Hoefer, J. Kumar, T. Udo, B. Hutton, and H. A. Zucker. 2020. Cumulative incidence and diagnosis of SARS-CoV-2 infection in New York. *Annals of Epidemiology* 48:23–29. doi: 10.1016/j.annepidem.2020.06.004.

[35] Bendavid, E., B. Mulaney, N. Neeraj Sood, S. Shah, E. Ling, R. Bromley-Dulfano, C. Lai, Z. Weissberg, R. Saavedra-Walker, J. Tedrow, D. Tversky, A. Bogan, T. Kupiec, D. Eichner, R. Gupta, J. Ioannidis, and J. Bhattacharya. 2020. COVID-19 antibody seroprevalence in Santa Clara County, California. *medRxiv* preprint. https://doi.org/10.1101/2020.04.14.20062463.

[36] Sood, N., P. Simon, P. Ebner, D. Eichner, J. Reynolds, E. Bendavid, and J. Bhattacharya. 2020. Seroprevalence of SARS-CoV-2-specific antibodies among adults in Los Angeles County, California, on April 10–11, 2020. *JAMA* 323(23):2425–2427. doi: 10.1001/jama.2020.8279.

[37] Stringhini, S., A. Wisniak, G. Piumatti, A. S. Azman, S. A. Lauer, H. Baysson, D. De Ridder, D. Petrovic, S. Schrempft, K. Marcus, S. Yerly, I. Arm Vernez, O. Keiser, S. Hurst, K. M. Posfay-Barbe, D. Trono, D. Pittet, L. Gétaz, F. Chappuis, I. Eckerle, N. Vuilleumier, B. Meyer, A. Flahault, L. Kaiser, and I. Guessous. 2020. Seroprevalence of anti-SARS-CoV-2 IgG antibodies in Geneva, Switzerland (SEROCoV-POP): A population-based study. *The Lancet* 396(10247):313–319. doi: 10.1016/S0140-6736(20)31304-0.

[38] Vogel, G. 2020. "These are answers we need." WHO plans global study to discover true extent of coronavirus infections. *Science*, April 2. www.sciencemag.org/news/2020/04/these-are-answers-we-need-who-plans-global-study-discover-true-extent-coronavirus (accessed September 1, 2020).

[39] Mostashari, F., and E. J. Emanuel. 2020. We need smart coronavirus testing, not just more testing. *STAT*, March 24. www.statnews.com/2020/03/24/we-need-smart-coronavirus-testing-not-just-more-testing (accessed September 1, 2020).

[40] Lipsitch, M., D. L. Swerdlow, and L. Finelli. 2020. Defining the epidemiology of COVID-19—studies needed. *New England Journal of Medicine* 382:1194–1196.

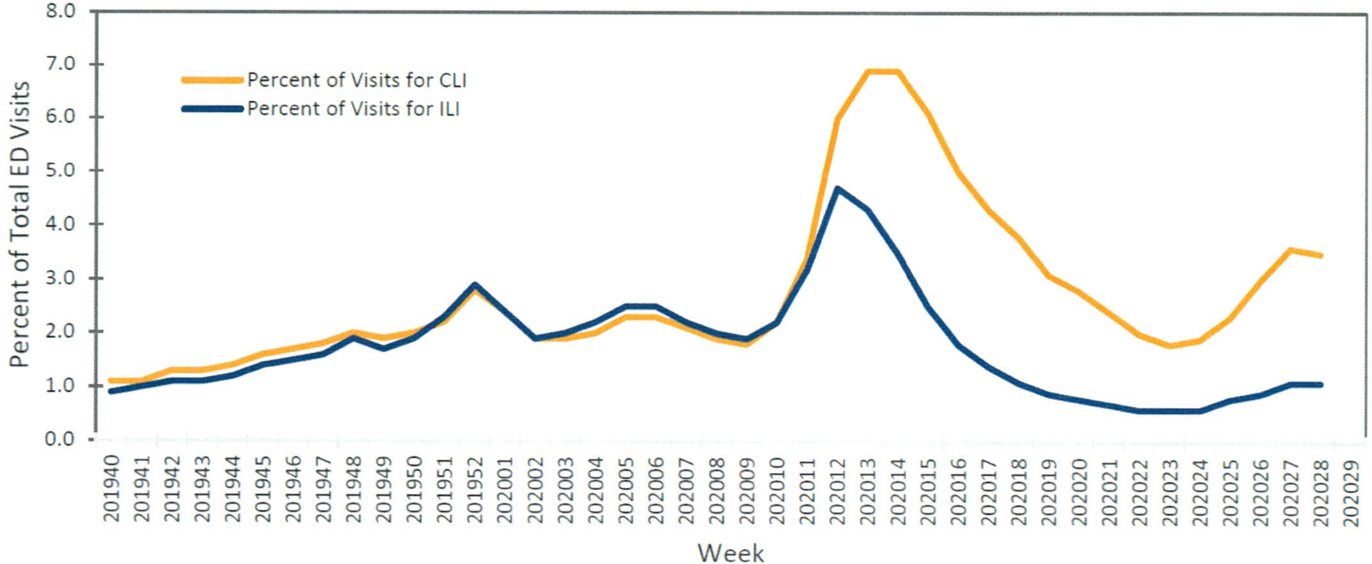

FIGURE C-1 National Syndromic Surveillance Program (NSSP): Percentage of emergency department visits for COVID-19-like illness or influenza-like illness, September 29, 2019–July 11, 2020.
NOTE: CLI = COVID-like illness; ED = Emergency Department; ILI = Influenza-like illness.
SOURCE: Centers for Disease Control and Prevention. 2020. COVIDView—A weekly surveillance summary of U.S. COVID-19 activity: Key updates for week 28, ending July 11, 2020. https://www.cdc.gov/coronavirus/2019-ncov/covid-data/pdf/covidview-07-17-2020.pdf (accessed September 1, 2020).

approximately 2,600 primary care providers, emergency departments, and urgent care centers throughout the United States. Because COVID-19 illness often presents with ILI symptoms, ILINet is being used to track trends and allows for comparison with prior influenza seasons. Also, the National Syndromic Surveillance Program (NSSP), which tracks emergency department visits in 47 states, has been extended to include COVID-19-like illness (fever and cough or shortness of breath or difficulty breathing). Figure C-1 displays the NSSP data through July 11, 2020,[41] suggesting a peak number of cases in early April and a re-emergence in June and July.

Several survey studies of COVID-19 have used data from quasi or non-random samples, which generally raise questions of bias and non-generalizability, but the pandemic has provided examples of how such studies can still provide useful information. For instance, SARS-CoV-2 testing was performed on 214 pregnant women who delivered infants at the NewYork-Presbyterian Allen Hospital and Columbia University Irving Medical Center during the height of New York's outbreak (between March 22 and April 4, 2020) and 33 tested positive (i.e., a prevalence rate of about 15 percent), but only 4 of these infected women (12 percent) had symptoms of COVID-19, suggesting very high rates of asymptomatic infection among pregnant women.[42]

COVID-19 also shows how population survey data can be used in combination with case count data to generate insights. For example, CDC is partnering with commercial laboratories to conduct sero-prevalence surveys using de-identified clinical blood specimens from people with blood drawn for reasons unrelated to COVID-19, aiming to test about 1,800 samples from 10 areas around the United States approximately every 3–4 weeks.[43] Initial results show the proportion of persons with COVID-19 antibodies ranged from 1.0 percent in the San Francisco Bay area (collected April 23–27) to 6.9 percent of persons in New York City (collected March 23–April 1). When compared to case count estimates, these data suggest that the number of total infections ranged from 6 to 24 times the number of

[41] Centers for Disease Control and Prevention. 2020. COVIDView—A weekly surveillance summary of U.S. COVID-19 activity: Key updates for week 28, ending July 11, 2020. https://www.cdc.gov/coronavirus/2019-ncov/covid-data/pdf/covidview-07-17-2020.pdf (accessed August 3, 2020).

[42] Sutton, D., K. Fuchs, M. D'Alton, and D. Goffman. 2020. Universal screening for SARS-CoV-2 in women admitted for delivery. *New England Journal of Medicine* 382:2163–2164.

[43] Centers for Disease Control and Prevention. 2020. Commercial laboratory seroprevalence survey data. https://www.cdc.gov/coronavirus/2019-ncov/cases-updates/commercial-lab-surveys.html (accessed September 1, 2020).

reported cases; for seven sites the total number of infections was estimated to be more than 10 times the number of reported cases.[44]

COVID-19 has also shown how surveys can be used to measure and track morbidity, such as mental health and other problems, by adding a disaster-specific module to an ongoing survey. For example, the weekly "pulse surveys" fielded by the U.S. Census Bureau were modified in response to the COVID-19 epidemic and are based on a representative sample of more than 1 million households.[45] Early results in May 2020, found that 34 percent of respondents showed symptoms of anxiety, depression, or both.[46] The results also show that many households have experienced a loss in employment income, are concerned about food security, and have deferred decisions to access health care.[47]

Despite the promise of these approaches, it must be noted that most of the survey-based methods described in this section were developed quickly to meet emergent needs. Methodological research to improve these approaches (Recommendation 4-1) and efforts to enhance the nation's capacity to conduct such research (Recommendation 4-2) would enhance the validity of survey results and facilitate their use and utility in future disasters.

Using Excess Mortality and Morbidity Methods in the COVID-19 Pandemic

Calculation of excess mortality and morbidity may provide the most complete, albeit often imprecise, estimates of the total impacts of disasters, including for infectious diseases. This has been illustrated by the experience with COVID-19, and it has been long-recognized for other infectious diseases. For instance, excess mortality is the standard way to determine the overall death toll for influenza each year. Because pneumonia is often

---

[44] Havers, F. P., C. Reed, T. Lim, J. M. Montgomery, J. D. Klena, A. J. Hall, A. M. Fry, D. L. Cannon, C.-F. Chiang, A. Gibbons, I. Krapiunaya, M. Morales-Betoulle, K. Roguski, M. Ata Ur Rasheed, B. Freeman, S. Lester, L. Mills, D. S. Carroll, S. M. Owen, J. A. Johnson, V. Semenova, C. Blackmore, D. Blog, S. J. Chai, A. Dunn, J. Hand, S. Jain, S. Lindquist, R. Lynfield, S. Pritchard, T. Sokol, L. Sosa, G. Turabelidze, S. M. Watkins, J. Wiesman, R. W. Williams, S. Yendell, J. Schiffer, and N. J. Thornburg. 2020. Seroprevalence of antibodies to SARS-CoV-2 in 10 sites in the United States, March 23–May 12, 2020. *JAMA Internal Medicine*. doi: 10.1001/jamainternmed.2020.4130.

[45] U.S. Census Bureau. 2020. Household pulse survey technical definition. https://www.census.gov/programs-surveys/household-pulse-survey/technical-documentation.html (accessed September 1, 2020).

[46] Fowers, A., and W. Wan. 2020. A third of Americans now show signs of clinical anxiety or depression, Census Bureau finds amid coronavirus pandemic. *The Washington Post*, May 26. www.washingtonpost.com/health/2020/05/26/americans-with-depression-anxiety-pandemic/?arc404=true (accessed September 1, 2020).

[47] U.S. Census Bureau. 2020. New household pulse survey shows concern over food security, loss of income. https://www.census.gov/library/stories/2020/05/new-household-pulse-survey-shows-concern-over-food-security-loss-of-income.html (accessed August 3, 2020).

the proximate cause of death for individuals with influenza, and laboratory testing for influenza is often not performed, CDC regularly tracks the number of deaths from either pneumonia or influenza as a proportion of all deaths recorded each week. These data are then compared to typical seasonal patterns and departures above this pattern, as in 2018, which indicate higher total mortality from flu (see Figure C-2). Recently, CDC added COVID-19 deaths to this analysis and found that almost 25 percent of all deaths occurring during the week ending April 11, 2020, were due to pneumonia, influenza, or COVID-19. This is far above the traditional epidemic threshold of 7.0 percent, with sharp weekly increases from the end of February through mid-April.[48] CDC also uses statistical modeling

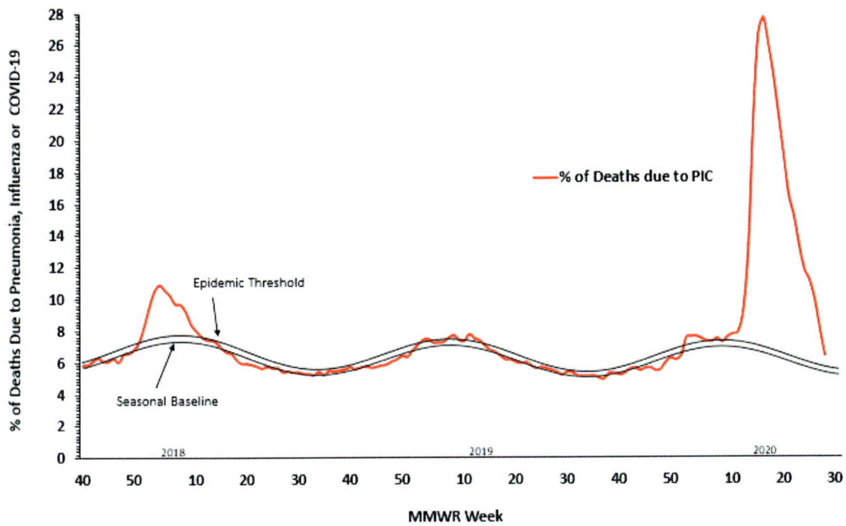

FIGURE C-2 Pneumonia, influenza, or COVID-19 mortality. Data through the week ending July 11, 2020, as of July 16, 2020.
NOTES: Data during recent weeks are incomplete because of the lag in time between when the death occurred and when the death certificate is completed, submitted to NCHS and processed for reporting purposes. MMRW = Morbidity and Mortality Weekly Report; PIC = Pneumonia, Influenza, or COVID.
SOURCE: Centers for Disease Control and Prevention. 2020. COVIDView—A weekly surveillance summary of U.S. COVID-19 activity: Key updates for week 28, ending July 11, 2020. https://www.cdc.gov/coronavirus/2019-ncov/covid-data/pdf/covidview-07-17-2020.pdf (accessed September 1, 2020).

[48] Centers for Disease Control and Prevention. 2020. COVIDView—A weekly surveillance summary of U.S. COVID-19 activity. https://www.cdc.gov/coronavirus/2019-ncov/covid-data/covidview/index.html (accessed August 3, 2020).

of background rates[49] to estimate the annual number of influenza-related deaths, which was about 80,000 in the 2018–2019 season, the disease's highest death toll in at least four decades.[50]

COVID-19 also illustrates that excess mortality methods are especially useful for assessing total deaths during an outbreak, including both direct and indirect causes. The initial efforts to describe excess mortality for COVID-19 were published in the media. For instance, *The Economist* found sharp increases in cardiac arrest 911 calls and deaths as well as confirmed COVID-19 deaths in March and early April 2020 in New York City (see Figure C-3).[51]

Similarly, based on data compiled by NCHS, *The New York Times* estimated that there had been 23,000 excess deaths in New York City between March 15 and May 2, 2020, leading to a total number of deaths that was more than three times the normal amount.[52] A more comprehensive analysis published by *The New York Times* estimated that by May 13, more than 100,000 Americans had already died as a result of the pandemic, rather than the 83,000 whose deaths had been directly attributed to the disease by that date.[53] *The Economist* maintains a comparison of excess deaths across countries.[54]

In May 2020 the New York City Department of Health and Mental Hygiene published a preliminary estimate of excess mortality in New York City from March 11 through May 2. As illustrated in Figure C-4, they estimated that out of a total of 32,107 reported deaths, 24,172 were in excess of the seasonal expected baseline. Of the excess, 13,831 (57 percent) were laboratory-confirmed COVID-19-associated deaths and 5,048 (21 percent) were probable COVID-19-associated deaths, leaving 5,293 (22 percent)

---

[49] Rolfes, M. A., I. M. Foppa, S. Garg, B. Flannery, L. Brammer, J. A. Singleton, E. Burns, D. Jernigan, S. J. Olsen, J. Bresee, and C. Reed. 2018. Annual estimates of the burden of seasonal influenza in the United States: A tool for strengthening influenza surveillance and preparedness. *Influenza and Other Respiratory Viruses* 12:132–137.

[50] CDC. 2020. COVIDView—A weekly surveillance summary of U.S. COVID-19 activity: Key updates for week 28, ending July 11, 2020. https://www.cdc.gov/coronavirus/2019-ncov/covid-data/pdf/covidview-07-17-2020.pdf (accessed September 1, 2020).

[51] *The Economist.* 2020. Deaths from cardiac arrests have surged in New York City. www.economist.com/graphic-detail/2020/04/13/deaths-from-cardiac-arrests-have-surged-in-new-york-city (accessed September 1, 2020).

[52] Katz, J., D. Lu, and M. Sanger-Katz. 2020. Tracking the real coronavirus death toll in the United States. *The New York Times*, May 6. www.nytimes.com/interactive/2020/05/05/us/coronavirus-death-toll-us.html?smid=em-share (accessed September 1, 2020).

[53] Kristof, N. 2020. America's true COVID toll already exceeds 100,000. *The New York Times*, May 14. www.nytimes.com/2020/05/13/opinion/coronavirus-us-deaths.html?smid=em-share (accessed September 1, 2020).

[54] *The Economist.* 2020. Tracking COVID-19 excess deaths across countries. www.economist.com/graphic-detail/2020/07/15/tracking-covid-19-excess-deaths-across-countries (accessed September 1, 2020).

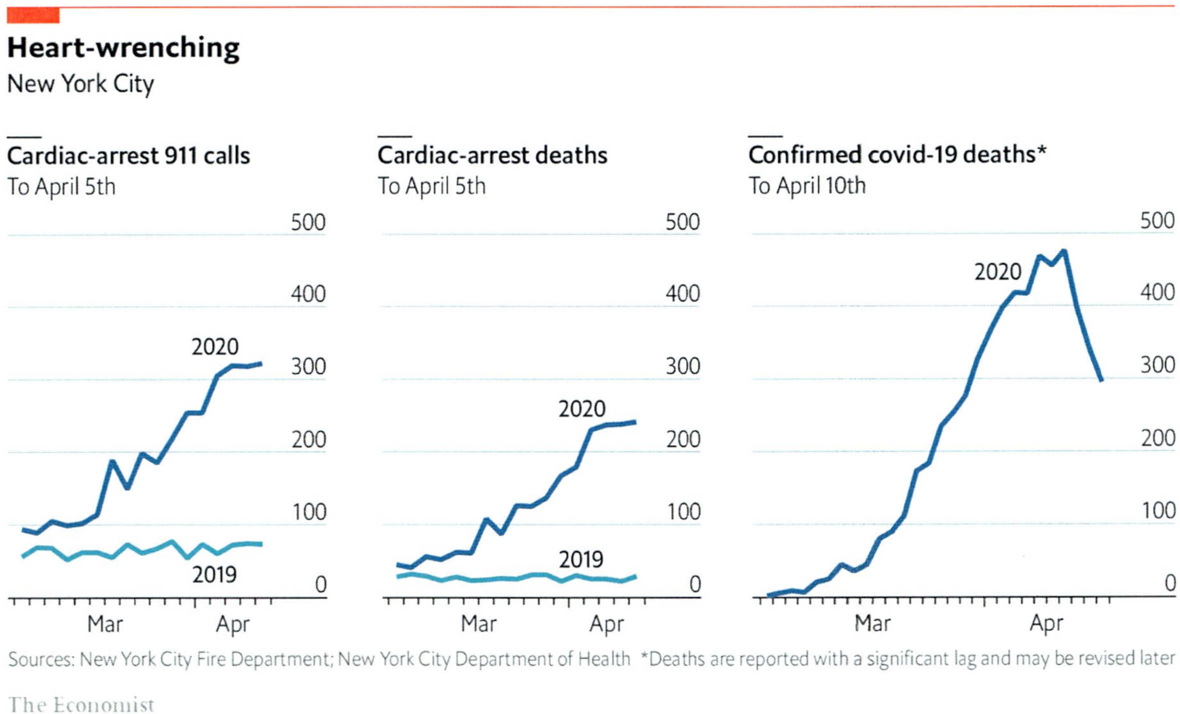

FIGURE C-3 Cardiac arrest 911 calls, cardiac arrest deaths, and confirmed COVID-19 deaths in New York City.
SOURCE: Reprinted with Permission: © The Economist Group Limited, London (April 13, 2020). *The Economist*. 2020. Deaths from cardiac arrests have surged in New York City. www.economist.com/graphic-detail/2020/04/13/deaths-from-cardiac-arrests-have-surged-in-new-york-city (accessed September 1, 2020).

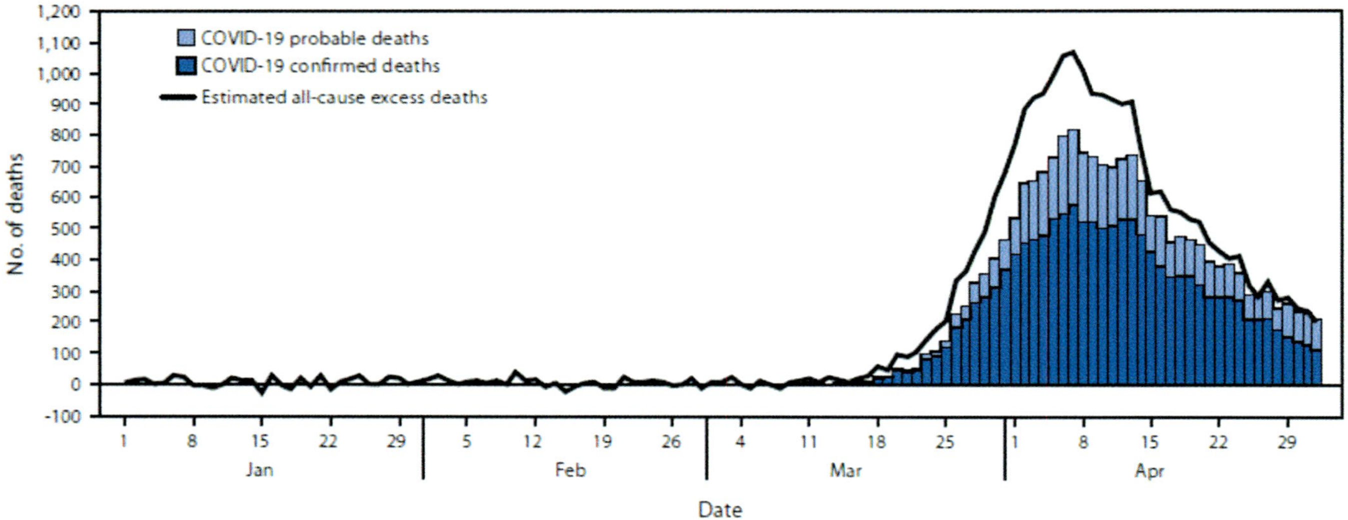

FIGURE C-4 Number of laboratory-confirmed* and probable† COVID-19-associated deaths and total estimated excess deaths§—New York City, March 11–May 2, 2020.

NOTES: * Death of a person with a positive laboratory test for SARS-CoV-2 RNA.

† Death in a person without a positive test for SARS-CoV-2 RNA but for whom COVID-19, SARS-CoV-2, or a related term was listed as an immediate, underlying, or contributing cause of death on the death certificate. § Total excess all-cause deaths were calculated as observed deaths minus expected deaths as determined by a seasonal regression model using mortality data from the period January 1, 2015–May 2, 2020.

SOURCE: New York City Department of Health and Mental Hygiene COVID-19 Response Team. 2020. Preliminary estimate of excess mortality during the COVID-19 outbreak—New York City, March 11–May 2, 2020. *Morbidity and Mortality Weekly Report* 69:603–605. http://dx.doi.org/10.15585/mmwr.mm6919e5.

excess deaths that were not identified as either laboratory-confirmed or probable COVID-19-associated deaths.[55]

In an analysis originally published in *The Washington Post*,[56] Weinberger et al. conducted a similar analysis for the entire United States from March 1 through May 30, 2020. They estimated that there were 122,300 more deaths than would typically be expected at that time of year, 28 percent higher than the official tally of COVID-19-reported deaths during that period based on case counts. The patterns varied substantially across geographical areas; Figure C-5 illustrates the results from New York City and State, the hardest hit areas during this period.[57]

The COVID-19 pandemic can be used to demonstrate that many of the deaths missed by case counting but captured using excess mortality methods are indirect deaths. For example, Woolf et al. analyzed mortality between March 1 and April 25, 2020, and estimated 87,001 excess deaths nationally, of which 65 percent were attributed directly to COVID-19. But the authors also identified substantial increases in mortality from heart disease, diabetes, and other causes, and few from non-COVID pneumonias or influenza as underlying causes.[58]

Corroborating evidence of indirect health effects has also been obtained during the COVID-19 pandemic. For example, 29 percent of adults in a recent survey said they have avoided medical care, fearing contracting the coronavirus,[59] and there has been a dramatic drop in the number of vaccines provided to children since the national emergency was declared on

---

[55] New York City Department of Health and Mental Hygiene COVID-19 Response Team. 2020. Preliminary estimate of excess mortality during the COVID-19 outbreak—New York City, March 11–May 2, 2020. *Morbidity and Mortality Weekly Report* 69:603–605. http://dx.doi.org/10.15585/mmwr.mm6919e5.

[56] Brown E., A. B. Tran, B. Reinhard, and M. Ulmanu. 2020. U.S. deaths soared in early weeks of pandemic, far exceeding number attributed to COVID-19. *The Washington Post*. https://www.washingtonpost.com/investigations/2020/04/27/covid-19-death-toll-undercounted/?p9w22b2p=b2p22p9w00098 (accessed September 1, 2020).

[57] Weinberger, D. M., J. Chen, T. Cohen, F. W. Crawford, F. Mostashari, D. Olson, V. E. Pitzer, N. G. Reich, M. Russi, L. Simonsen, A. Watkins, and C. Viboud. 2020. Estimation of excess deaths associated with the COVID-19 pandemic in the United States, March to May 2020. *JAMA Internal Medicine* 180(10):1336–1344. doi: 10.1001/jamainternmed.2020.3391.

[58] Woolf, S. H., D. A. Chapman, R. T. Sabo, D. M. Weinberger, and L. Hill. 2020. Excess deaths from COVID-19 and other causes, March–April 2020. *JAMA*. doi: 10.1001/jama.2020.11787.

[59] Kacik, A. 2020. Nearly a third of Americans have put off healthcare during COVID-19. *Modern Healthcare*. https://www.modernhealthcare.com/patient-care/nearly-third-americans-have-put-healthcare-during-covid-19 (accessed August 3, 2020).

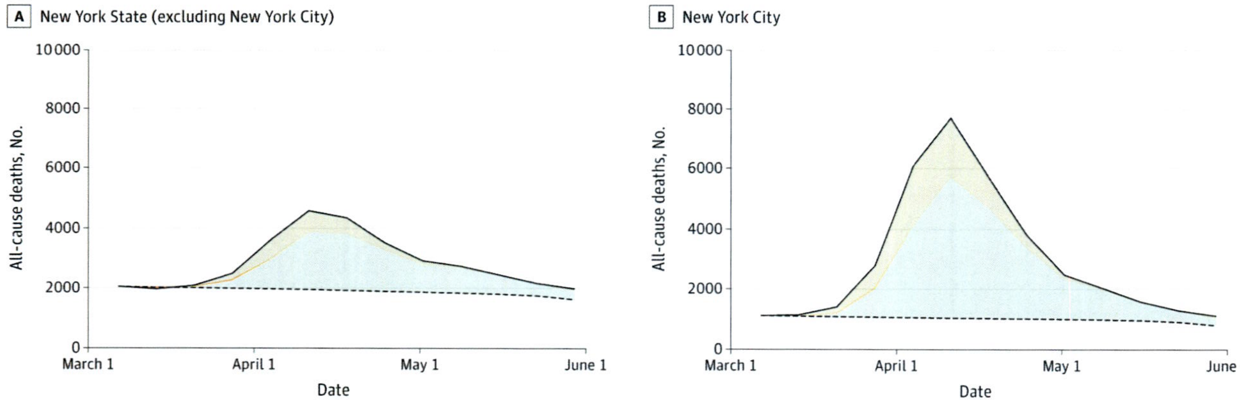

FIGURE C-5 Excess deaths in New York State (excluding New York City) and in New York City from March 1 through May 30, 2020.

NOTES: The observed number of deaths is indicated by the solid line, and the expected number of deaths, adjusting for seasonality, influenza epidemics, and reporting delays, is indicated by the dashed line. The area between these two lines represents the total number of excess deaths: blue-gray (bottom), deaths recorded as due to COVID-19; orange (narrow middle section), additional pneumonia and influenza excess deaths not coded as due to COVID-19; and beige (top), deaths that were not attributed to COVID-19, pneumonia, or influenza.

SOURCES: Reproduced with permission from JAMA Internal Medicine. 2020;e203391. doi: 10.1001/jamainternmed.2020.3391. Weinberger, D. M., J. Chen, T. Cohen, F. W. Crawford, F. Mostashari, D. Olson, V. E. Pitzer, N. G. Reich, M. Russi, L. Simonsen, A. Watkins, and C. Viboud. 2020. Estimation of excess deaths associated with the COVID-19 pandemic in the United States, March to May 2020. *JAMA Internal Medicine*. doi: 10.1001/jamainternmed.2020.3391.

March 13, 2020.[60] Researchers at the Well Being Trust and the Robert Graham Center have estimated that COVID-related unemployment, social isolation, and uncertainty could result in as many as 75,000 "deaths of despair" from suicide or alcohol and other substance abuse.[61] On the other hand, social distancing might also result in fewer traffic accidents and deaths caused by pollution. All of these indirect effects of the pandemic will be best assessed using population estimations.

As with individual counts, population estimation methods require a number of judgments about definition, statistical methods, data, and other assumptions. For instance, increases in cardiac mortality are common following natural disasters,[62] so the increases being documented now are plausibly related to stress caused by the pandemic. Whether these excess deaths should be regarded as "caused by" the pandemic is a matter of definitional dispute, and an illustration of how population estimation methods require judgments to interpret as well as judgments to carry out. The methods research described under Recommendation 4-1 would address these issues and help to ensure the validity and utility of excess mortality estimates in future disasters.

Lessons from Interpreting Data on Mortality and Morbidity in the COVID-19 Pandemic

In a crisis, the public wants to know what is happening and policy makers want good data for decisions. However, the COVID-19 pandemic shows how the availability of different approaches for assessing morbidity and mortality can create confusion. In particular, the availability of different methods generating widely differing estimates creates opportunities for manipulation or the appearance of manipulation. In addition, COVID-19 has shown that the lack of standards for who gathers and analyzes the data, definitions and processes used, and how they are reported can create further confusion and opportunities for intentional or inadvertent selective use of data to support a point of view. The pandemic also illustrates that the precision of the "death toll" based on case counting methods holds enormous

---

[60] Santoli, J. M., M. C. Lindley, M. B. DeSilva, E. O. Kharbanda, M. F. Daley, L. Galloway, J. Gee, M. Glover, B. Herring, Y. Kang, P. Lucas, C. Noblit, J. Tropper, T. Vogt, and E. Weintraub. 2020. Effects of the COVID-19 pandemic on routine pediatric vaccine ordering and administration—United States, 2020. *Morbidity and Mortality Weekly Report* 69:591–593. http://dx.doi.org/10.15585/mmwr.mm6919e2.

[61] Well Being Trust. 2020. The COVID pandemic could lead to 75,000 additional deaths from alcohol and drug misuse and suicide. https://wellbeingtrust.org/areas-of-focus/policy-and-advocacy/reports/projected-deaths-of-despair-during-covid-19 (accessed August 3, 2020).

[62] Hayman, K. G., D. Sharma, R. D. Wardlow, and S. Singh. 2020. Burden of cardiovascular morbidity and mortality following humanitarian emergencies: A systematic literature review. *Prehospital and Disaster Medicine* 30(1):80–88. doi: 10.1017/S1049023X14001356.

appeal for policy makers and the public, despite agreement among experts that these are an underestimate of the full impacts of the pandemic.

Case counting and statistical estimation methods have different strengths and weaknesses and generally produce different but complimentary information (see Table C-1), but the COVID-19 pandemic also shows that there are special risks of generating misleading numbers when using these methods in combination. In particular, case count and population estimation methods predictably lead to lower and higher numbers, respectively. So, use of population estimation methods such as serological surveys to assess infection rates will predictably generate higher estimates than case counting methods, while using individual case counts to assess mortality will predictably generate low estimates. Doing so in combination will therefore suggest large numbers of non-fatal infection (i.e., generating an artificially low case fatality rate). Using data obtained through different methods to obtain a falsely low case fatality rate is inappropriate, but such calculations could easily be carried out from naiveté rather than malice. In the end, data obtained from these different methods should be regarded as pieces of a puzzle that, when used in appropriate combinations, can help create a clearer picture of how the disease is spreading and its severity.[63] Thus, as suggested in Recommendation 2-2, both counts and estimates should be used and reported.

The major difference between pandemics and other natural disasters is the matter of temporality; hurricanes and wildfires occur over a period of days or weeks (although recovery can take much longer), while the COVID-19 pandemic has already stretched into months and could last years. In all disasters, attributed mortality and morbidity counts and estimates change over time for two reasons: some long-term consequences take time to occur and all data systems have lags, which vary over time. In pandemics, both of these factors apply, but there is an additional dynamic: the continued infection of new cases. Indeed, questions about the evolution of the pandemic itself—where the number of new cases is growing or shrinking in response to control efforts—are critical. For instance, real-time estimates of incidence are used as triggers to decide whether certain non-pharmaceutical measures—such as social distancing or mask wearing—can be relaxed. For this purpose, it is critical to know whether a decrease in the number of new reported cases reflects decreased incidence or simply less testing being done, as noted earlier.

For many disasters, case-based death counts are the focus of attention during the response phase, often because nothing else is available in the short term. While case counts have some lag associated with them,

[63] NASEM. 2020. *Evaluating data types*: A *guide for decision makers using data to understand the extent and spread of COVID-19*. Washington, DC: The National Academies Press. https://doi.org/10.17226/25826.

survey-based estimates and excess mortality calculations often take much longer (though one could imagine better data infrastructure alleviating some of these delays). But with COVID-19, the time frame is extended, meaning that statistical estimation methods have the potential to provide a more complete and accurate characterization of the COVID-19 pandemic in time to inform policy and practice decisions. The COVID-19 pandemic also reminds us that "death toll" estimates based on case counts are often misleading. To avoid both confusion and manipulation, statistics derived from case counts should be referred to as "reported infections" and "reported deaths" from COVID-19 rather than as "total infections" or the "death toll." These counts should include suspected and probable cases, though these should also be reported separately from confirmed cases.

Total mortality, or the "death toll" from COVID-19, should only be reported using population estimation approaches, preferably using the same methods as are used for seasonal influenza. These methods produce a more complete picture of the consequences of the pandemic and are preferable for guiding policy decisions, such as about reopening strategies and targeting aid to areas and populations most affected.

Finally, though disease surveillance is primarily a state responsibility, CDC should not only issue standard case definitions, but also recommend common processes for reporting cases and deaths and metrics that state and local health departments report to help ensure that comparisons among states and other population groups are more meaningful. In this spirit, a group of public health experts recently published a list of 15 key metrics with standardized definitions that states and communities can use so that health departments, decision makers, and the public can get a clearer picture of how the response to the pandemic is working in their area.[64,65] Standardizing mortality data and reporting (Recommendation 3-2) and strengthening systems to improve the quality of these data (Recommendation 3-1) would address these issues and improve future policy makers' ability to manage pandemics and other disasters.

---

[64] Arnold, C. 2020. How scientists know COVID-19 is way deadlier than the flu. *National Geographic.* https://www.nationalgeographic.com/science/2020/07/coronavirus-deadlier-than-many-believed-infection-fatality-rate-cvd (accessed September 1, 2020).

[65] Tracking COVID-19 in the United States. 2020. Prevent epidemics. https://preventepidemics.org/covid19/resources/indicators (accessed August 3, 2020).

Appendix D

Integrating Community Vulnerabilities into the Assessment of Disaster-Related Morbidity and Mortality: Two Illustrative Case Studies

Authored by Emma Fine, National Academies staff, July 31, 2020

INTRODUCTION

The report of the Committee on Best Practices for Assessing Mortality and Significant Morbidity Following Large-Scale Disasters describes the lack of coordination across stakeholders; the absence of a standardized approach and terminology for estimating morbidity and mortality; and extreme variation in practices for collecting, recording, reporting, and using disaster-related mortality and morbidity data. The main chapters of the report address issues such as (1) describing the current architecture, methodologies, and information systems currently in use by state, local, tribal, and territorial (SLTT) public health agencies; (2) identifying barriers to collecting, recording, and reporting mortality and morbidity data; and (3) reviewing analytical approaches and statistical methods for estimating mortality and morbidity at a population level. Early in the committee's deliberation the committee acknowledged that the social determinants of health (SDOH) contribute in known and less well-defined ways to disaster-related mortality and morbidity; however, they were bound by the limitations of the report's scope from conducting an in-depth review of these critical socio-environmental dimensions and how those relate to community vulnerabilities and mortality and morbidity assessment.

In response, this appendix paper was drafted to provide two high-level case studies summarizing the inextricable link between the SDOH and mortality and morbidity related to two disasters—Hurricane Katrina and the early months of the coronavirus disease 2019 (COVID-19) pandemic. These case studies will also reflect on how these dimensions may relate to the collection, reporting, and recording of morbidity and mortality data.

Ultimately, efforts to explore the intersection of these issues inform our collective understanding of the factors underlying a community's resilience and vulnerability to disasters.

The Value of Multidimensional Mortality and Morbidity Data

As described in the committee's report, mortality and morbidity data represent a wide variety of uses and values. These data, if accurate and complete, can be used to identify at-risk populations, among other uses, and respond with appropriate actions to support recovery, mitigate root vulnerabilities, and prepare to prevent future harm, which represent great value to the field of disaster management. Critically, mortality and morbidity data alone represent just one category of data, and further contextualization of these data with other rich data points, such as race and ethnicity, socioeconomic status, among others, provides for a multidimensional understanding of those same mortality and morbidity data. The integration of these data represent real opportunities to identify the underlying causal pathways and sub-population inequities existing at the intersection of the SDOH, disaster exposure, and disaster-related mortality and morbidity, which could in turn allow for the improved design and targeting of resources and programs to the sub-populations in greatest need. The contextualization of morbidity and mortality using SDOH data adds additional value and evidence to foster a stronger and more responsive disaster management enterprise that prioritizes community resilience (see Figure D-1).

While the SDOH operate at a subpopulation level, the contributory role of these factors on vulnerability should not be de-emphasized. For example, as Thomas-Henkel and Schulman (2017) write, "SDOH can account for up to 40% of individual health outcomes, particularly among low-income populations, [and] their providers are increasingly focused on strategies to address patients' unmet social needs (e.g. food insecurity, housing, transportation, etc.)." Co-morbidities are one significant consequence of these unmet social needs (Valderas et al., 2009), which add distinct complexity to the assessment and use of disaster-related mortality and morbidity data. Certain socio-environmental factors—population density, exposure to pollution, outdoor manual labor—are known to increase biological susceptibility to disease, and those impacts seep into individual treatment and care of various medical conditions (McKibben, 2020). During and after a disaster, these influences are even more pronounced. Other SDOH, such as race and economic status, and other well-established determinants are known to be associated with persistent inequities in health and further indicate that the vulnerabilities as they relate to the SDOH are critical to understand alongside disaster-related mortality and morbidity data to provide a foundation of evidence for promoting community resilience.

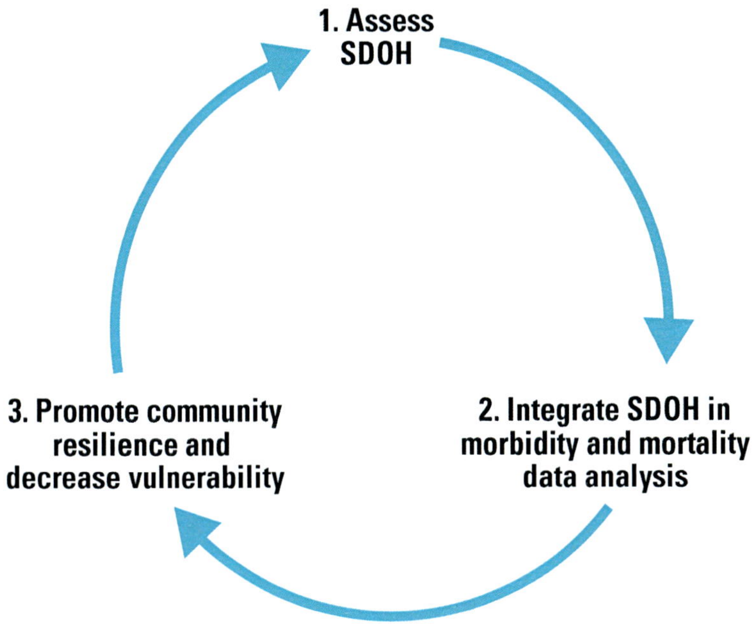

FIGURE D-1 Causal pathway.
NOTE: SDOH = social determinants of health.

Because a body of literature already exists around how the SDOH relate to health disparities, and how disaster exposures further heighten these vulnerabilities and inequalities within marginalized populations (Healthy People 2020, 2017; NASEM, 2019), this appendix will not attempt to summarize this body of work. There are many different definitions for SDOH, as well as many various elements that comprise these determinants. For this appendix, the following definition of SDOH (see Box D-1) will be used, along with the following six key social capital elements (see Figure D-2).

SOCIAL DETERMINANTS OF HEALTH AND DISASTER-RELATED MORTALITY AND MORBIDITY

Post-Hurricane Maria Puerto Rico: A Case Study

1. Natural (or environmental)

Hurricane Maria made landfall in Puerto Rico on September 20, 2017, just 2 weeks after Hurricane Irma stuck the island and had already caused damage to roads, water supply, and access to medical care (Kishore et al., 2018). When Hurricane Maria hit the island, the storm was tracked as a "Category 4" and, over the past century, Maria was the strongest recorded

BOX D-1
Definition of Social Determinants of Health

Social determinants of health are the conditions in the environments in which people are born, grow, live, learn, work, play, worship, and age that affect a wide range of health, functioning, and quality-of-life outcomes and risks. The circumstances are shaped by the distribution of money, power, and resources at global, national, and local levels.

1. Natural (or environmental)
2. Built (infrastructure)
3. Financial (economic)
4. Social/psychosocial
5. Human and cultural
6. Political (institutional or governance)

SOURCES: Healthy People 2020, 2017; NASEM, 2019; WHO, 2020.

hurricane to hit Puerto Rico (Michaud and Kates, 2017). Widespread physical and infrastructural damage occurred as a result, the total number of deaths is still unknown, and the impact of the storm continues to have short- and long-term impacts on population health (Michaud and Kates, 2017). Kishore et al. (2018) write that damages from Hurricane Maria reached approximately $90 billion, ranking it as the third costliest hurricane in the United States since 1900 and resulted in the displacement of thousands of individuals and families from their homes (Kishore et al., 2018). The natural effects of the hurricane had large impacts on the population and migration of those in Puerto Rico. Data indicate that an estimated 114,000–213,000 (or between 2–4 percent) of the population left Puerto Rico in the year after the hurricane, often heading to places such as Florida or even as far away as Hawaii and Alaska (DeWaard et al., 2020). DeWaard et al. (2020) highlight that those who migrated out of Puerto Rico were commonly of school or working ages. This population drain from the island will have lasting impacts on the schooling, labor market, economy, and public service sectors and their trajectories within both Puerto Rico and the United States (DeWaard et al., 2020).

With regard to the environment, Hurricane Maria had strong impacts on the overall air quality and air pollution within Puerto Rico. Some of the most significant infrastructure damage caused by the hurricane was the destruction of the island's electrical grid, which left many communities without power for months on end (ACS, 2018). In fact, 3 months after

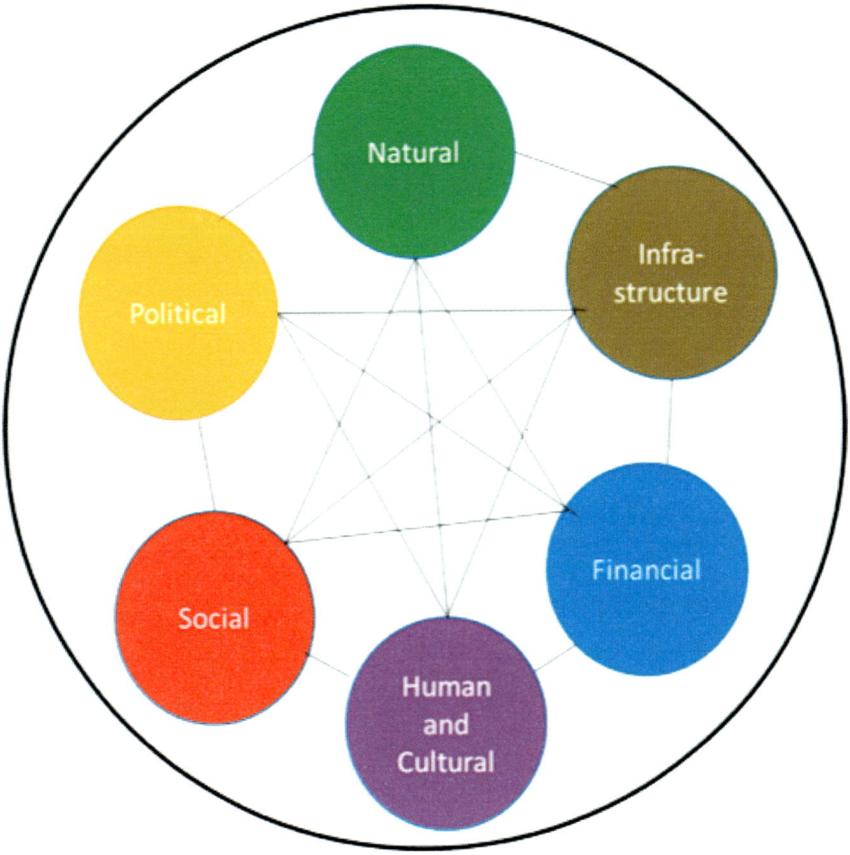

FIGURE D-2 Interconnectedness of the six elements of the social determinants of health.
SOURCE: NASEM, 2019.

Hurricane Maria struck, 50 percent of Puerto Rico still lacked electricity, and even those who did not lack access to electricity experienced ongoing power outages (ACS, 2018). As a consequence, many communities began to rely on backup generators that run on gasoline or diesel, leading to increased air pollution in communities where generators were widely used (ACS, 2018). During the period that the quality of the air was being monitored, 80 percent of those days showed sulfur dioxide levels that exceeded the Environmental Protection Agency's air quality standards, and in many other places air quality could not be measured due to such significant damage (ACS, 2018). Population exposure to these higher levels of air pollution have lasting impacts on the respiratory health of those residing in Puerto Rico, especially in areas where the levels of pollution were extreme.

2. Built (infrastructure)

Even today, the exact number individuals who died as a result of Hurricane Maria remains unknown, illustrating a persistent shortcoming in disaster management and part of the impetus for the committee's authoring of this report. The official death toll of Hurricane Maria remains 64. However, researchers from the Harvard T.H. Chan School of Public Health, via survey data, argue that a more accurate estimate of all-cause mortality due to Hurricane Maria is 4,645 dead as a result of the storm (Kishore et al., 2018). This mortality estimate is more than 70 times the official estimate and represents a 62 percent increase in mortality compared to a similar time frame in 2016. However, even this is still likely to be an under-representation of the true impact of the disaster on human life (Kishore et al., 2018). Part of the higher mortality estimate exists due to the researchers' integration of population displacement, loss of services, and excess deaths into the overall toll. For example, researchers found that on average, households impacted by the hurricane went 84 days without electricity, 68 days with no water, and just more than 40 days with no cellular service, with a disproportionate impact on those residing in more remote regions (Kishore et al., 2018). In terms of disruption to services, 31 percent of households surveyed reported an issue—14.4 percent of households were unable to access medications, 9.5 percent were unable to access electricity to operate respiratory equipment, 8.6 percent reported closed medical facilities, 6.1 percent were patients of absent doctors, and even 8.8 percent were unable to reach 911 (Kishore et al., 2018). After 3 weeks, nearly 94 percent of the island lacked power, 43 percent lacked potable water, and only 30 percent of the hospitals could provide services (Lybarger, 2018). All of these losses of services and interruption in care can lead to cases of morbidity and mortality that may not be captured in the overall estimate of reported mortality based on individual counts of deaths directly attributed to the disaster. The accuracy of the death count was also impacted by the rise of uncounted bodies (Dyer, 2017). *BMJ* reports that during the hurricane, hospitals and hospital morgues were overcrowded and that triaging and communication were major challenges. Even more so, morgues were so full that only those who had death certificates were added to the official mortality count, and morgues had the policy of not releasing bodies until the death certificate had been issued. This was compounded by the fact that some individuals responsible for issuing death certificates were themselves unaccounted for (Dyer, 2017), creating a cyclical problem.

Hurricanes are capable of extensive destruction of buildings and structures, including infrastructure that facilitates essential needs such as access to shelter, food, water, electricity, transportation, and communication, which all have impacts on a community's public health (Michaud and Kates, 2017). Even prior to Hurricane Maria, the effects of SDOH were clear for many individuals residing there. Nearly 44 percent of Puerto Rico's residents live at or below the poverty level—compared to just under 13 percent in the United States—and the unemployment rate hovers around 10 percent (Michaud and Kates, 2017). In terms of overall health prior to the hurricane, nearly 34 percent of the population reported having fair or poor general health, 15.4 percent live with a disability, and the prevalence of diabetes was 50 percent higher when compared to that in the United States (Michaud and Kates, 2017). After the hurricane, the physical impacts on the built environment had significant impacts on the health of residents. Many were unable to access grocery stores or fresh food and had to rely on the nearly 1 million meals provided each day from emergency first responders even 1 month after the hurricane (Michaud and Kates, 2017). This lack of adequate food is tied to other health conditions and can result in malnutrition, which can both cause and exacerbate other co-morbidities (Michaud and Kates, 2017). Puerto Rico also saw an increase in conditions related to the consumption of unclean water as some communities were left without access to safe water and had to result to natural freshwater sources, subject to human and environmental contamination (Michaud and Kates, 2017). Hospitals also suffered infrastructural damage to the extent that only three of the island's major hospitals were functioning 3 days after the hurricane. One month later, 40 percent of tracked hospitals were still running on backup generators. Running on generators was also a significant problem for those relying on dialysis centers to treat the high burden of diabetes in Puerto Rico (Michaud and Kates, 2017). These examples illustrate how the infrastructure of Puerto Rico was significantly damaged by the 2017 hurricane, and how certain populations, such as those with diabetes, were at an increased risk for mortality or morbidity related to the hurricane as a result of the storm's impacts to the built environment.

3. Financial (economic)

Puerto Rico faced public health challenges both before and after the arrival of Hurricane Maria. The financial status of many hospitals, after suffering severe structural damage, remained an issue at least through 2018, when Chowdhury et al. (2019) conducted interviews in Puerto Rico. Hospital employees in 2018 reported that structural damage from the hurricane damaged a cardiac catheterization lab and a cancer institute and described how many hospitals experienced flooding that damaged x-ray and other imaging technology. Chowdhury et al. (2019, p. 1727) writes

> Financially, the hospital was already short of funds for needed improvements before the hurricanes. After the hurricanes, the hospital had accrued hundreds of millions of dollars in damages, and substantial questions re-

main about the best way to move forward, weighing the relative benefits of rebuilding, replacing, or accepting the loss of facilities.

Financial debt has led to the loss of treatment centers for various diseases, likely impacting the number of patients who can be treated, which exacerbated risks for mortality and morbidity.

However, these financial strains did not just impact large buildings and structures, but also the communities and individuals residing within Puerto Rico. Rodriguez-Diaz (2018) explains that the under-resourced communities experienced exacerbated public health effects due to inadequate health systems and lack of sufficient humanitarian disaster relief, which led to "outbreaks of infectious diseases, limited access to clean water, and malnutrition, among other problems." Additionally, the slow and limited federal response to the hurricane disaster highlighted the impact of poverty on many communities. Indeed, Rodriguez-Diaz (2018, p. 31) indicates that "poverty has the largest impact in terms of health inequities after the hurricane and magnif[ies] the impact of social determinants of Puerto Ricans' health (e.g., housing, health care services, access to clear water and sanitation." The SDOH, such as financial capital, have clear implications for the ability of a locality to recover from adversity and also for its most financially vulnerable populations.

4. *Social/Psychosocial*

Hurricanes not only damage the natural and built environments but they can also negatively impact mental health. Hurricanes can lead to an increased risk for conditions such as anxiety, depression, and posttraumatic stress disorder (Scaramutti et al., 2018). Within 2 months of the hurricane's arrival, the demand for mental health services increased sharply and individuals were reporting anxiety and depression more frequently, even among those who had never experienced these previously (Michaud and Kates, 2017). Chowdury et al. (2019, p. 1728) write of other alarming events such as "perceived amplified behavioral and mental health issues on the island such as thefts resulting in gunshot wounds, domestic violence, alcohol use disorders, and depression." These mental health impacts are not thought to exist only in the short term. Kaiser Family Foundation reported that, in fact, adverse mental health conditions may even increase over the following months and years after the hurricane. For example, those affected similarly by Hurricane Katrina saw elevated rates of mental illness that were sustained for more than 1 year after the event (Michaud and Kates, 2017). Hurricane Maria undoubtedly had impacts on the mental health of the residents of Puerto Rico (Lybarger, 2018), and the lasting structural damage alongside increased demand for mental health services likely compounded the impact this SDOH capital on morbidity and mortality.

5. Human and Cultural

While the hurricane had impacts on the physical environment and health of Puerto Rico's citizens, it also created profound damage on some of society's most vulnerable—children. A study, which was also the largest sample ever of Hispanic youth impacted by disaster, indicated just some of these consequences on children. Nearly 50 percent of children's family homes were damaged and nearly 84 percent of children witnessed damaged homes; 24 percent of children helped rescue others; 25.5 percent of children were forced to evacuate; 32 percent experienced shortages of food and water; and nearly 17 percent still did not have electricity between 5 to 9 months after the hurricane. Additionally, nearly 58 percent had a family member or friend leave Puerto Rico (Orengo-Aguayo et al., 2019). The cultural and social implications of what these children faced may have long-term consequences, and stress the need for disaster management to include the SDOH in policy and practice.

6. Political (institutional or governance)

Puerto Rico provides appropriations to the Federal Emergency Management Agency annually in order to utilize their disaster relief management efforts; however, the arrival and subsequent damage that Hurricane Maria caused exposed colonial laws that limit Puerto Rico's abilities to recover from natural disasters (Rodriguez-Diaz, 2018). Two of these significant laws are the Merchant Marine Act of 1920 (commonly known as the Jones Act) and the Puerto Rico Oversight, Management, and Economic Stability Act (PROMESA) (Rodriguez-Diaz, 2018). The Jones Act ensures that the "maritime waters and ports of Puerto Rico are controlled by U.S. agencies," which, downstream, means that "under this kind of control, the cost of consumer goods arriving to Puerto Rico can be higher than in the Continental U.S. ... and [it] restrains the ability of non-U.S. vessels and crews to engage in commercial trade with Puerto Rico" (Rodriguez-Diaz, 2018, p. 30), which ultimately serves to restrict the economic independence of this territory. Additionally, PROMESA "limits the Puerto Rican government's disaster response by restricting the amount of resources the state can mobilize locally in attending to the crises brought by the 2017 hurricane season" (Rodriguez-Diaz, 2018, p. 30). The natural disaster and the burden of political and economic restraints resulting from these two laws (Rodriguez-Diaz, 2018) made managing post-disaster response and recovery extremely challenging. The prolonged delay in receiving the materials and supplies needed may have further impacted morbidity and mortality caused by this natural disaster.

Early Months of the COVID-19 Pandemic: A Case Study

Substantial evidence exists demonstrating the impact of social determinants on the vulnerabilities of certain communities and populations to the adverse outcomes of disasters. For example, "social determinants exert a powerful influence on different elements of risk, principally vulnerability, exposure and capacity and thus, on people's health" (Nomura et al., 2016). Vincent Lafronza and Natalie Burke write that

> social conditions are major determinants of health" with "social forces acting at a collective level shaping individual biology, individual risk behaviors, environmental exposures, and access to resources that promote health ... and while public health programs alone cannot ameliorate the social forces that are associated with poor health outcomes, developing a better understanding of the social determinants of health is critical to reducing health disparities. (Lafronza and Burke, 2007, p. 12)

Using the SDOH definition, the six elements that comprise it (see Box D-1), and the global pandemic of COVID-19, examples will be provided to show exactly how influential the SDOH are in the outcomes of morbidity and mortality during a disaster, specifically in reference to the COVID-19 pandemic.

Severe acute respiratory syndrome coronavirus 2 (SARS-CoV-2) is a virus that typically manifests in respiratory illness along with other symptoms such as fever, shortness of breath, and unexplained loss of taste or smell (Sauer, 2020). In March 2020, the World Health Organization (WHO) declared the coronavirus disease 2019 (COVID-19) outbreak a global pandemic (Cucinotta and Vanelli, 2020) as the virus continued to spread across every continent except Antarctica (Sikorska, 2020). As of July 2020, the United States has seen more than 135,991 deaths from COVID-19 with more than 3.4 million total cases (CDC, 2020). Unprecedented measures such as school, work, and restaurant closures; legal requirements to wear face masks; and social distancing policies have been implemented worldwide in efforts to reduce the spread of this potentially fatal virus. However, through our understanding of the SDOH, the coronavirus and its implications for morbidity and mortality do not impact all individuals or communities equally.

1. Natural (or environmental)

One of the key ways coronavirus transmits is through air droplets—meaning proximity to and density of people, especially when indoors—is extremely important to transmission of the infection. A study of overcrowding in housing found that, for those that had one or more persons per room, only 1 percent of non-Hispanic whites fell into this category compared to 12 percent of Hispanics. Even when looking at overcrowding in housing based on citizenship, only 1 percent of those born in the United States had one or more persons per room while 15 percent of foreign-born (not a U.S. citizen) individuals had one or more persons per room. Therefore, natural or environmental factors such as overcrowding in housing can be, at times, directly related to social factors such as race or nationality, which, in the case of COVID-19, can have direct implications for infection and transmission, and ultimately mortality. If Hispanic populations, compared to non-Hispanic whites, are more likely to experience overcrowding in housing, they are also more likely to be at greater risk for COVID-19, which is more easily transmitted among individuals in dense indoor environments (Benfer and Wiley, 2020).

Redlining, defined as "a discriminatory practice by which banks, insurance companies, etc., refuse or limit loans, mortgages, insurance, etc., within specific geographic areas, especially inner-city neighborhoods" (Dictionary.com, 2020), commonly practiced in the 1930s, is not a vestige of the past. A study conducted by the National Community Reinvestment Coalition in 2018 indicated that a majority of the homes that were redlined, or marked as "hazardous" by the federal Home Owners' Loan Corporation during the period from 1935 to 1939, are today "much more likely than other areas to comprise lower-income, minority residents" (Jan, 2018). These dated policies have stagnated and stunted economic growth where three out of four redlined neighborhoods still struggle economically 80 years later (Jan, 2018; Mitchell and Franco, 2018). This result of concentrated poverty ultimately puts low-income communities of color in less safe areas geographically and they are often at higher risks for co-morbidities. According to research by the Tulane University School of Public Health & Tropical Medicine, minority groups are at highest risk for COVID-19 due to their higher rates of co-morbidities such as heart disease and obesity, they have higher rates of multigenerational household units, and compared to their White counterparts they face a greater difficulty in access to the necessary testing. These minority communities also experience barriers to health and economic opportunity and, often due to their employment, are unable to comply with social distancing guidelines meant to protect them from COVID-19 itself (Patel et al., 2020; Raifman and Raifman, 2020).

The natural environment, such as housing or zip code, can greatly influence or sway the likelihood that certain individuals or populations will be at increased risk for contracting and transmitting COVID-19, which directly impacts morbidity and mortality and clearly shows how these rates are impacted by the SDOH.

2. Built (infrastructure)

A consequence of the COVID-19 pandemic has been the alteration of work environments—many individuals found themselves working full time at home while other workers, often those serving low-wage jobs such as restaurant workers or grocery store cashiers, were unable to remain protected at home as their work became deemed "essential" (Burkholder et al., 2020). These essential workers were forced to either show up to their workplaces—increasing their own exposure to COVID-19—or face potentially losing their jobs. Amid this disaster, Congress passed the Families First Coronavirus Response Act, part of which served to make it easier for workers to receive paid sick leave if they contract COVID-19 or are responsible for caring for out-of-school children (Khazan, 2020). This act established a 2-week period of paid sick leave for quarantined or symptomatic individuals as well as 12 weeks of paid leave at a rate of two-thirds of their salary if they are taking care of a child (Khazan, 2020). However, many employees are not eligible to receive these protections—this law exempts employers with more than 500 employees, and those with fewer than 50 employees are eligible to file for an exemption (e.g., local grocery stores, restaurants, or Amazon employees). The Center for American Progress found that "only 47% of private-sector workers will have guaranteed access to coronavirus-related sick leave" (Khazan, 2020). Policies such as these serve to reinforce the difficult decision many essential employees face to either stay home when sick or lose their job. The Center for Economic and Policy Research found that "the United States is the only 1 of 22 rich countries that fails to guarantee workers some form of paid sick leave" and that the United States is also "1 of only 3 countries that does not provide paid sick days for a worker missing 5 days of work due to the flu" (CEPR, 2020). Infrastructural challenges such as relying on essential business coupled with the lack of protections for these essential workers and low-wage nature of these jobs means that low-wage workers are more exposed and more susceptible to contracting COVID-19. Additionally, the U.S. Bureau of Labor Statistics Job Flexibilities and Work Schedules Summary shows that 37 percent of Asians, 30 percent of non-Hispanic or non-Latinos, 29.9 percent of Whites, 19.7 percent of Blacks, and just 16.2 percent of Hispanic or Latino populations are eligible to work from home (U.S. Bureau of Labor Statistics, 2019). These infrastructural inequities ensure that the risk of COVID-19 exposure and infection does not impact all persons equally and illustrates the reality that minority populations and low-wage workers bear the brunt of the potential morbidity and mortality.

Beyond employee paid sick leave, other built or infrastructural elements also impact morbidity and mortality. According to Tulane University, minority groups face greater difficulty in accessing COVID-19 testing when compared to their White counterparts (Lieberman-Cribbin et al., 2020).

Many of the first testing sites established were drive-through only, excluding access to testing for those who did not have vehicles (Griffith et al., 2017). Black, indigenous, and other populations of people of color are also less likely to be insured compared to their White counterparts. Ellis (2020) argues that "structural inequalities have kept black Americans significantly poorer than their white counterparts, and economic disparity creates health disparities, especially during a pandemic," which is strongly supported by research from the Centers for Disease Control and Prevention, which cites discrimination (including racism) as having an impact on overall well-being and health (CDC, 2020c). The built or infrastructural elements of SDOH have clear and lasting implications for disease prevalence and incidence and thus morbidity and mortality.

3. Financial (economic)

An important indicator of health, as well as an SDOH, is the level of wealth of an individual or community. COVID-19 presents a key example of how rich individuals and families were able to flee New York City, a virus hotspot, to safer areas throughout the United States. Data show that between March 1 and May 1, 2020, about 5 percent of New York City residents (approximately 420,000 people) left the city. Extremely affluent neighborhoods, such as the Upper East Side or SoHo, however, saw their residential populations decrease by 40 percent or more, with the overall trend indicating that "the higher-earning a neighborhood is, the more likely it is to have emptied out," where out of all of the neighborhoods to see population dips, the highest-earning ones emptied out first (Quealy, 2020). The populations of the neighborhoods that did empty are mostly White, have lower poverty rates, and are more likely to be able to walk or bike to work or work from home; and more than half of the residents of these neighborhoods have incomes that exceed $100,000, with one in three earning more than $200,000 (Quealy, 2020). This example exposes how the SDOH, particularly financial wealth, can provide an opportunity for escaping a disaster or a sentencing to experience it personally. As the wealthy flee the viral hot spot, they are able to reduce their likelihood of infection and transmission—their financial status serving protections that are not afforded to others. This ultimately creates a situation where those with less financial security are simultaneously forced to face the brunt of COVID-19 morbidity and mortality—"the lower a person's socioeconomic status, the more limited their resources and ability to access essential goods and services, and the greater their chance of suffering from chronic disease, including conditions like heart disease, lung disease, and diabetes that may increase the mortality risk of COVID-19" (Benfer and Wiley, 2020).

4. Social/Psychosocial

A recent survey conducted by the Kaiser Family Foundation found that nearly half of all Americans (45 percent) indicate that, due to stress and worry related to COVID-19, their mental health has been negatively impacted (Panchal et al., 2020). Compounding the anxiety individuals feel while facing the pandemic, policies such as sheltering in place can exacerbate feelings of negative mental health or stress. The same study showed that 47 percent of individuals sheltering in place reported negative mental health effects compared to 37 percent of those not sheltering in place (Panchal et al., 2020). Another consequence of COVID-19, job loss, may at first appear to have exclusively economic implications but this has psychological impacts as well. Recent polls show that more than half of those who have lost their job or experienced reduced income report higher rates of major mental health issues than high-income, employed individuals. Additionally, job loss is "associated with increased depression, anxiety, distress, and low self-esteem and may lead to higher rates of substance use disorder and suicide" (Panchal et al., 2020). By gender, 24 percent of females compared to 15 percent of males feel that the coronavirus has had a negative impact on their mental health (Kirzinger et al., 2020). By race, 17 percent of Whites compared to 24 percent of Blacks and Hispanics feel that their mental health has been majorly impacted by the pandemic (Kirzinger et al., 2020). These rates of increased mental health distress among certain populations have key implications for morbidity and mortality outcomes, showing once again the role that the SDOH have in managing disaster-related morbidity and mortality.

Certain populations also face increased susceptibility to mental health issues amplified by COVID-19. Older adults are not only more likely to develop serious illness if they contract COVID-19 but they are also at high risk of poor mental health due to loneliness and bereavement. According to research by *JAMA*, adolescent populations are also at risk for either worsening existing mental health or creating new mental health issues (Golberstein et al., 2020). Nearly 55 million students ranging from kindergarten to high school seniors were impacted by COVID-19-related school closures. This is not only a consequence for their learning but schools are often major sources of nutrition as well as providers of health care and mental health services—in fact, from 2012 to 2015, 35 percent of students received mental health services exclusively from school (Golberstein et al., 2020). In the absence of resources such as community for elders or mental health services for adolescent populations, COVID-19 has implications on mental health, one of the key pillars of the SDOH. Mental health, exacerbated by COVID-19, clearly has implications for morbidity and mortality for more than half of Americans, specifically populations more vulnerable to psychological issues and stress.

5. Human and Cultural

The nature of the spread of COVID-19, originating in late 2019 in Wuhan, China, created stigma about the coronavirus to certain subsets of the population such as those of Asian descent, individuals who had traveled, and even first responders and health care workers (CDC, 2020b). Additionally, policies implemented to diminish the spread of the virus may actually further stigmatize already stigmatized populations who cannot comply with the policies (Logie and Turan, 2020). For example, COVID-19-related policies included travel bans, social distancing, and quarantines. These movement-related guidelines further stigmatize already stigmatized populations such as homeless persons, racial minorities, migrants, and refugees (Logie and Turan, 2020). Importantly, this has strong implications for morbidity and mortality. Individuals or populations facing stigmatization may face social avoidance or rejection, refusal of service for health care, education, housing, or employment, and may also be subject to or targets of physical violence (CDC, 2020b). A joint statement released by the International Federation of Red Cross and Red Crescent Societies, the United Nations Children's Fund, and WHO warns that stigmatization can actually enhance the spread of the virus, not hamper it, and it can lead to infected individuals hiding their illness, prevent people from seeking care right away, and can even discourage the exhibition and practice of healthy behaviors (IFRC et al., 2020).

Alongside stigma, race, another SDOH, plays a significant role in COVID-19-related morbidity and mortality. According to patient analysis of a health care system in Northern California, Black patients were hospitalized at nearly three times the rate of White and Hispanic patients when seeking medical care for COVID-19 (Azar et al., 2020). This study also found that Black patients may experience limited access to care or delayed seeking help until the disease had clinically advanced and were also less likely to have been tested for the virus prior to seeking treatment when compared to White, Hispanic, or Asian patients (Azar et al., 2020; Rabin, 2020). An especially important finding showed that the disparity exists even after "differences in age, sex, income, and the prevalence of chronic health problems that exacerbate COVID-19, such as hypertension and Type 2 diabetes" (Rabin, 2020) were taken into account, indicating that race itself is a large factor when evaluating rates of morbidity and mortality.

6. Political (institutional or governance)

As COVID-19 began to spread across the United States, the implementation of policies such as stay-at-home orders were not issued federally, but at the state level. This state-by-state nature allowed governors and mayors to decide for their constituents how, when, and to what degree they would establish, maintain, and enforce these policies as well as when they would allow their states to begin to reopen. By allowing states to autonomously operate, differences in shutdown and reopening timelines can be seen across all 50 states. For instance, Alabama saw their stay-at-home order expire on April 30, 2020, with many businesses able to open that day and all business allowed to open by May 22, 2020. Arkansas, on the other hand, did not have a statewide stay-at-home order in place at any time, with a phased reopening beginning May 6, 2020. New Hampshire's stay-at-home order was initiated March 27, 2020, and expired June 15, 2020, with some businesses opening May 11, 2020. California, one of the earliest states to enact stay-at-home orders on March 19, 2020, has still not issued a formal closure of that policy but has created their own phased reopening starting May 12, 2020 (Lee et al., 2020). These variable reopening times staggering through April, May, and June 2020—along with staggered start times, if implemented at all, for the initial stay-at-home orders—means that the United States is seeing inconsistent patterns in cases and overall spread. The likelihood of increased or decreased exposure to COVID-19 could ultimately be left up to state leaders and significantly impact the number of COVID-19 cases in a first and potential second wave. The politics of one's zip code, a clear SDOH, in this case, can be clearly tied to the incidence and prevalence of COVID-19, which directly links to its related morbidity and mortality.

SOCIAL DETERMINANTS OF HEALTH AND MORTALITY AND MORBIDITY ASSESSMENT: IMPLICATIONS FOR THE FUTURE

As highlighted throughout the report, the absence of the systematic collection of disaster-related morbidity and mortality data, variation in SLTT data collection and recording systems, and the wide range of stakeholders involved only complicate the assessment and use of data to the benefit of the disaster management enterprise. These data are crucial for guiding response and recovery priorities, ensuring a common operating picture and real-time situational awareness across stakeholders, and protecting vulnerable populations and settings at heightened risk. While mortality and morbidity data hold immense potential value, the lack of incorporation of the SDOH into the collection and assessment of these data limits the degree to which these data can inform changes in policy, practice, and behavior.

The incorporation of SDOH data into morbidity and mortality assessment for the purpose of informing the disaster management enterprise will require improvements in data collection, recording, reporting, and use if these data are to be used in collaboration to identify groups most at risk and can help target public health efforts more successfully. For example,

> despite widespread public perception that the federal government and the private sector collect vast amounts of data, the availability of racial and ethnic data in the health care system itself is quite limited. A variety of government sources include data on race and ethnicity, but the utility of these data is constrained by ongoing problems with reliability, completeness, and lack of comparability across data sources. (NRC, 2004, p. 203)

Many barriers persist for gathering the data related to the SDOH, which transcend law, policy, regulation, and ethics such as patient privacy, confidentiality, civil rights laws, and the administrative burden imposed on various organizations and entities (NRC, 2004). Despite these barriers, the integration of SDOH into the measures of morbidity and mortality data will be critical to mitigate the impact of disasters, especially on those living in disaster-prone areas, and to set priorities for targeting health and other disaster management resources. For example, there is increasing awareness that policies and resources are needed to address mental health, trauma, and chronic illness as the primary morbidities related to disasters. The National Research Council (2001, p. 24) writes, "measuring only mortality during an emergency says nothing about sequelae of complex emergency that may have profound effects on the population." Therefore, SDOH data hold intrinsic value, which can be tapped to more accurately interpret mortality and morbidity data following disasters and target the root causes of community vulnerabilities to disasters—a value that will likely expand as certain disasters grow in frequency and severity.

REFERENCES

ACS (American Chemical Society). 2018. *Monitoring air pollution after Hurricane Maria.* https://www.acs.org/content/acs/en/pressroom/presspacs/2018/acs-presspac-october-31-2018/monitoring-air-pollution-after-hurricane-maria.html (accessed September 1, 2020).

Azar, K., Z. Shen, R. Romanelli, S. Lockhart, K. Smits, S. Robinson, S. Brown, and A. Pressman. 2020. Disparities in outcomes among COVID-19 patients in a large health care system in California. *Health Affairs* 39(7):1253–1262. doi: 10.1377/hlthaff.2020.00598.

Benfer, E., and L. Wiley. 2020. Health justice strategies to combat COVID-19: Protecting vulnerable communities during a pandemic. *Health Affairs.* https://www.healthaffairs.org/do/10.1377/hblog20200319.757883/full (accessed October 1, 2020).

Burkholder, S., S. Eldred, K. Harrison Belz, N. Keppler, M. Kreidler, M. Majchrowicz, B. Martin, S. Wang, J. Eilperin, D. Santamariña, and R. Fischer-Baum. 2020. What counts as an essential business in 10 U.S. cities. *The Washington Post*, March 25. https://www.washingtonpost.com/graphics/2020/national/coronavirus-esssential-businesses (accessed September 1, 2020).

CDC (Centers for Disease Control and Prevention). 2020a. *Coronavirus disease 2019: Cases & deaths in the US.* https://www.cdc.gov/coronavirus/2019-ncov/cases-updates/us-cases-deaths.html (accessed September 1, 2020).

CDC. 2020b. *Coronavirus disease 2019: Reducing stigma.* https://www.cdc.gov/coronavirus/2019-ncov/daily-life-coping/reducing-stigma.html (accessed September 1, 2020).

CDC. 2020c. *Health equity considerations and racial and ethnic minority groups*. https://www.cdc.gov/coronavirus/2019-ncov/community/health-equity/race-ethnicity.html?CDC_AA_refVal=https%3A%2F%2Fwww.cdc.gov%2Fcoronavirus%2F2019-ncov%2Fneed-extra-precautions%2Fracial-ethnic-minorities.html (accessed September 1, 2020).

CEPR (Center for Economic and Policy Research). 2020. *United States lags world in paid sick days for workers and families*. https://cepr.net/documents/publications/psd-summary.pdf (accessed September 1, 2020).

Chowdhury, M., A. J. Fiore, S. A. Cohen, C. Wheatley, B. Wheatley, M. Puthucode Balakrishnan, M. Chami, L. Scieszka, M. Drabin, K. A. Roberts, A. C. Toben, J. A. Tyndall, L. M. Grattan, and J. G. Morris, Jr. 2019. Health impact of Hurricanes Irma and Maria on St Thomas and St John, US Virgin Islands. *American Journal of Public Health* 109(12):1725–1731. https://ajph.aphapublications.org/doi/pdf/10.2105/AJPH.2019.305310 (accessed September 1, 2020).

Cucinotta, D., and M. Vanelli. 2020. WHO declares COVID-19 a pandemic. *Acta Biomedica* 91(1):157–160. doi: 10.23750/abm.v91i1.9397.

DeWaard, J., J. Johnson, and S. Whitaker. 2020. Out-migration and return migration to Puerto Rico after Hurricane Maria: Evidence from the consumer credit panel. *Population and Environment* 42:28–42. https://doi.org/10.1007/s11111-020-00339-5.

Dictionary.com. 2020. Redlining. https://www.dictionary.com/browse/redlining (accessed September 1, 2020).

Dyer, O. 2017. Puerto Rico's morgues full of uncounted bodies as hurricane death toll continues to rise. *BMJ* 359:j4648. https://doi.org/10.1136/bmj.j4648.

Ellis, E. G. 2020. COVID-19 is killing black people unequally—don't be surprised. *Wired Magazine*. https://www.wired.com/story/covid-19-coronavirus-racial-disparities (accessed September 1, 2020).

Golberstein, E., H. Wen, and B. Miller. 2020. Coronavirus disease 2019 (COVID-19) and mental health for children and adolescents. *JAMA Pediatrics* 174(9):819–820. doi: 10.1001/jamapediatrics.2020.1456.

Griffith, K., L. Evans, and J. Bor. 2017. The Affordable Care Act reduced socioeconomic disparities in health care access. *Health Affairs* 36(8):1503–1510. doi: 10.1377/hlthaff.2017.0083.

Healthy People 2020. 2017. Chapter 39: *Social determinants of health (SDOH)*. https://www.cdc.gov/nchs/data/hpdata2020/HP2020MCR-C39-SDOH.pdf (accessed September 1, 2020).

IFRC (International Federation of Red Cross and Red Crescent Societies), United Nations Children's Fund (UNICEF), and WHO (World Health Organization). 2020. Social stigma associated with COVID-19. https://www.unicef.org/sites/default/files/2020-03/Social%20stigma%20associated%20with%20the%20coronavirus%20disease%202019%20%28COVID-19%29.pdf (accessed September 1, 2020).

Jan, T. 2018. Redlining was banned 50 years ago. It's still hurting minorities today. *The Washington Post*. https://www.washingtonpost.com/news/wonk/wp/2018/03/28/redlining-was-banned-50-years-ago-its-still-hurting-minorities-today (accessed September 1, 2020).

Kirzinger, A., A. Kearney, L. Hamel, and M. Brodie. 2020. *KFF health tracking poll—early April 2020: The impact of coronavirus on life in America*. Kaiser Family Foundation. https://www.kff.org/coronavirus-covid-19/report/kff-health-tracking-poll-early-april-2020 (accessed September 1, 2020).

Kishore, N., D. Marqués, A. Mahmud, M. V. Kiang, I. Rodriguez, A. Fuller, P. Ebner, C. Sorensen, F. Racy, J. Lemery, L. Maas, J. Leaning, R. A. Irizarry, S. Balsari, and C. O. Buckee. 2018. Mortality in Puerto Rico after Hurricane Maria. *New England Journal of Medicine* 379:162–170. doi: 10.1056/NEJMsa1803972.

Lafronza, V., and N. Burke. 2007. *Katrina and social determinants of health: Toward a comprehensive community emergency preparedness approach*. http://cretscmhd.psych.ucla.edu/nola/volunteer/FoundationReports/CHA_KatrinaSocialDet.pdf (accessed September 1, 2020).

Lee, J., S. Mervosh, Y. Avila, B. Harvey, and A. Leeds Matthews. 2020. See how all 50 states are reopening (and closing again). *The New York Times*. https://www.nytimes.com/interactive/2020/us/states-reopen-map-coronavirus.html (accessed September 1, 2020).

Lieberman-Cribbin, W., S. Tuminello, R. M. Flores, and E. Taioli. 2020. Disparities in COVID-19 testing and positivity in New York City. *American Journal of Preventive Medicine* 59(3):326–332. doi: 10.1016/j.amepre.2020.06.005.

Logie, C., and J. Turan. 2020. How do we balance tensions between COVID-19 public health responses and stigma mitigation? Learning from HIV research. *AIDS and Behavior* 24:2003–2006. doi: 10.1007/s10461-020-02856-8.

Lybarger, J. 2018. Mental health in Puerto Rico. *American Psychological Association* 49(5):20. https://www.apa.org/monitor/2018/05/puerto-rico (accessed September 1, 2020).

McKibben, B. 2020. Racism, police violence, and the climate are not separate issues. *The New Yorker*. https://www.newyorker.com/news/annals-of-a-warming-planet/racism-police-violence-and-the-climate-are-not-separate-issues (accessed September 1, 2020).

Michaud, J., and J. Kates. 2017. *Public health in Puerto Rico after Hurricane Maria*. Kaiser Family Foundation. https://www.kff.org/other/issue-brief/public-health-in-puerto-rico-after-hurricane-maria (accessed September 1, 2020).

Mitchell, B., and J. Franco. 2018. HOLC "Redlining" maps: The persistent structure of segregation and economic inequality. National Community Reinvestment Coalition. https://ncrc.org/wp-content/uploads/dlm_uploads/2018/02/NCRC-Research-HOLC-10.pdf (accessed September 1, 2020).

NASEM (National Academies of Sciences, Engineering, and Medicine). 2019. *Building and measuring community resilience: Actions for communities and the Gulf Research Program*. Washington, DC: The National Academies Press. https://doi.org/10.17226/25383.

Nomura, S., A. Parsons, M. Hirabayashi, R. Kinoshita, Y. Liao, and S. Hodgson. 2016. Social determinants of mid- to long-term disaster impacts on health: A systematic review. *International Journal of Disaster Risk Reduction* 16:53–67. https://doi.org/10.1016/j.ijdrr.2016.01.013.

NRC (National Research Council). 2001. *Forced migration and mortality*. Washington, DC: National Academy Press. https://doi.org/10.17226/10086.

NRC. 2004. *Eliminating health disparities: Measurement and data needs*. Washington, DC: The National Academies Press. https://doi.org/10.17226/10979.

Orengo-Aguayo, R., R. Stewart, M. de Arellano, J. Suarez-Kindy, and J. Young. 2019. Disaster exposure and mental health among Puerto Rican youths after Hurricane Maria. *JAMA Network Open* 2(4):e192619. doi: 10.1001/jamanetworkopen.2019.2619.

Panchal, N., R. Kamal, K. Orgera, C. Cox, R. Garfield, L. Hamel, C. Munana, and P. Chidambaram. 2020. *The implications of COVID-19 for mental health and substance use*. Kaiser Family Foundation. https://www.kff.org/coronavirus-covid-19/issue-brief/the-implications-of-covid-19-for-mental-health-and-substance-use (accessed September 1, 2020).

Patel, J. A., F. B. H. Nielsen, A. A. Badiani, S. Assi, V. A. Unadkat, B. Patel, R. Ravindrane, and H. Wardle. 2020. Poverty, inequality and COVID-19: The forgotten vulnerable. *Public Health* 183:110–111. https://doi.org/10.1016/j.puhe.2020.05.006.

Quealy, K. 2020. The richest neighborhoods emptied out most as coronavirus hit New York City. *The New York Times*. https://www.nytimes.com/interactive/2020/05/15/upshot/who-left-new-york-coronavirus.html (accessed September 1, 2020).

Rabin, R. 2020. Black coronavirus patients land in hospitals more often, study finds. *The New York Times*. https://www.nytimes.com/2020/05/23/health/coronavirus-black-patients.html (accessed September 1, 2020).

Raifman, M. A., and J. R. Raifman. 2020. Disparities in the population at risk of severe illness from COVID-19 by race/ethnicity and income. *American Journal of Preventive Medicine* 59(1):137–139. doi: 10.1016/j.amepre.2020.04.003.

Rodriguez-Diaz, C. 2018. Maria in Puerto Rico: Natural disaster in a colonial archipelago. *American Journal of Public Health* 108(1):30–31. doi: 10.2105/AJPH.2017.304198.

Sauer, L. 2020. *What is coronavirus?* Johns Hopkins Medicine. https://www.hopkinsmedicine.org/health/conditions-and-diseases/coronavirus (accessed September 1, 2020).

Scaramutti, C., C. Salas-Wright, S. Vos, and J. Schwartz. 2019. The mental health impact of Hurricane Maria on Puerto Ricans in Puerto Rico and Florida. *Disaster Medicine and Public Health Preparedness* 13(1):24–27. doi: 10.1017/dmp.2018.151.

Sikorska, K. 2020. Coronavirus disease 2019 as a challenge for maritime medicine. *International Maritime Health* 71(1):4. doi: 10.5603/IMH.2020.0002.

Thomas-Henkel, C., and M. Schulman. 2017. Screening for social determinants of health in populations with complex needs: Implementation considerations. Center for Health Care Strategies, Inc. https://www.chcs.org/media/SDOH-Complex-Care-Screening-Brief-102617.pdf (accessed September 1, 2020).

U.S. Bureau of Labor Statistics. 2019. *Job flexibilities and work schedules summary*. https://www.bls.gov/news.release/flex2.nr0.htm (accessed September 1, 2020).

Valderas, J., B. Starfield, B. Sibbald, C. Salisbury, and M. Roland. 2009. Defining comorbidity: Implications for understanding health and health services. *Annals of Family Medicine* 7(4):357–363. https://www.ncbi.nlm.nih.gov/pmc/articles/PMC2713155/pdf/0060357.pdf (accessed September 1, 2020).

WHO (World Health Organization). 2020. *Social determinants of health*. https://www.who.int/social_determinants/sdh_definition/en (accessed September 1, 2020).

Appendix E

Committee and Staff Biographical Sketches

Ellen J. MacKenzie, Ph.D., Sc.M. (*Chair*), is the 11th dean of the Johns Hopkins Bloomberg School of Public Health. An expert on improving trauma care systems and policy, a nationally renowned researcher, and a respected academic leader, Dr. MacKenzie brings wide experience to her role as dean. After earning graduate degrees from the Bloomberg School, Dr. MacKenzie joined the school's health policy and management faculty in 1980, with a joint appointment in the Department of Biostatistics. A Bloomberg Distinguished Professor, she holds faculty appointments in the school of medicine's departments of orthopaedic surgery, emergency medicine, and physical medicine and rehabilitation. In 2018 she was elected to the National Academy of Medicine. Dr. MacKenzie founded and leads the Major Extremity Trauma Research Consortium, a collaboration of more than 50 U.S. trauma centers and military treatment facilities. As the former director of the Johns Hopkins Center for Injury Research and Policy, she has shaped the field of trauma services and outcomes research, leading to improved quality of life for trauma survivors. As a professor, department chair, and senior associate dean for academic affairs at the Bloomberg School, Dr. MacKenzie has distinguished herself as an inspired leader. As the health policy and management chair, Dr. MacKenzie enhanced practice as a part of the department's mission, established a faculty development program that has served as a model for other departments, and facilitated the development of a core curriculum in policy. She also helped establish the Dr.P.H. cohort programs in Taiwan, Abu Dhabi, the Pacific Rim, the United Arab Emirates, and China.

Sue Anne Bell, Ph.D., FNP-BC, NDHP-BC, is a nurse scientist and an assistant professor at the University of Michigan, with expertise in disaster response and emergency care. Her program of research examines the health effects of disasters and the impact of climate change on human health within a health equity framework. She is particularly interested in the long-term impact of disasters on human health, in developing policy that protects and promotes health throughout the disaster management cycle, and in the relationship among community resilience, health disparities, and disasters. Dr. Bell is clinically active in disaster response through the Department of Health and Human Services' National Disaster Medical System with recent deployments to Hurricane Irma, Hurricane Maria, and the California wildfires.

H. Russell Bernard, Ph.D., is the director of the Institute for Social Science Research at Arizona State University and an emeritus professor of the University of Florida. He is a cultural anthropologist specializing in technology and social change, language death, and social network analysis. His work in network analysis includes helping to develop the network scale-up method for estimating the size of uncountable populations. Dr. Bernard has done research or taught at universities in Germany, Greece, Japan, Mexico, and the United States. He is a former editor of *Human Organization* and the *American Anthropologist* and is the founder and the editor of the journal *Field Methods*. Dr. Bernard's books include *Social Research Methods: Qualitative and Quantitative Approaches*, *Analyzing Qualitative Data: Systematic Approaches* (with Gery Ryan), and *Native Ethnography* (with Jesús Salinas Pedraza). Dr. Bernard was the 2003 recipient of the Franz Boas Award from the American Anthropological Association and is a member of the National Academy of Sciences.

Aram Dobalian, Ph.D., J.D., M.P.H., is a professor in and the director of the Division of Health Systems Management and Policy at The University of Memphis. His research and consulting focus on access and quality of care during disasters and other crises, including work on community health resilience, crisis leadership, inpatient and outpatient quality metrics, health care facility evacuation, information technology in disasters, disaster behavioral health, and workforce readiness. He is a member of the Standing Committee on Medical and Public Health Research During Large-Scale Emergency Events of the National Academies of Sciences, Engineering, and Medicine. Dr. Dobalian led the development of the first Department of Veterans Affairs (VA) Comprehensive Emergency Management Program Evaluation and Research agenda in 2007–2008. In 2010 he became the founding director of the Veterans Emergency Management Evaluation Center, the only national research center focused on VA's emergency management responsibilities to ensure timely access to high-quality care for veterans during crises and to improve the nation's health preparedness for response to national emergencies, natural disasters, and terrorism. Dr. Dobalian has also examined end-of-life decision making and resource use in nursing homes, the role of pain in health care use, nursing home malpractice, the Nationwide Health Information Network Trial Implementation, veteran reintegration into civilian life, institutional review board quality, and nursing education. He led the national program evaluation of the VA Nursing Academy (VANA), a 5-year program consisting of 15 partnerships between VA hospitals and nursing schools. VANA, now named the Enhancing Academic Partnerships Program, promotes innovations in clinical nursing education and practice. He has taught classes on the U.S. health care system, health law, health policy, and health ethics and is a member of the State Bar of California.

Marcella F. Fierro, M.D., Diplomate, ABP, AP, CP, FP, is the chief medical examiner emerita for the Commonwealth of Virginia. She was responsible for the oversight of medical examiner investigations of all violent, suspicious, and unnatural deaths in Virginia. She also served as a professor of pathology and a professor and the chair of the Department of Legal Medicine at the Virginia Commonwealth University School of Medicine from 1994 to 2008. She is a fellow and the past president of the National Association of Medical Examiners and served on its board of directors and the executive committee. Dr. Fierro is a fellow of the American Academy of Forensic Sciences and was a member of the Forensic Science Board for the Commonwealth. She has served as a consultant to the Federal Bureau of Investigation on the National Crime Information Center Unidentified and Missing Persons Files, and on federal panels and committees developing best practices in forensic identification and forensic medicine. Dr. Fierro served on the National Academies' Committee on Science, Technology, and Law, which authored the report *Strengthening Forensic Science in the United States: A Path Forward*. Dr. Fierro served on the board of directors of the Virginia Institute of Forensic Science and Medicine. She has published in professional journals, has edited texts, contributed chapters to several books, and presented at national and international meetings. Dr. Fierro serves as a reviewer for *The American Journal of Forensic Medicine and Pathology*. In retirement, Dr. Fierro continues to consult on forensic death-related matters with a special passion for reuniting the many unidentified dead in our nation with their searching families. She also consulted with the Virginia Institute on a grant for developing tools for recruiting physicians to enter forensic pathology as a career choice.

Elizabeth Frankenberg, Ph.D., is the Cary C. Boshamer Distinguished Professor of Sociology and the director of the Carolina Population Center at the University of North Carolina. Dr. Frankenberg's research focuses on individual and family response to change and the role of community, broadly construed, in individual behaviors and outcomes across the life course. In addition to these substantive interests, two crosscutting themes are inherent in her research: health status as a critical dimension of well-being and the close integration of methods and data. She has developed and implemented innovative and ambitious designs for data collection to support her own research and that of the scientific and policy communities more broadly. One of these projects, the Study of the Tsunami Aftermath and Recovery, which is ongoing, assesses the social, economic, demographic, and health impacts of the December 26, 2004, earthquake and tsunami in Indonesia. It provides unique data measuring population-level response to a disaster over a long period of time. Dr. Frankenberg is trained in demography, sociology, and public policy. She has held social science staff positions at RAND, faculty appointments in the departments of sociology and community health sciences at the University of California, Los Angeles, and faculty appointments in the Sanford School of Public Policy and in sociology at Duke University.

John L. Hick, M.D., is a faculty emergency physician at Hennepin Healthcare and a professor of emergency medicine at the University of Minnesota. He serves as the deputy medical director for Hennepin County emergency medical services and the medical director for Emergency Preparedness at the Hennepin County Medical Center. He served the Minnesota Department of Health as the medical director for the Office of Emergency Preparedness until becoming an advisor to the director of occupational and environmental medicine at the Office of the Assistant Secretary for Preparedness and Response at the Department of Health and Human Services, where he is the lead editor for the TRACIE health care disaster preparedness website. He is the founder and past chair of the Minneapolis/St. Paul Metropolitan Area Hospital Compact, a 32-hospital mutual aid and planning group active since 2002. Dr. Hick is a national speaker on hospital preparedness issues and has published numerous papers dealing with hospital preparedness for contaminated casualties, personal protective equipment, crisis standards of care, and surge capacity. He was honored to serve the Institute of Medicine/National Academies on the Crisis Standards of Care projects as well as the Forum on Medical and Public Health Preparedness for Disasters and Emergencies.

Ali S. Khan, M.D., M.P.H., M.B.A., is the dean of the College of Public Health at the University of Nebraska Medical Center. Dr. Khan is a retired assistant surgeon general and the former director of the Centers for Disease Control and Prevention's (CDC's) Center for Preparedness and Response. He has served on several key CDC leadership positions overseeing programs including pandemic influenza, special pathogens, malaria, and other infectious diseases. Dr. Khan led the development of a number of innovative information projects including BioFusion, Red Sky, Dragon Fire, and the national health security preparedness index. He has had extensive national and global public emergency response leadership experience for Hurricane Katrina, severe acute respiratory syndrome, the Asian tsunami, anthrax, Rift Valley Fever, and influenza. Dr. Khan has served on White House committees on food safety and health security and serves on the steering committee for the World Health Organization Global Outbreak Alert and Response Network. As part of that network he most recently was called on to help the Pacific Island nations respond to a measles outbreak with prior deployments for Ebola in West Africa and the Rohingya humanitarian crisis in Bangladesh. Apart from being an author of more than 100 scientific articles and many policy briefs, Dr. Khan is known to the public for his recent book *The Next Pandemic* where he describes his firsthand experience with deadly infectious disease. He is an expert on health systems and politics surrounding these systems and on anticipating prevention and treatment of emerging and re-emerging infectious disease.

Maureen Lichtveld, M.D., M.P.H., is a professor and the Freeport McMoRan Chair on Environmental Policy at the Tulane University School of Public Health & Tropical Medicine, as well as the director of the Center for Gulf Coast Environmental Health Research, Leadership, and Strategic Initiatives, and a member of the National Academy of Medicine. Her research focuses on environmentally induced disease, health disparities, environmental health policy, disaster preparedness, public health systems, and community resilience. With more than 35 years of environmental public health experience, Dr. Lichtveld carries out national and global environmental health research that examines the cumulative impact of chemical and non-chemical stressors on communities facing environmental health threats, disasters, and health disparities. Dr. Lichtveld is a member of the National Academies' Roundtable on Environmental Health Sciences, Research, and Medicine; National Academies' Board on Global Health; and National Academies' Climate Communications Initiative Advisory Board. She was elected to the Board of the Consortium of Universities for Global Health and serves on the National Advisory Environmental Health Sciences Council at the National Institutes of Health. Dr. Lichtveld was a member of the Environmental Protection Agency's scientific advisory board and the health disparities subcommittee at the Centers for Disease Control and Prevention (CDC); the past chair of the editorial board of the *American*

Journal of Public Health; and past president of Hispanic-Serving Health Professions Schools. Other recognitions include the Johns Hopkins University Society of Scholars, CDC's Environmental Health Scientist of the Year, and Woman of the Year, New Orleans.

Charles Rothwell, M.S., M.B.A. (retired), formerly served as the director for the National Center for Health Statistics (NCHS). He came to federal government service in 1987 as the associate director of NCHS responsible for information technology (IT) and information services of the center, and in 2003 he became the center's director of vital statistics. Before entering federal service, Mr. Rothwell spent 13 years in the state health department in North Carolina and became the first director of the State Center for Health Statistics. He was responsible for health statistics, public health IT, and statewide public health planning activities, and he served as an adjunct assistant professor of biostatistics at the University of North Carolina Gillings School of Global Public Health and the Cecil G. Sheps Center for Health Services Research. Over the years, he has been involved with health statistics and IT activities of the U.S. Agency for International Development, the United Nations, the Robert Wood Johnson Foundation, the National Science Foundation, and the National Institute of Standards and Technology. He also served as a legislative assistant for Senator Lieberman, working health and education issues. Mr. Rothwell served as an officer in the U.S. Marine Corps, reaching the rank of captain. He received his B.S. in physics from the Virginia Military Institute, an M.S. in operations research and systems analysis from the University of North Carolina at Chapel Hill, and an M.B.A. from the University of Maryland. Mr. Rothwell is a fellow of the American Statistical Association and in February 2013 was selected as one of the five Top Leaders in Federal Service.

Richard Serino is the former deputy administrator of the Federal Emergency Management Agency (FEMA) and former chief of Boston Emergency Management Services (EMS), and is currently a distinguished senior fellow among the Harvard University National Preparedness Leadership Initiative (NPLI) faculty. In this role he participates in the NPLI's education and research initiatives. Mr. Serino also serves as a senior advisor at the Massachusetts Institute of Technology Urban Risk Lab. Mr. Serino brings more than 40 years of experience in disaster preparedness, response, and recovery as well as mass casualty incidents and leadership and innovation in government. He has received more than 35 local, national, and international awards for public service and innovation, including the NPLI's Meta-Leader of the Year Award for his work in the response to Superstorm Sandy. At FEMA, Mr. Serino worked directly with Administrator Craig Fugate to build, sustain, and improve the department's capacity to prepare for, protect against, respond to, recover from, and mitigate all hazards. Mr. Serino has more than 35 years of state and local emergency management and emergency medical services experience. Prior to his appointment to FEMA, he served as the chief of Boston EMS and the assistant director of the Boston Public Health Commission. In that role he bolstered the city's response plans for major emergencies, including chemical, biological, and radiological attacks. He also led citywide planning for H1N1 influenza. Mr. Serino has served as an incident commander for more than 35 mass casualty incidents and for all of Boston's major planned events, including the Boston Marathon, Boston's Fourth of July celebration, First Night, and the 2004 Democratic National Convention. He began working for Boston EMS in 1973; over the years, he rose through the ranks, and in 1999 became chief of the department. During his tenure as chief he has seen the agency expand and improve to become nationally recognized for the first-rate services provided by the agency's emergency medical technicians and paramedics. Since 1998 Mr. Serino has been a national faculty member for the Domestic Preparedness Program. He was an original contributing member for the Defense Department's Domestic Preparedness Training Program and Metropolitan Medical Response System. Mr. Serino has been involved, since its inception, with the Lessons Learned Information Sharing network for emergency responders. As a consultant to the Pentagon and the defense department, he served on the 9/11 after-action team to assess medical consequence management policies and procedures. Mr. Serino attended Harvard University's Kennedy School Senior Executives in State and Local Government program in 2000, completed the Kennedy School's National Preparedness Leadership Initiative in 2005, and graduated from the Executive Leadership Program, Center for Homeland Defense and Security at the Naval Postgraduate School.

Michael A. Stoto, Ph.D., is a professor of health systems administration and population health at Georgetown University as well as a statistician, epidemiologist, and health services researcher. He also holds adjunct faculty appointments in the Department of Family Medicine, the Georgetown University Law Center, and the Harvard T.H. Chan School of Public Health. Dr. Stoto's research includes methodological topics in epidemiology and statistics including systematic reviews/meta-analysis and other analytical methods for comparative effectiveness research, community health assessment, evaluation methods, and performance measurement. His substantive research interests include public health practice, especially with regard to emergency preparedness; drug and vaccine safety; infectious disease policy; and ethical issues in research and public health practice. Dr. Stoto is an expert on population health and public health assessment and the associate director of the population health scholars program in the Georgetown

University School of Medicine. His work in this area has included systems-oriented evaluations of public health surveillance systems at the local to global level, addressing both statistical methods and public health practice issues. Dr. Stoto has developed methods for evaluating community health assessments and performance measures and helped to develop community health needs assessments (CHNAs) in MedStar Georgetown University Hospital and the other hospitals in the MedStar system as well as state and local health departments in the Washington, DC, metropolitan area. Dr. Stoto is currently working on a national study to identify best practices for hospital and community CHNAs. Dr. Stoto is also an expert in public health systems research (PHSR), focusing on applying and developing rigorous mixed-methods approaches to studying and evaluating federal, state, and local public health systems. Much of Dr. Stoto's recent PHSR work has focused on public health emergency preparedness, and he was the co-principal investigator of the Centers for Disease Control and Prevention–funded Preparedness and Emergency Response Research Center based at the Harvard T.H. Chan School of Public Health. Dr. Stoto's work in this area has focused on regionalization in public health, the evaluation of biosurveillance methods, and the development of methods for assessing emergency preparedness capabilities based on exercises and actual events. Dr. Stoto is currently working with the European Centre for Disease Prevention and Control and the University of Bologna to develop a competency-based training program for public health emergency preparedness in the European Union.

W. Craig Vanderwagen, M.D., is a member as well as a manager of East West Protection, LLC. Dr. Vanderwagen served for 28 years as a uniformed officer in the U.S. Public Health Service, retiring with the rank of rear admiral (upper half). He served for 25 years in the Indian Health Service. His last assignment was as the presidentially appointed and Senate-confirmed Assistant Secretary for Preparedness and Response (ASPR) at the Department of Health and Human Services. He also serves as a senior partner with Martin, Blanck & Associates, a professional consulting firm located in Alexandria, Virginia. As the founding ASPR, he implemented federal legislation that established the ASPR as the principal leader for all federal public health and medical response activities to any deliberate or natural disasters in the United States. The legislation established a federal role in the development and use of human and other material assets in preparedness and response and also established systems for deploying and managing these assets in emergency situations. His position also gave him authority and oversight of the federal effort to develop and support a wide range of medical countermeasures (diagnostics, vaccines, therapeutic drugs and biologics) against chemical, biological, radiological, and nuclear as well as pandemic influenza threats. This oversight responsibility included scientific discovery, product development, licensure, acquisition, and deployment. Dr. Vanderwagen was responsible for the creation of operational plans to address 15 national threats (including biological threats such as anthrax, smallpox, and plague as well as threats from nuclear, radiation, and chemical devices and natural disasters such as hurricanes and earthquakes) supported by appropriate situational awareness, logistics, planning, training, and exercises coordinated through the Department of Health and Human Services' Secretary's Command Center, an emergency operations center linked to all other federal, state, and local command centers. Dr. Vanderwagen received his doctor of medicine degree from the Michigan State University College of Human Medicine. He completed his residency in family medicine at The University of New Mexico and is board certified in family practice medicine. He received his bachelor's degree from Calvin University.

Daniel Wall, RN, M.P.P.A., B.S.N., currently works for the City of Ventura as the emergency manager and was previously at the Ventura County Health Care Agency as a manager for 11 years. Mr. Wall recently finished a master's degree in public policy and administration. He has been a registered nurse for 15 years and has been working in the medical field for more than 30 years. He is a veteran of the U.S. Army and was a combat medic. Mr. Wall's primary career experience has been in the field of emergency medicine as a nurse.

Matthew Wynia, M.D., M.P.H., is the director of the University of Colorado Center for Bioethics and Humanities. His career has included developing a research institute and training programs focusing on bioethics, professionalism, and policy issues (the American Medical Association's [AMA's] Institute for Ethics) and founding AMA's Center for Patient Safety. His research has focused on novel uses of survey data to inform and improve the practical management of ethical issues in health care and public policy. He has led projects on a wide variety of topics related to ethics and professionalism, including understanding and measuring the ethical climate of health care organizations and systems; ethics and quality improvement; communication, team-based care, and engaging patients as members of the team; defining physician professionalism; public health and disaster ethics; medicine and the Holocaust (with the U.S. Holocaust Memorial Museum); and inequities in health and health care. He has served on committees, expert panels, and as a reviewer for the National Academies, The Joint Commission, The Hastings Center, the American Board of Medical Specialties, federal agencies, and other organizations. Dr. Wynia is the author of more than 150 published articles, chapters, and essays; co-editor of several books; and co-author of a book on fairness in health care benefit design. He is a past president of the American Society for Bioethics and Humanities, and has chaired the ethics forum of the American Public Health Association and the ethics committee of the Society of General Internal Medicine.

STAFF

Scott H. Wollek, M.P.A., is a senior program officer with the Board on Health Sciences Policy at the National Academies of Sciences, Engineering, and Medicine, where he serves as the director of the Forum on Medical and Public Health Preparedness for Disasters and Emergencies. Since joining the National Academies staff in 2015, Mr. Wollek has worked on a range of projects focused on medical countermeasures, civilian biodefense, workforce resilience, health care capacity building, and other health security topics. Prior to joining the National Academies, Mr. Wollek served as the senior disaster program manager at the American Red Cross in the National Capital Region (NCR). In that role he was responsible for the management of preparedness, response, and recovery programs throughout the NCR, including the response to more than 500 local disasters each year. During his 11 years with the Red Cross, Mr. Wollek held a variety of paid and volunteer staff positions involving local disaster response, training, exercises, plans, and operations. Mr. Wollek served in leadership positions during disasters and special events including the 2009 and 2013 presidential inaugurations, 2010 blizzard, and the NCR response to Hurricane Irene, Tropical Storm Lee, the 2012 derecho, Hurricane Sandy, and the shootings at the Washington Navy Yard. Mr. Wollek earned a bachelor's degree in emergency health services from The George Washington University and a master's degree in public administration, with a concentration in homeland security and emergency management, from George Mason University.

Michelle Mancher, M.P.H., was a program officer on the Board on Health Sciences Policy. She served as a staff co-director for the *Integrating Clinical Research into Epidemic Response: The Ebola Experience* report and as a liaison for the Sharing Clinical Trial Data Action Collaborative. Ms. Mancher joined the National Academies of Sciences, Engineering, and Medicine in 2009 and worked on many consensus studies and workshops related to health care services delivery, clinical trial data sharing, and medical product research and development, including *Initial National Priorities for Comparative Effectiveness Research*; *Clinical Practice Guidelines We Can Trust*; *Variation in Health Care Spending: Target Decision Making, Not Geography*; *Sharing Clinical Trial Data: Maximizing Benefits, Minimizing Risk*; and *Global Health Risk Framework: Research and Development of Medical Products: Workshop Summary*. Prior to joining the National

Academies, Ms. Mancher held positions at the Arthritis Foundation: Metro DC Chapter, Clinton Foundation Alliance for a Healthier Generation, and the New York City Health + Hospitals Corporation's office of managed care. Ms. Mancher holds a master's degree in public health in health care management and policy from Columbia University and a bachelor of arts in international relations from The George Washington University.

Daniel L. Cork, Ph.D., is a senior program officer for the Committee on National Statistics (CNSTAT). He has served as a study director or a program officer for nearly all of the committee's studies or workshops related to the U.S. decennial census and the American Community Survey since joining the CNSTAT staff in 2000, including the Panels on Residence Rules in the Decennial Census, Research on Future Census Methods (2010 Planning panel), Review of the 2000 Census, and Review of the 2010 Census, and the Standing Committee on Reengineering Census Operations. He also directed the Panel on Modernizing the Nation's Crime Statistics and the Panel to Review the Programs of the Bureau of Justice Statistics (in cooperation with the Committee on Law and Justice) and was the senior program officer for the Panel on the Feasibility, Accuracy, and Technical Capability of a National Ballistics Database (joint with the Committee on Law and Justice and the National Materials Advisory Board). His research interests include quantitative criminology, geographical analysis, Bayesian statistics, and statistics in sports. He has a B.S. in statistics from The George Washington University and an M.S. in statistics and a joint Ph.D. in statistics and public policy from Carnegie Mellon University.

Olivia C. Yost, M.Sc., is a program officer with the Board on Health Sciences Policy. She has supported multiple consensus study and workshop committees related to the topics of respiratory protection, preparedness, and occupational health—most recently, the Committee on Best Practices for Assessing Mortality and Significant Morbidity Following Large-Scale Disasters, the Committee on Current Issues in the Assessment of Respiratory Protective Devices, and the Committee on the Use of Elastomeric Respirators in Health Care. Prior to joining the National Academies in 2015, Ms. Yost worked as a research officer for ARCHIVE Global, a global health organization based in New York City, where she managed evaluation activities for disease control programs in the Caribbean, West Africa, and South Asia. Ms. Yost received her M.Sc. in the Control of Infectious Diseases from the London School of Hygiene & Tropical Medicine, where her graduate research focused on developing rapid, low-cost testing methodologies to identify failing wastewater infrastructure. She received her B.A. in history and communications from Franklin University Switzerland.

Michael Berrios, M.A., is a research associate with the Board on Health Sciences Policy. He has worked on several previous National Academies of Sciences, Engineering, and Medicine reports, most recently with the Committee on Medication-Assisted Treatment for Opioid Use Disorder and the Committee on Clinical Trials During the 2014–2015 Ebola Outbreak. He has an M.A. in Asian studies from The George Washington University.